HEAD TRAUMA SOURCEBOOK

Health Reference Series

Volume Twenty-three

HEAD TRAUMA SOURCEBOOK

Basic Information for the Layperson about Open-Head and Closed-Head Injuries, Treatment Advances, Recovery, and Rehabilitation, along with Reports on Current Research Initiatives

Edited by
Karen Bellenir

Omnigraphics, Inc.

Penobscot Building / Detroit, MI 48226

BIBLIOGRAPHIC NOTE

This volume contains publications issued by the following government agencies: National Institutes of Health (NIH), National Institute of Neurological Disorders and Stroke (NINDS), National Institute on Disability and Rehabilitation Research (NIDRR), and National Institute on Alcohol Abuse and Alcoholism; the Food and Drug Administration (FDA); and the U.S. Consumer Product Safety Commission. It also contains copyrighted documents from the following organizations: Brain Injury Association, Inc., Children's National Medical Center, HDI Publishers, Institute for Highway Safety, National Conference of State Legislatures, The National Foundation for Brain Research, and the National Rehabilitation Information Center (NARIC). Copyrighted articles from the following journals are also included: *Journal of the American Medical Association, Journal of Head Trauma and Rehabilitation, Journal of Trauma Injury and Infection, Mayo Clinic Health Letter, Patient Care,* and the *Southern Medical Journal.* All copyrighted material is reprinted with permission. Document numbers where applicable and specific source citations are provided on the first page of each chapter. Every effort has been made to secure all necessary rights to reprint the copyrighted material. If any omissions have been made, contact Omnigraphics to make corrections for future editions.

Edited by Karen Bellenir

Peter D. Dresser, Managing Editor, *Health Reference Series*

Omnigraphics, Inc.

Matthew P. Barbour, *Production Manager*
Laurie Lanzen Harris, *Vice President, Editorial*
Peter E. Ruffner, *Vice President, Administration*
James A. Sellgren, *Vice President, Operations and Finance*
Jane J. Steele, *Marketing Consultant*

Frederick G. Ruffner, Jr., *Publisher*

Copyright © 1997, Omnigraphics, Inc.

Library of Congress Cataloging-in-Publication Data

Head trauma sourcebook : basic information for the layperson about
    open-head and closed-head injuries, treatment advances, recovery,
    and rehabilitation, along with reports on current research
    initiatives / edited by Karen Bellenir.
        p. cm. -- (Health reference series ; v. 23)
      I n cludes bibliographical reference series and index.
      ISBN 0-7808-0208-X
      1. Head--Wounds and injuries--Popular works. 2. Brain damage
    --Popular works. I. Bellenir, Karen. II. Series.
    RD521,H46 1997
    617.4'81044--dc21

∞

This book is printed on acid-free paper meeting the ANSI Z39.48 Standard. The infinity symbol that appears above indicates that the paper in this book meets that standard.

Printed in the United States

Contents

Part III: Rehabilitation and Research

Part IV: Special Concerns Faced by Family Members and Other Survivors

Part V: Further Help and Information

Preface

About This Book

Every year in the United States head trauma leaves up to 90,000 victims permanently disabled, results in 5,000 cases of seizure disorders, puts 2,000 people into a vegetative existence, and claims as many as 100,000 lives—including 10 of every 100,000 children. Nearly one in every three traumatic brain injuries is the result of a motor vehicle accident. Perhaps the saddest statistic is that in many instances head trauma could have been prevented by using simple techniques—most notably seat belts and bike helmets.

This book presents information about head trauma both for the patient and for family members and others whose lives have been impacted by head trauma. The documents selected for inclusion were produced by a wide variety of government and private agencies and organizations and were chosen to help provide answers to some difficult questions.

How to Use this Book

This book is divided into parts and chapters. Parts focus on broad areas of interest. Chapters are devoted to single topics within a part.

Part I: Overview of Head Trauma and Prevention Issues includes basic information about the brain and its functions. Statistical data about head trauma and its impact on society along with important safety tips are presented.

Part II: Types, Causes, and Consequences of Head Trauma defines the difference between open- and closed-head injuries, explains the distinction between mild, moderate, and severe head trauma, presents information about the consequences of head trauma, and describes the different methods used to evaluate a patient's potential for improvement. Because brain-related medical interventions are so complex, some readers may find Chapter 13 (describing hearing loss and dizziness after head trauma) and Chapter 17 (reporting on potential outcomes for patients in comas, vegetative states, or minimally responsive states) more difficult to understand than others. The editor suggests that these chapters be reviewed with a physician.

Part III: Rehabilitation and Research begins with a look at brain injury from a recovering patient's perspective. Additional chapters provide information about rehabilitation services and procedures along with common problems encountered.

Part IV: Special Concerns Faced by Family Members and Other Survivors provides encouragement and hope to family members and other people whose lives have been impacted as a result of head trauma in a spouse, child, other relative, or acquaintance. Family guides provide information on what to expect and how to make appropriate care decisions. To help smooth the transition when people with head injuries are ready to return to work, one chapter is devoted to employment issues. Information about financial assistance and government programs is also provided.

Part V: Further Help and Information includes answers to basic questions about disability following a head injury and lists several different types of available resources. A glossary of medical terms related to head trauma offers easy-to-understand definitions of the sometimes complex terms used throughout this book.

Acknowledgements

This book was prepared with the help of many people and organizations. The editor wishes to thank the Brain Injury Association, Inc. and HDI Publishers for contributing information from their collections of educational materials. The editor also gratefully acknowledges the contributions of the Children's National Medical Center, the Institute for Highway Safety, the National Conference of State Legislatures, The National Foundation for Brain Research, and the National Rehabilitation Information Center (NARIC). In addition, thanks go to Margaret Mary Missar for obtaining the documents reproduced in this volume, and to Bruce the Scanman for making its production a reality.

Note from the Editor

This book is part of Omnigraphics' *Health Reference Series*. The series provides basic information about a broad range of medical concerns. It is not intended to serve as a tool for diagnosing illness, in prescribing treatments, or as a substitute for the physician/patient relationship. All persons concerned about medical symptoms or the possibility of disease are encouraged to seek professional care from an appropriate health care provider.

Dedication

This book is dedicated in memory of the editor's father, Paul E. Chanley (1931-1996). Although his brain injury prevented him from finishing many of the things he wanted to do during his sojourn in this world, it did not stop him from being loved. His desire was that in some small way his life and experiences would benefit someone else. If you find any hope, help, or comfort in the pages of this book, his legacy lives on.

Part One

Overview of Head Trauma and Prevention Issues

Chapter 1

Exploring the Brain

Almost everything you do, from simple physical things like walking the dog, throwing a ball, or picking up a pen to write, to more complex emotional states, such as anger or falling in love, starts in the brain. Through an infinite repertoire of chemical and electrical signals, the brain is the control center of our bodies.

Anatomy

The average adult brain weighs just three pounds. It is contained in a bony vault called the skull, and it has been described as resembling a wrinkled walnut or even a mushroom.

The wrinkled grayish tissue that could be considered the "cap" of the mushroom is actually the uppermost, 80 percent of the brain. It is called the cerebral cortex, and it is a recent brain part in the history of evolution. It is responsible for what we call "brain work"—thinking, perceiving, and producing and understanding language. Underlying the cerebral cortex are many other structures that help us to move, wake, sleep, breathe, smell, see, hear, taste and eat. For reasons we do not yet fully understand, we really have two parts to our brain, the left and right cerebral hemispheres. The corpus callosum, a highway of nerve fibers, joins the cerebral hemispheres, the two halves of your brain, allowing for the transfer of information across both hemispheres.

Excerpted from *Exploring the Brain*, a publication of the National Foundation for Brain Research, nd; reprinted with permission.

While the cerebral hemispheres appear to be mirror images of each other, detailed inspection reveals they are not truly identical. In most people, language abilities are found in the left hemisphere, as are capabilities for reasoning and logic. On the other hand, appreciation of shapes and textures, recognition of voice, ability to orient yourself in space, and musical talent and appreciation are housed in the right hemisphere. For these reasons the right hemisphere is often called the "artistic brain," and the left the "analytical brain."

Each hemisphere is divided into four lobes, set apart by noticeable folds in the surface. Although there is some overlap of tasks among them, each lobe specializes in a particular area of functioning.

Together, these and the other parts of your brain and the spinal cord make up the central nervous system. About a cup of fluid, called cerebrospinal fluid, fills the spaces in the brain (in and around the lobes) and spinal cord. All the nerve cells that lie outside the brain or spinal cord, such as those in the foot or hand, make up the peripheral nervous system. Information about the outside world is brought into the central nervous system via the peripheral nervous system, which is made up of two sets of nerves: somatic nerves keep the body in touch with the outside world, and autonomic nerves control the internal environment, such as blood pressure and heart rate.

The frontal lobes control movement. The premotor cortex controls complex motor movements. The prefrontal fibers exert control over our actions (such as telling us not to talk in class or the movies). The olfactory bulb, which processes smell, is just under the frontal lobes.

The parietal lobes contain the sensory cortex, the part of the brain interpreting touch, pain and temperature. This lobe is linked to each part of the body, telling us when we burn our finger, and that it is our finger and not our foot that has been burned.

The temporal lobes are involved in hearing and memory. The sense of who we are as an individual is also located here. The sensation that you are reliving something that already happened (called deja vu) can occur by electrically stimulating this lobe.

The occipital lobes contain the vision center. If you bump the back of your head hard enough, it may affect the occipital lobes, and can cause you to "see stars."

The brainstem is where the spinal cord enters the brain. A one-inch part of the brainstem, called the medulla, controls swallowing, vomiting and breathing and is partly involved in the control of blood pressure, balance, and heart rate.

The cerebellum represents only one-eighth the total weight of the brain. Yet without it, you could not hold this book, walk out the door,

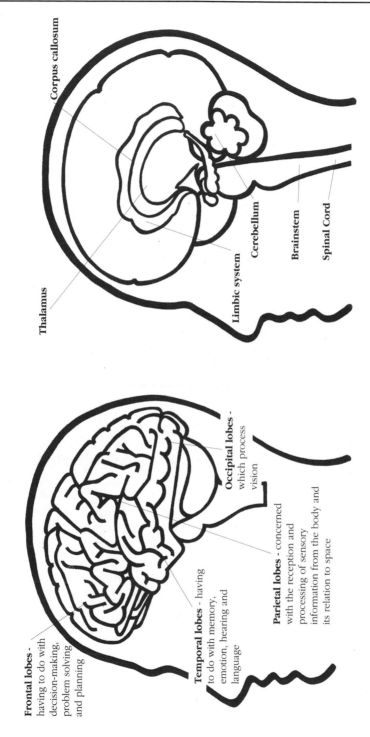

Corpus callosum

Thalamus

Limbic system

Cerebellum

Brainstem

Spinal Cord

Frontal lobes - having to do with decision-making, problem solving and planning

Temporal lobes - having to do with memory, emotion, hearing and language

Parietal lobes - concerned with the reception and processing of sensory information from the body and its relation to space

Occipital lobes - which process vision

Figure 1.1. The human brain.

or write a sentence. It coordinates the brain's instructions for skilled repetitive movements (such as swimming and running) and for maintaining posture and balance.

The thalamus, which in Greek means "couch," sits under the cerebral hemispheres. Most sensory information must pass through the thalamus before reaching the cerebral cortex. The sense of smell sends signals directly to the cerebral cortex.

The limbic system, a group of structures surrounding the brainstem, contains the mechanisms that make mammals warm-blooded, and processes many of our emotional reactions—especially life-sustaining ones dealing with sex and aggression. A part of the limbic system called the hippocampus is responsible for memory. Certain chemicals, such as the active ingredient in marijuana, temporarily weaken short-term memory. The hypothalamus, which is only the size of a thumbnail, is the control center for food intake, hormone levels and motivational states, and orchestrates the behavior that accompanies emotions.

Neurons: Building Blocks of the Brain

Even the world's greatest engineers could not have conceived of and built the human brain. You are born with all the neurons you will ever have. To arrive at the more than 100 billion neurons found in a human newborn, the brain must grow at an average rate of 250,000 neurons per minute throughout the course of a pregnancy. Not only is the number staggering, but the great number of tasks that each cell undertakes in the assembling and functioning of the nervous system is mind-boggling. Nothing comes close to approaching the efficiency and complexity of such a plan.

Each neuron has thousands of connections leading to other neurons. And, like snowflakes, no two neurons are identical in shape, although they share common features. Neurons are distinctively shaped cells containing a long, single fiber (the axon) to transmit impulses; numerous short fibers (the dendrites) to receive impulses; and a unique structure, the synapse, for transferring information from one neuron to the next. These billions of cells make up an exquisitely organized society of totally separate nerve cells that each have a particular function and form and, most importantly, a particular set of connections to other neurons. In the brain, neurons that are close to each other and share the same function—for example, sensory perception or muscle control—are assembled into groups called nuclei. The brain contains hundreds of nuclei.

Communication between brain cells is fundamental to the mechanism by which neurons generate brain functions. This communication occurs mainly through the release of chemical substances. This is what happens when neurons communicate: a message, traveling as an electrical impulse, moves down an axon and towards the synapse. There, it triggers the release of molecules called neurotransmitters. The neurotransmitter diffuses across the synapse as a chemical signal, traveling towards the receiving neuron, where it stimulates or inhibits an electrical response in the receiving neuron's dendrites. Many axons are covered with insulation, called myelin. Nodes along the myelin allow the electrical signals to jump from one node to another, racing at a speed as fast as 400 feet per second. Axons without myelin conduct signals at much slower speeds.

How the Brain Learns, Sees and Remembers

There's more going on in your brain than you might think. How we learn, see and remember are complex processes based as much on previous experience as current information that we receive from our senses. Even simple daily tasks, both physical and intellectual, are actually complicated maneuvers involving perception, comprehension and cognition. Your brain juggles and combines a variety of sensory information in order to make sense of the world around you.

Sensation and Perception

You do not see solely with your eyes, but rather with a combination of your eyes and brain. The eyes pick up impressions from the outside world and send messages to the brain for interpretation. If the primary visual region of your brain were damaged, but your eyes were not, you still would be unable to see. The eyes and brain work in sync to provide visual perception—the ability to analyze sensory information. Besides visual images, the sensory stimulus can also be an odor, sound, touch, or flavor.

Vision is easy for the brain to process, but difficult for us to understand because the brain receives, stores and processes images so rapidly. An intricate system of neurons and light receptors transmits images to the brain. The retina, a sheet of light receptors, contains 125 million specialized vision neurons called rods and cones that line the back of the eye. Rods and cones convert light stimuli into electrical signals which are transmitted via the optic nerve, through a relay station in the thalamus, to the primary visual cortex at the back of your head. Images in the left field of vision from both the eyes transmit to the right brain, and images in the right field of vision transmit to the left.

It is in the visual cortex of the occipital lobe that the brain first begins to assemble something resembling an image. At the same time, this part of the brain sends signals to neighboring areas, each of which relays the signals to several other areas to compare new visual images with ones already in our memory. The brain uses this storehouse of data to interpret images and even allows us to see more than is actually visible.

Sometimes, however, our brains draw the wrong conclusions from what our eyes tell us. This phenomenon, called "optical illusion," challenges our expectations because the brain tries to interpret what it sees based on past experience as opposed to what is truly there. Some optical illusions, containing two images in one, confuse the brain because your brain tends to oscillate from one image to the other.

Hearing allows us to communicate with each other by receiving sounds and interpreting speech. The brain's analysis of sound follows a pattern similar to that of vision. When the signals from the neurons reach the auditory cortex in the temporal lobe, they are sent to the left hemisphere for processing in the language center. The thalamus also is involved in hearing, in the sense that it plays a leading role in such things as our interpretation and appreciation of music and speech.

Smell and taste work together. Taste allows us to distinguish between something sweet or bitter. Smell is closely linked to taste; if you lose your sense of smell, you also lose much of what you think of as taste.

Touch helps us determine size, shape, and texture. Touch receptors are located in the skin and are connected to sensory nerves that lead to the spinal cord, thalamus, and finally the sensory cortex. Sensations perceived at certain points within these regions correspond to the parts of the body from which the signals came. These regions are so exact that sometimes when somebody has lost an arm or leg, they can continue to feel pain in the "phantom limb" even though it is no longer there—the perception of pain results from dozens of chemical and electrical processes. Injury results in the release of these chemicals which enhance the sensitivity of receptors that send messages to the brain. In the case of pain in phantom limbs, the nerves in the remaining part of the limb continue to fire, generating impulses to the brain.

Learning, Thinking, and Memory

We all know that thinking hard can be as fatiguing as extreme physical exertion. But what is thinking—a kind of silent talking to yourself? A collection of images and pictures put together? What is learning? Everyone is familiar with these terms, but they are difficult to define. Learning is normally a change that occurs, as a result of experience, that allows you to do something you never did before, or to do it better. You can learn facts like people's names, or general concepts like addition and multiplication, or habits or skills, like driving a car. Learning enables us to continually adapt to our environment.

The study of thinking, learning and memory is based on the idea that thinking relies on the interpretation of symbols, which provide us with a kind of shorthand, both saving time and space and providing a logic and organization which our brains can handle. The ability to create and use symbols in order to understand, store, and recall things about the world is the essential feature of intelligence.

One of the most prominent intellectual activities that depends on symbols, as well as memory, is language. Scientists believe that when we hear a word, the sound is received in the auditory cortex and then transferred to the left hemisphere to be understood. When we read a word, the information passes through the visual cortex to the left brain, where it is processed. Scientists have learned a great deal about the brain and language from studies of people who have lost speech or language because of a stroke or other brain injury.

Your Brain in Sickness and in Health

Your brain is as individual as your fingerprint. Everything you do affects the brain and the way it functions. Genetics, life experiences, our social environment, aging, disease, physical damage, and drugs— all of these alter your brain structure and influence the way you interact with the world.

Fifty million Americans are afflicted with brain illness or injury. Because the brain is where our imagination and intelligence lie, it is especially tragic when illness or injury strikes; brain disorders rob us of our essential human qualities.

Abnormalities in the process of sending and receiving messages can contribute to mental disorders. Some networks of neurons are especially relevant to mental disorders, such as the neurons controlling cognition—the process of knowing—or those associated with behavior and emotions. If these areas are not functioning properly, they are

9

likely to be involved in the thinking and mood disturbances found in severe mental disorders.

Until recently, the causes of these conditions remained largely locked within the brain. In the past two decades, scientists have been able to "map" the chemistry, circuitry, and anatomy of the human brain in minute detail using brain imaging techniques, which have resulted in our ability to understand and help alleviate the effects of brain disorders previously thought to be untreatable.

Special care is used in research on brain disorders, particularly when it comes to experimental treatments. Patients with head injuries or brain disorders often are not capable of making decisions about their own participation in research. Numerous government and scientific regulations have been created to protect patients who are candidates for scientific research, but there is a continual concern about how to conduct effective research while protecting the rights of the individuals involved.

Head Injury and Trauma

For all its resilience, the brain is a fragile thing. The injured brain does not heal the same way other parts of our bodies heal. A broken arm can mend; a broken brain does not.

Damage to the brain can occur from head injuries, strokes, substance abuse, or neurotoxic agents from the environment, such as lead poisoning. A brain injury can impair our ability to think, talk, see, walk, hear, feel emotions, learn and recall. One thing that distinguishes these types of brain injuries and trauma from other brain diseases and disorders is that many of them are preventable to some degree.

Here are some facts about head injuries: over two million people suffer head injuries each year. Of these, 100,000 die and 500,000 require hospitalization. Motor vehicle accidents cause half of all such injuries, falls cause 21 percent, and 12 percent are the result of violence. Over 5,000 survivors of brain injuries develop epilepsy and many experience profound changes in personality.

Researchers have been encouraged by recent experimental results in which the brain cells of animals have regenerated, findings which may some day lead to the possibility of recovering functions lost due to brain damage. Currently, however, treatment of most head injury consists of long-term rehabilitation. Wearing helmets, using seat belts, driving sober, avoiding dangerous situations and other preventative methods will significantly reduce the risk of head injury.

Chapter 2

The Incidence of Traumatic Brain Injury in the United States

An estimated 1.9 million Americans experience traumatic brain injury (TBI) each year.[1] About half of these cases result in at least short-term disability, and 52,000 people die as a result of their injuries.[2] The direct medical costs for treatment of TBI have been estimated at more than $4 billion annually.[3]

This text summarizes data on the incidence and causes of TBI, the populations it affects, and the degree of disability it causes. Estimates are based on three years (1985-87) data from the National Health Interview Survey (NHIS), a household survey of the non-institutionalized U.S. population. In the NHIS, respondents are asked about injuries they received during a two-week period prior to the interview, and their answers are used to provide annual incidence estimates. In addition, they are questioned about restrictions in their normal activities during the same two-week reference period, caused by injuries received during the previous three months. For the purposes of this text, injuries classified as "skull fractures and intracranial injuries" are considered TBI, corresponding to the International Classification of Diseases (ICD-9) codes 800-804 and 850-854.

Incidence Rates

The incidence rate for TBI is 0.8 percent, meaning that 8 out of every 1,000 persons experience a skull fracture or intracranial injury

Disability Statistics Abstract, Number 14, November 1995. Published by the U.S. Department of Education, National Institute on Disability and Rehabilitation Research (NIDRR).

in any given year. The incidence rate is higher for men than women (0.9 versus 0.7 percent). Age is an even more significant factor in incidence rates, with the highest rates among youth (1.1 percent) and younger adults (0.9 percent).

Young males have the highest incidence rates of any group, with those under 18 having a 1.6 percent chance of experiencing TBI in each year. Those between 18 and 44 years of age have an incidence rate of 0.8 percent.

Annual Number and Incidence Rate of TBI Cases, by Gender and Age, 1985

Total
  Number: 1,931,000
  Incidence rate: 0.8 percent

Gender

Male
  Number: 1,058,000
  Incidence rate: 0.9 percent

Female
  Number: 872,000
  Incidence rate: 0.7 percent

Age

0-18 years
  Number: 685,000
  Incidence rate: 1.1 percent

18-44 years
  Number: 881,000
  Incidence rate: 0.9 percent

44-64 years
  Number: 205,000[*]
  Incidence rate: 0.5 percent[*]

65+ years
  Number: 159,000[*]
  Incidence rate: 0.6 percent[*]

*Estimate has low statistical reliability—standard error exceeds 30 percent of estimate.

Source: 1985-87 National Health Interview Survey, tabulated in Collins, J.G., Types of Injuries by Selected Characteristics: United States, 1985-87. National Center for Health Statistics. Vital Health Stat 10(175). 1990.

Causes of TBI

An estimated 31.0 percent of traumatic brain injuries involve moving motor vehicles, making traffic accidents the largest single cause of TBI. Household accidents are the second leading cause, accounting for 26.3 percent of cases. Workplace accidents are much less frequently cited.

Statistics on place of injury reveal the same pattern, with streets and highways (including sidewalks and adjacent area) accounting for 33.1 percent of cases and private residences accounting for 26.3 percent. Schools, places of recreation, and industrial sites accounted for most of the remaining cases.

Annual Number and Incidence Rate of TBI Cases, by Class and Place of Accident, 1985-87

Total
Number: 1,931,000
Incidence rate: 0.8 percent

Class of Accident

Moving motor vehicle
Number: 599,000
Incidence rate: 0.3 percent

Household
Number: 507,000
Incidence rate: 0.2 percent

Workplace
Number: 164,000*
Incidence rate: 0.1 percent*

Other
    Number 730,000
    Incidence rate: 0.3 percent

Place of Accident

Street or highway
    Number: 640,000
    Incidence rate: 0.3 percent

Residence
    Number: 507,000
    Incidence rate: 0.2 percent

School
    Number: 259,000*
    Incidence rate: 0.1 percent*

Place of recreation
    Number: 176,000*
    Incidence rate: 0.1*

Industrial site
    Number: 73,000*
    Incidence rate: 0.0 percent*

Other
    Number: 276,000*
    Incidence rate: 0.1 percent*

*Estimate has low statistical reliability—standard error exceeds 30 percent of estimate.

Source: 1985-87 National Health Interview Survey, tabulated in Collins, J.G., Types of Injuries by Selected Characteristics: United States, 1985-87. National Center for Health Statistics. Vital Health Stat 10(175). 1990.

TBI As a Cause of Disability

While almost all (99.3 percent) of the reported cases of skull fractures and intracranial injuries are medically attended, only about half

14

(49.2 percent) result in limitations in activity and about a third (36.8 percent) cause the person to be restricted to bed for at least half a day. Thus, only half of TBI cases are severe enough to cause any disability at all.

Nonetheless, TBI does cause significant short-term disability. On average, a traumatic brain injury causes 7.4 days of restricted activity, of which 3.0 are spent in bed. These figures rank TBI fourth among the most disabling categories of injury reported: only fractures of the neck, trunk or upper limbs, fractures of the lower limbs, and dislocations cause more days of restricted activity and bed disability, per injury, than TBI.

Although the NHIS does not permit analysis of long-term disability caused by TBI, it does indicate that a substantial number of Americans—nearly 1 million each year who experience short-term activity limitation—are at risk for lingering and possibly disabling effects from their injuries.

Types of Injury Causing Greatest Activity Limitation, 1985-87

Fractures of lower limb
    Average number of restricted-activity days: 24.1
    Average number of bed-disability days: 9.5

Fractures of neck, trunk, and upper limb
    Average number of restricted-activity days: 11.6
    Average number of bed-disability days: 3.1

Dislocations
    Average number of restricted-activity days: 10.2
    Average number of bed-disability days: 4.0

Skull fractures and intracranial injuries
    Average number of restricted-activity days: 7.4
    Average number of bed-disability days: 3.0

Sprains and strains
    Average number of restricted-activity days: 6.6
    Average number of bed-disability days: 1.7

Source: 1985-87 National Health Interview Survey, tabulated in Collins, J.G., Types of Injuries by Selected Characteristics: United States, 1985-87. National Center for Health Statistics. Vital Health Stat 10(175). 1990.

Reducing the Incidence of TBI

The high incidence rates of TBI among youth and younger adults, especially males, suggests that strategies to reduce TBI should concentrate on that population. In addition, the large number of cases caused by traffic accidents points toward reducing such accidents and their severity. Other studies[4] have concluded that one of the most significant causes of injury and fatality among those aged 15-24 is motor vehicle accidents related to alcohol consumption. A reduction in the number of young adults who drink and drive would therefore result in a reduced incidence of TBI among that population.

Recent data indicate that firearms are the most common cause of fatality due to TBI[5]. This phenomenon also disproportionately affects young males, suggesting another strategy for reducing the incidence of TBI.

The large proportion of cases occurring in the home and at school suggests that falls are a significant cause of TBI. Prevention and education efforts could also focus on improving home and school safety. In addition, a substantial number of cases are associated with recreational activities (possibly including those occurring on roadways but not involving motor vehicles), suggesting that the safety of such activities as bicycling, skating, and contact sports could be improved.

Notes

1. TBI incidence data in this abstract are obtained from Collins, J.G., Types of Injuries by Selected Characteristics: United States, 1985-87. National Center for Health Statistics. Vital Health Stat 10(175). 1990.

2. Daniel Sosin, Joseph Sniezek, and Richard J. Waxweiler, Trends in Death Associated with Traumatic Brain Injury, 1979 Through 1992. JAMA 272:1778, 1995.

3. Wendy Max, Ellen J. MacKenzie, and Dorothy P. Rice, Head Injuries: Costs and Consequences. J. Head Trauma Rehab. 6:76, 1991.

4. Richard J. Waxweiler, David Thurman, Joseph Sniezek, Daniel Sosin, and Joann O'Neil, Monitoring the Impact of Traumatic

Brain Injury: A Review and Update. J. of Neurotrauma 2:509, 1995.

5. Daniel Sosin, Joseph Sniezek, and Richard J. Waxweiler, Trends in Death Associated with Traumatic Brain Injury, 1979 Through 1992. JAMA 272:1778, 1995.

— by Joel Anton Forkosch,
H. Stephen Kaye, and
Mitchell P. LaPlante

Disability Statistics Rehabilitation Research and Training Center, University of California, San Francisco.

Chapter 3

Why Should Legislators Be Concerned about Traumatic Brain Injury?

As medical research allows more lives to be saved, legislators are faced with the public policy problem of supporting growing numbers of people with traumatic brain injury. Legislators are concerned about the high cost to society, the high cost of inappropriate care, the inability of existing service systems to meet the needs, aging caregivers, the growth of advocacy groups, national initiatives, and the availability of better data.

High Cost to Society

The catastrophic costs of traumatic brain injury exact a heavy toll on society. The economic costs alone approach $7.6 billion a year, $2.9 billion in direct costs and $4.7 billion in indirect cost, including lost wages and productivity. The costs ripple through society and assume a number of forms. A person with a severe brain injury faces $436,000 of medical costs, and annual costs of $32,000 to 63,000 dollars. Because people with brain injuries are typically young adults, the loss of productivity and jobs over the normal life span is enormous. In addition, family members often have to give up full-time jobs to take care of loved ones, resulting in a further loss of tax revenues. The ripple effect of reduced earnings of family members leads to a reduction in savings, which affects the long-term growth of the economy.

Excerpted from *What Legislators Need to Know about Traumatic Brain Injury*, ©1993 National Council of State Legislatures, reprinted with permission.

The costs of caring for people with traumatic brain injury are borne by various types of payers—federal, state, and local governments; private insurance; worker's compensation; and private individuals. However, the public sector bears a large part of the responsibility since young adults, who make up a majority of people with brain injuries, frequently do not have adequate private insurance coverage and must tap public assistance to help pay for their extensive care.

Although nationwide statistics do not exist, Missouri, through its Head and Spinal Cord Injury Registry, determined that more than half the people with brain injuries had government insurance or no insurance at all. The Rehabilitation Research and Training Center on Community Integration of Persons with Traumatic Brain Injury at the State University of New York at Buffalo estimates that 20 percent of brain injury patients nationwide are eligible for Medicaid at the time of the injury, and that 50 percent of people currently disabled by brain injury are living below the poverty line. Federal and state governments are absorbing the costs of caring for people with brain injury. The important question is, are the dollars being spent wisely?

High Cost of Inappropriate Care

Most states do not have the existing rehabilitation services to care for people with brain injuries and end up sending the people to out-of-state facilities at often exorbitant costs to the state. Also, many states have no way of determining that the care is appropriate.

A study by the New York State Department of Health found that of the 511 people with traumatic brain injuries placed in out-of-state facilities, approximately 411 were inappropriately placed, at a cost of $46.5 million a year, including $18.6 million in state money and $4.65 million in local dollars. If those individuals were brought back to the state and placed in community settings (or, in the case of persons in coma for more than a year, in nursing homes in their community), the estimated savings would be $27.3 million. This would amount to a direct savings to the state of $10.9 million and a $1.4 million saving to local government.

States do not necessarily have to spend more money on people with traumatic brain injury if they spend it wisely. Across the country, as states face tight budgets, lawmakers will be under enormous pressure to get the most for their money. Increasingly, advocates and professionals are finding that people who reside in institutions can be cared for at an equal or lesser cost in the community. Community alternatives not only save money, they provide the chance for people with brain injuries to live a life like other people, with a job, a house, friends, dignity, and self-esteem. States that lack appropriate outpatient and community reintegration programs are forced to care for individuals in more costly inpatient programs because there are no other alternatives.

Inability of Existing Service Systems to Meet Needs

In most states, traumatic brain injury has no commonly identified home in the bureaucracy. This is a major problem as states look to develop policies that would more appropriately meet the needs of people with brain injuries. These people have diverse needs that make it difficult for them to fit easily into existing service systems. State delivery systems tend to be based on diagnosis (developmental disabilities, mental illness, special health care needs) or on financial need, such as Medicaid. These services are not always available or appropriate for people with brain injuries. Federal funding streams have shaped state services, making it sometimes difficult to restructure or expand existing services to include people with traumatic brain injuries. Legislators need to pay attention to the special needs of people with brain injuries.

Aging Caregivers

Approximately 80 percent of people with brain injuries discharged from acute rehabilitation facilities return to be cared for by family members. The average family caregiver is 50 years old. In the next 10 to 20 years, as these caregivers become elderly or die, government agencies will experience an alarming demand for housing, supervision, and case management services for these people.

Growth of Advocacy Groups

Until recently, people with brain injuries and their families have been a disorganized and weak lobbying group, often at odds with the private insurance system. But today, across the country family members and people with brain injuries are finding their voice. The National Head Injury Foundation now has 45 state associations. The National Survivors' Council reaches a large number of people with traumatic brain injuries and their families through its newsletter. Most are of voting age. The state brain injury foundations are sharing information and learning effective lobbying from each other. Advocacy leaders in many states have influenced and worked with their governors, legislators, and key agency administrators. It is no accident that the states with the strongest brain injury foundations tend to be the states most responsive to the needs of people with brain injuries. Increasingly, state legislatures will be hearing from constituents about the staggering problems families encounter when they try to care for a family member without any public support. Advocates will be lobbying state legislators to take a more proactive stand for people with brain injuries.

National Initiatives

Three proposed pieces of legislation before Congress will help raise awareness about traumatic brain injury and put it on the national agenda:

Brain Injury Rehabilitation Quality Act of 1992 (H.R. 4243)

Introduced by Congressman Ron Wyden of Oregon, this bill results from a congressional investigation into waste and patient abuse in rehabilitation care for people with traumatic brain injuries. The bill encourages states, through the Medicaid option, to develop individualized patient management plans to maximize the quality and cost effectiveness of treatment. Home- and community-based settings are emphasized. The bill includes a declaration of individual rights and a national system of standards and oversight of treatment. The legislation will be reintroduced in the 103rd Congress.

Traumatic Brain Injury Act of 1992 (S. 2949)

This bill introduced by Senator Edward Kennedy of Massachusetts will define traumatic brain injury in the federal, state, and local data collection agencies as a specific and reportable condition at the direction of the Centers for Disease Control. The act will study the effectiveness of brain injury interventions, develop special community-based projects, improve due process through protection and advocacy, and empower people with brain injuries and their families to actively participate in the establishment of state policies through consumer-controlled state advisory boards. Hearings on the legislation have been held by the Senate Committee on Labor and Human Resources.

Brain Injury Rehabilitation Quality Act of 1992 (S. 3002)

Introduced by Senators John D. Rockefeller IV of West Virginia and Dave Durenberger of Minnesota, this legislation would allow optional Medicaid coverage of case management services for people with traumatic brain injury as long as the total cost of the new program did not exceed current state expenditures for the care of brain-injured individuals. Greater emphasis would be placed on home- and community-based settings, rather than more costly and sometimes inappropriate residential care settings. A central registry would be established through the Centers for Disease Control. This act would be administered through the General Accounting Office, so it would not have to be renewed each year. In the 102nd Congress, the bill was not reported out of the Senate Committee on Finance. A decision has not yet been made on whether to reintroduce the legislation in the 103rd Congress.

Availability of Better Data

To make good policy decisions, legislators need data about the numbers of people with traumatic brain injury in their states, what services these people need, and how much the services cost. Until recently these data have been in short supply, but things are changing. A growing number of states have established state brain injury registries that collect data on people with brain injuries. The Centers for Disease Control, appointed the lead federal agency to coordinate services for people with traumatic brain injury, is moving forward to establish traumatic brain injury as a category in reporting systems, such as the Health Care Financing Administration and Social Security Administration records, to ensure identification and epidemiologic assessment of people with brain injuries and their needs, to document the relative priority of traumatic brain injury, and to provide a basis for allocating resources. Central reporting systems are included in legislation now before Congress. As better data become available, advocates will be able to back up their demands with more convincing figures, and public policymakers can bolster their decisions with good data.

—by Barbara Wright

23

Chapter 4

Prevention of Pediatric Mortality from Trauma: Are Current Measures Adequate?

Abstract: Trauma accounts for nearly half of pediatric deaths in the United States. We reviewed all pediatric trauma-related deaths that occurred over a 5-year period at two Georgia trauma centers to determine the number of trauma deaths in children, mechanism of injury, cause of death, and compliance with safety standards. Of the 69 fatalities, 31 were caused by motor vehicle accidents. Twenty-five of these victims (81%) were unrestrained; 17 were 4 years old or less, and only 1 of them was restrained in a car seat. Pedestrian versus vehicle accidents resulted in 19 deaths, 10 of the victims being 4 years old or less. Bicycle versus vehicle accidents resulted in 4 deaths, 2 of them due to closed head injury; none of the victims wore headgear. All-terrain vehicle accidents resulted in 2 deaths from massive head injury; neither victim wore a helmet. One death occurred from bicycle handlebar injury; 12 deaths resulted from causes other than vehicle accidents. Major causes of pediatric fatalities were motor vehicle accidents (45%), pedestrian-vehicle accidents (28%), and bicycle accidents (6%). This study indicates that when safety measures such as restraint systems, helmets, or proper supervision are ignored, children may die as a result of trauma.

Trauma is the cause of 44% of deaths in children 4 years old or less.[1] Automobile accidents are responsible for about half of all trauma-related mortality, and one child of every 60 living today is

Southern Medical Journal, Vol. 89, No. 2, February 1996; reprinted with permission.

expected to die in a traffic accident.[1,2] Even with these alarming statistics, many children are not properly restrained when traveling in motor vehicles.[3] In addition, more than 1,200 bicycle-related deaths occur each year in the United States. The majority are from head injury, but the use of bicycle helmets remains optional in most states.[4]

Better preventive measures have been shown to save four times as many lives as improved posttrauma management.[5] Legislation has been enacted regarding mandatory use of seat belts, car seats, and bicycle helmets for young children. These laws have helped to reduce morbidity and mortality in the pediatric age group; however, noncompliance with these laws and its effect on trauma outcome have not been well established. We reviewed all pediatric trauma deaths at two metropolitan Level I trauma centers in the state of Georgia over a 5-year period to determine the number of deaths, mechanisms of injury causing death, and whether preventive measures or protective devices were used.

Methods

A retrospective review of all pediatric trauma deaths that occurred between January 1, 1987, through September 30, 1992, was conducted at Scottish Rite Children's Medical Center, Atlanta, Georgia, and at Memorial Medical Center, Savannah, Georgia. Both are designated trauma centers. Information was obtained from admission histories and physical examinations and from the Department of Human Resources Emergency Medical Service Trip Reports, which identified the mechanisms of injury and, when applicable, the use of protective devices (e.g., seat belts, helmets). All trauma-related deaths in patients aged 14 or less were reviewed, including victims who were dead on arrival.

Results

During the study period, 69 trauma deaths occurred—43 at Scottish Rite Children's Hospital and 26 at Memorial Medical Center. Fifty-seven deaths resulted from motor vehicle accidents and 12 from other causes (Table 4.1). Seven of the victims were dead on arrival. Age of victims ranged from 2 weeks to 14 years.

Table 4.1. Trauma-Related Deaths

Mechanism of Injury	No. of Victims
Motor vehicle accident	31
Pedestrian vs vehicle	19
Bicycle vs vehicle	4
Bicycle	1
All-terrain vehicle	2
Gunshot	3
Child abuse	4
Fall	3
Diving accident	1
Compressed air tank explosion	1
Total	69

Thirty-one deaths resulted from motor vehicle accidents in which all victims were passengers (Table 4.2). Twenty-five (81%) of the victims were unrestrained; the restraint status of four victims was unknown. Seventeen (55%) of the victims were aged 4 or less; only one in that age group was properly restrained in a car seat. One of the remaining 16 in that age group was improperly secured in a car seat, ejected with the car seat, and fatally injured. Eight of the unrestrained victims were ejected. Severe head injury that resulted in subsequent brain death accounted for 17 (55%) of the 31 deaths. The remaining deaths resulted from multiple injuries.

Table 4.2. Motor Vehicle Trauma Deaths

Restraint Status	No. of Victims
Unrestrained	25
Restrained	2
Unknown	4
Total*	31

Cause of Death	No. of Victims
Head injury	17
Multiple injuries	14
Total	31

*Seventeen victims were aged 4 or less; 8 victims were ejected.

Nineteen trauma deaths (28%) resulted from pedestrian versus motor vehicle accidents (Table 4.3). The age range of those victims was 2 to 13 years. Ten victims (53%) were aged 4 or less. Severe head injury with subsequent brain death was the cause of death in 68% of these victims.

Bicycle versus motor vehicle accidents resulted in 4 deaths. None of the victims was wearing protective headgear. Closed head injury with subsequent brain death occurred in 2 of the 4 deaths. One death resulted from a handlebar injury with blunt abdominal trauma due to a fall from a bicycle; death was attributed to delay in seeking treatment and thus was preventable.

Two deaths resulted from all-terrain vehicle (ATV) accidents. One accident occurred on a three-wheeler, and one occurred on a four-wheeler. Neither victim was wearing a helmet; both sustained massive head injuries that resulted in subsequent brain death.

Table 4.3. Pedestrian vs Motor Vehicle Accident

Age	No. of Victims
2	4
3	3
4	3
5	1
7	2
8	1
10	2
11	1
12	1
13	1
Total*	19

Cause of Death	No. of Victims
Head injury	17
Multiple injuries	14
Total	31

*Ten victims were aged 4 or less.

Discussion

Motor vehicle accidents remain the leading cause of death of children in the United States.[3] Despite the mandatory child restraint legislation enacted in all 50 states, an estimated 40% to 60% of young children are unrestrained when traveling in vehicles.[3] When child seats are used, nearly 75% are used incorrectly.[6] Early studies showed that the use of seat belts reduced injury severity by 55% to 60% and fatalities by 43%.[6-10] A 1991 epidemiologic study in Washington State, which evaluated the morbidity and mortality of unrestrained versus restrained children in motor vehicle accidents, concluded that restraints were 70% effective in reducing injuries and 90% effective in reducing the number of deaths.[11] The chance of death in a car accident is 25 times greater for victims thrown from the vehicle. Thirty-five percent of unrestrained children are ejected from motor vehicles in accidents.[2,3,12] Restraint systems are clearly invaluable in preventing death and morbidity in children who are auto crash victims.

In this study, pedestrian versus motor vehicle accidents accounted for 28% of trauma mortality. More than half of the victims (52%) were 4 years old or less, an age group that is at great risk and in need of close supervision.

Head trauma occurs in approximately one third of all bicycle accidents and results in approximately 85% of all fatalities from bicycle accidents.[4,5,13,14] Head trauma is responsible for nearly two thirds of all hospital admissions.[4,14] Five of the victims in this study died as a result of bicycle accidents (four bicycle versus motor vehicle accidents and one bicycle accident). Two of the five deaths were due to massive head injury. None of the victims was wearing protective headgear.

An Australian study of head injuries in bicyclists and motorcyclists showed that head injury rates were significantly higher among bicyclists than among motorcyclists—despite the lower speed of bicycles—because bicyclists were not legally required to wear helmets, whereas motorcyclists were.[5,15,16] Numerous studies show the effectiveness of bicycle helmets in reducing the number and severity of head injuries from bicycle accidents,[13,14,16] yet no national and few state laws mandate bicycle helmet use.

Two of the victims in this study died of massive head injuries sustained in all-terrain vehicle accidents. Studies have shown that ATVs are a significant cause of pediatric trauma.[17,18] Headgear has been proved to protect against intracranial and facial injuries.[19,20] Non-helmeted patients have higher mean injury severity scores, greater number of injuries per patient, and higher proportion of head and facial injuries. An estimated 60% of fatalities from ATV accidents might be prevented by the use of helmets.[21] All-terrain vehicles are banned from public roads; therefore, laws regarding protective devices and minimum age limits are difficult to enforce.

The 12 nonvehicular pediatric deaths in the study were associated with inadequate parental supervision and were potentially preventable. In this study, an average of 14 pediatric trauma deaths occurred each year. Compliance with national mandatory seat belt and helmet laws could potentially have protected these children. Lack of compliance with these laws endangers a child and could be considered neglect, and, consequently, child abuse.

Stronger legislation would be unlikely to change the pediatric trauma death rate, and adequate enforcement is logistically difficult. To protect children from serious injury and death from vehicular and other accidents, safety awareness and compliance with safety measures should be promoted by the educational systems, news media, medical community, and law enforcement agencies.

Further studies would be helpful in determining the role of noncompliance with safety laws in pediatric trauma morbidity and mortality. A multicenter analysis that includes survivors as well as nonsurvivors and focuses on mechanisms of injury, injury severity, outcome, and use or nonuse of protective devices would be valuable.

References

1. Hamilton SM: Coalition on trauma—trauma prevention and trauma care: Presidential Address, Trauma Association of Canada. *J Trauma* 1991; 31:951-957

2. Governor's Office of Highway Safety Belt Fact Sheet. Georgia Department of Human Resources and Division of Public Health, 1990

3. Wagenaar AC, Webster DW, Maybee RG: Effects of child restraint laws on traffic fatalities in eleven states. *J Trauma* 1987; 27:726-731

4. Bicycle-related injuries. Data from the National Electronic Injury Surveillance System. *JAMA* 1987; 257:3334

5. Browne GJ, Cass D, Ross F: Prevention in paediatric injury, Westmead Hospital (1982-87). *Prevention Coalition Report.* Westmead, NSW, Australia, 1987, p 65

6. Shelness A, Jewett J: Observed misuse of child restraints. SAE/NHTSA Child Restraint and Injury Conference Proceedings. San Diego, Calif, October 17-18, 1983. Society for Automotive Engineers, Warrendale, Pa, 1983, 831665, pp 207-215

7. Cynecki MJ, Goryl ME: The incidence and factors associated with child safety seat misuse. U.S. Department of Transportation, National Highway Traffic Safety Administration. Springfield, Va, National Technical Information Service, 1984, DOT publication HS-806-676

8. Evans L: Fatality risk reduction from safety belt use. *J Trauma* 1987; 27:746-749

9. Orsay EM, Turnbull TL, Dunne M, et al.: Prospective study of the effect of safety belts on morbidity and health care costs in vehicle accidents. *JAMA* 1988; 260:3598-3603

10. Peterson TD, Royer K: Motor vehicle crash injury: mechanisms and prevention. *Am Fam Physician* 1991; 44:1307-1314

11. Sherg RG: Fatal motor vehicle accidents of child passengers from birth through four years in Washington State. Proceedings of the National Conference on Child Passenger Protection. Washington, DC, December 10-12,1991

12. Paulson JA: The case for mandatory seat restraint laws. *Clin Pediatr* 1981; 20:285-290

13. Spaite DW, Murphy M, Criss EA, et al.: A prospective analysis of injury severity among helmeted and nonhelmeted bicyclists involved in collisions with motor vehicles. *J Trauma* 1991; 31:1510-1516

14. Fife D, Davis J, Tate L, et al.: Fatal injuries to bicyclists: the experience of Dade County, Florida. *J Trauma* 1983; 23:745-755

15. Wood T, Milne P: Head injuries to pedal cyclists and the promotion of helmet use in Victoria, Australia. *Accid Anal Prev* 1988; 20:177-185

16. McDermott FT, Klug GL: Differences in head injuries of pedal cyclist and motorcyclist casualties in Victoria. *Med J Aust* 1982; 2:30-32

17. Golladay ES, Slezak JW, Mollitt DL, et al.: The three wheeler — a menace to the preadolescent child. *J Trauma* 1985; 25:232-233

18. Stevens WS, Rodgers BM, Newman BM: Pediatric trauma associated with all-terrain vehicles. *J Pediatr* 1986; 109:25-29

19. Pollack CV Jr, Pollack SB: Injury severity scores in desert recreational all-terrain vehicle trauma. *J Trauma* 1990; 30:888-892

20. Friedman R, Harris JP, Sitzer M, et al.: Injuries related to all-terrain vehicular accidents: a closer look at head and neck trauma. *Laryngoscope* 1988; 98:1251-1254

21. Smith SM, Middaugh JP: Injuries associated with three-wheeled, all-terrain vehicles, Alaska, 1983 and 1984. *JAMA* 1986; 255:2454-2458

— by William C. Boswell, MD,
Carl R. Boyd, MD,
Savannah, Ga;

Donald Schaffner, MD,
Atlanta, Ga;

James S. Williams, MD,
and Elaine Frantz, RN, MA,
Savannah, Ga.

Chapter 5

To the Parent of a Young Bike Rider

Anyone Can Get Hurt

It's easy to crash on your bicycle. Each year, over half a million bicyclists visit the doctor when they do just that.

These injuries can happen anytime, anywhere. You may think your child is safe because he or she just rides around the neighborhood. Think again. Most serious bicycle crashes occur on quiet neighborhood streets. This is especially true for young children.

Head Injury: Not Just a Broken Bone

Broken bones can heal. But, often, a head injury can lead to death or permanent disability. One common result is epilepsy.

Each year, nearly 50,000 bicyclists suffer serious head injuries. Many never fully recover. It can happen to anyone.

Your child needs the protection that a good bicycle helmet provides.

Bicycle Helmets Can Help

Of course, a bicycle helmet can't keep your child from falling off a bike. But it can cut the chances of serious brain injury.

This chapter contains information from "Lou and His Friends Have Something Important to Tell You..." produced by the Brain Injury Association, nd; and "Helmet Laws," Insurance Institute for Highway Safety, August 1995; reprinted with permission.

Researchers say that bicycle helmets could prevent the vast majority of head injuries to bike riders. That's a worthwhile investment for any bicyclist, young or old.

What Price, Protection?

There's no getting around it. Bicycle helmets cost money. But what they protect is priceless: your child's life and future. For those who have suffered brain injuries, rehabilitation is a very costly and difficult challenge. Compare that with the cost of a helmet and you will see just how good a bargain one is.

Remember that a good helmet will last for years, as long as it's never crashed. That's more than you can say for a pair of sneakers!

Will Kids Wear Helmets?

Starting a new safety habit can be hard, both for the individual and for the group. That was true when they brought in hockey helmets, football helmets, motorcycle helmets, and many other protective measures. And it's true now of bicycle helmets.

But times are changing. Several million bicyclists now own and wear helmets when they ride their bicycles. With the right kind of gentle but firm encouragement from you, your child will join the growing helmet movement.

The New Helmets Look Great

Time was, bicycle helmets looked like buckets. They were hot, often uncomfortable, and they weighed a ton! But times have changed. With today's modern plastics, manufacturers have designed protective helmets that look great, feel light and cool...and protect better, too!

They come in all sorts of fashion colors and there's a style to suit everyone. You'll find one that's just right for your son or daughter.

Today's High-Tech Bicycle Helmets

They're tough. Most modern bicycle helmets meet or exceed either of two strict testing standards. These tests were created by the Snell Memorial Foundation and the American National Standards

Institute (ANSI). Only buy a bicycle helmet that has one of these stickers inside.

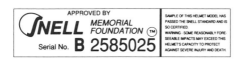 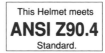

Figure 5.1. Snell Memorial Foundation and American National Standard Institute (ANSI) stickers.

They're light. Today's helmets weigh between 7 and 14 ounces—about as much as a wool sweater. This is much lighter than helmets sold only a few years ago. Weight is particularly important for young children riding in child seats; their necks have a hard time supporting heavy helmets. For older kids, weight isn't quite as critical as durability.

They're cool. Since bicyclists are their own engines and produce heat, helmet ventilation is important—especially on long rides on hot days. If your child will be doing more than neighborhood cruising or riding to school, look closely at how well the helmet cools. Some use slots or holes to let in air; others suspend the shell away from the head.

The Anatomy of a Modern Helmet

Every approved helmet contains a dense liner made from stiff polystyrene. This liner crushes and absorbs most of the impact in a crash. Many helmets protect this liner with a hard shell; some lightweight models, however, harden the liner itself to do the same thing. The straps and buckle keep the helmet from flying off during a crash. All parts of the helmet work together to prevent injury.

Fitting Your Child's Helmet

First, get the right sized helmet. Helmets come in sizes from Small to Extra Large. Each size fits a range of head sizes. Find one that fits comfortably and doesn't pinch. Let your child try the helmets on.

Next, use the sizing pads for a comfortable fit. Most helmets come with different sized foam pads. Use these to "fine tune" the helmet's fit. You can add thicker pads to the sides and thinner pads to front and back if your child's head is narrow, for example.

Finally, adjust the straps for a snug fit. The helmet should cover the top of the forehead and not rock back and forth or side to side. Helmets have adjustable straps to help you get them level and snug.

Taking Care of Your Child's Helmet

Be careful using paint or stickers on a helmet. Some paints and stickers can damage your bicycle helmet. Don't use anything on it unless you are sure it's safe. Some bike shops sell bright reflective stickers that are safe on helmets. Check them out!

Clean it with gentle soap and warm water. A helmet gets pretty dirty over time and it's nice to clean it up. But don't use solvents or cleansers! These can damage the helmet, even though the damage might not be visible.

Treat it with respect and care. While a helmet is made to take knocks, excessive abuse can damage it. It's best not to waste its strength by tossing it around or kicking it. This is particularly true of the new lightweight soft-shell helmets. If your child is hard on toys and equipment, consider one of the hard-shell helmets instead.

How to Get Your Child to Wear It

Helmets may take some getting used to at first. These tips may help you encourage the helmet habit.

Let your child help pick out the helmet. After all, he or she is the one who will be wearing it. Helmet straps may be difficult for young fingers. Help your child practice until he or she can buckle them easily.

Always insist your child wear the helmet. Anyone can get hurt anywhere.

When you ride together, wear your own helmet. Your own good example can make a big difference in encouraging your child to wear one.

Praise and reward each time he/she wears it. Your youngster may feel strange at first; take away some of the discomfort with words of support.

Begin the helmet habit with the first bicycle. Then, it'll become a natural habit as your child grows.

Encourage other parents to buy helmets. Making helmets common is the best way to eliminate the discomfort of being "different."

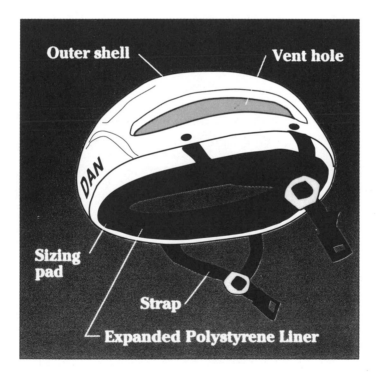

Figure 5.2. The anatomy of a modern helmet.

Helmet Laws

Bicycle helmets prevent injuries, but no state has a universal bicycle helmet law. Only 13 states have statewide bicycle helmet laws applying to young riders. Local ordinances in a few states require bicycle helmets for some or all riders. These and other differences among helmet laws in the 50 states as of July 1995 are summarized below.

Alabama—all riders younger than 16 (eff. 9/19/95)
California—all riders younger than 18
Connecticut—operator younger than 12
Delaware—all riders younger than 16 (eff. 4/1/96)
Georgia—all riders younger than 16
Maryland—all riders younger than 16 (eff. 10/1/95)
Massachusetts—all riders older than 1 and younger than 13[1]
New Jersey—all riders younger than 14
New York—all riders older than 1 and younger than 14[1]
Oregon—all riders younger than 16
Pennsylvania—passengers younger than 12
Rhode Island—all riders younger than 9 (eff. 7/1/96)
Tennessee—all riders younger than 12

[1]Bicycle helmet use laws in Massachusetts and New York prohibit people from transporting passengers younger than age 1.

Chapter 6

Motorcycle Helmet Laws

Compared with cars, motorcycles are especially dangerous. Per mile traveled, the number of deaths on motorcycles is about 20 times the number in cars. Motorcycles often have excessive performance capabilities, including especially rapid acceleration and high top speeds. They're less stable than cars in emergency braking and less visible. Motorcyclists are more prone to crash injuries than car drivers because motorcycles are unenclosed, leaving the rider vulnerable to contact hard road surfaces. This is why wearing a helmet is so important. Helmets are the principal countermeasure for reducing crash related head injuries, the leading cause of death among unhelmeted riders.

How effective are helmets?

Helmets decrease the severity of injury, the likelihood of death, and the overall cost of medical care. They're designed to cushion and protect riders' heads from the impact of a crash. Just like safety belts in cars, helmets can't provide total protection against head injury or death, but they do reduce the incidence of both. Studies show helmets are about 29 percent effective in preventing motorcyclist deaths. An unhelmeted rider is 40 percent more likely to suffer a fatal head injury and 15 percent more likely to incur a nonfatal head injury than

This chapter contains information from "Motorcycles," January 1996 and "Helmet Laws," August 1995, publications produced by Insurance Institute for Highway Safety; reprinted by permission.

a helmeted motorcyclist, the National Highway Traffic Safety Administration (NHTSA) estimates. Helmets are even more effective in preventing brain injuries. NHTSA estimates helmets are 67 percent effective in preventing this injury type.

Are there drawbacks to helmet use?

Claims have been made that helmets increase the risk of neck injuries and reduce peripheral vision and hearing, but there's no credible evidence to support these arguments. A study by J.P. Goldstein is often cited by helmet opponents as evidence that helmets cause neck injuries, allegedly by adding to head mass in a crash. More than a dozen studies have refuted Goldstein's findings. A study reported in the *Annals of Emergency Medicine* in 1994 analyzed 1,153 motorcycle crashes in four midwestern states and determined that "helmets reduce head injuries without an increased occurrence of spinal injuries in motorcycle trauma."

Regarding claims that helmets obstruct vision, studies show full-coverage helmets provide only minor restrictions in horizontal peripheral vision—less than 3 percent from that of an unhelmeted rider. A 1995 study by A. James McKnight analyzed the effects of motorcycle helmet use on seeing and hearing. The study found that wearing helmets "restricts neither the ability to hear horn signals nor the likelihood of visually detecting a vehicle in an adjacent lane prior to initiating a lane change." To compensate for any restrictions in lateral vision, riders increased their head rotation prior to a lane change. Subjects in the hearing study showed no differences in hearing thresholds under three helmet conditions: no helmet, partial coverage, and full coverage. The noise generated by a motorcycle is such that any reduction in hearing capability that may result from wearing a helmet is inconsequential. Sound loud enough to be heard above the engine can be heard within a helmet, a NHTSA study concluded.

How many motorcyclists wear helmets when not required by law to do so?

Without a helmet law only about 50 percent of motorcyclists wear helmets. Helmet use is near 100 percent when a law requiring all motorcyclists to wear helmets is implemented.

What is the history of helmet use laws in the United States?

Before 1967, only three states had motorcycle helmet use laws. The federal government in 1967 began requiring states to enact motorcycle helmet use laws in order to qualify for certain federal safety program and highway construction funds. Thirty-seven states enacted helmet use laws between 1967 and 1969. By 1975, all but three states mandated helmets for all motorcyclists.

As the Department of Transportation in 1976 moved to assess financial penalties on states without helmet laws, Congress responded to state pressure by revoking the department's authority to assess penalties for noncompliance. Between 1976 and 1978, 19 states weakened their helmet use laws to apply only to young riders, usually under age 18. Seven states repealed helmet use requirements for all motorcyclists.

Then, in the 1980s and early 1990s, several states reinstated laws applying to all riders. Congress in the 1991 Intermodal Surface Transportation Efficiency Act created incentives for states to enact helmet use and safety belt use laws. States with both laws were eligible for special safety grants, but states without them by October 1993 had up to 3 percent of their federal highway allotment redirected to highway safety programs.

Four years after establishing the incentives, Congress again reversed itself. In the fall of 1995, Congress lifted federal sanctions against states without helmet use laws, paving the way for state legislatures to repeal helmet laws. As of January 1, 1996, 25 states and the District of Columbia have helmet laws covering all riders, and 22 states have laws covering some riders, usually those under 18. Colorado, Illinois, and Iowa don't have helmet laws.

How do helmet laws affect motorcyclist deaths and injuries?

In the states that either reinstated or enacted a motorcycle helmet law in the past decade, helmet use has dramatically increased, and motorcyclist deaths and injuries have decreased:

California's use law covering all riders took effect January 1, 1992. Helmet use jumped from about 50 percent prior to the law to 99 percent afterward. During the same period, the number of motorcycle fatalities decreased 38 percent, from 523 in 1991 to 327 in 1992.

Nebraska reinstated a helmet law January 1, 1989 after repealing an earlier law in 1977. As a result, the state saw a 20 percent reduction in motorcyclist head injuries.

Texas from 1968 to 1977 had a universal helmet use law estimated to have saved 650 lives, but the law was amended in 1977 to apply only to riders younger than 18. The weakened law coincided with a 35 percent increase in motorcyclist fatalities. Texas reinstated its helmet law for all motorcyclists in September 1989. The month before the law took effect, the helmet use rate was 41 percent. The rate jumped to 90 percent during the first month of the law and had risen to 98 percent by June 1990. Serious injury crashes per registered cycle decreased 11 percent.

What other benefits result from helmet use laws?

Helmet use laws may also lead to a decline in motorcycle thefts, possibly because some potential thieves don't have helmets, and not wearing a helmet would attract police notice. After Texas enacted its universal helmet law, motorcycle thefts in 19 Texas cities decreased 44 percent from 1988 to 1990, according to the Texas Department of Public Safety. Motorcycle thefts dropped dramatically in three European countries after the introduction of laws that fined motorcyclists for failure to wear helmets. In London, motorcycle thefts fell 24 percent after Great Britain enacted a helmet law in 1973. The Netherlands saw a 36 percent drop in thefts in 1975 when its law was enacted. And in former West Germany, where on-the-spot fines were introduced in 1980, motorcycle thefts plummeted 60 percent.

How do motorcycle helmet use laws impact health care costs?

Unhelmeted riders have higher health care costs as a result of their crash injuries, and many lack health insurance. Results of NHTSA's Crash Outcome Data Evaluation System study released in April 1995 show average inpatient hospital charges for unhelmeted motorcycle crash victims were 25 percent higher than for helmeted riders— $15,447 compared with $12,374. After California introduced a helmet use law in 1992, studies show health care costs associated with head-injured motorcyclists declined. Average charges for head-injured motorcyclists admitted to hospitals in San Diego County fell 32 percent from 1991 to 1992, from $53,875 to $36,744, and average charges for all injured motorcyclists fell 17 percent. For head-injured patients treated and released from emergency rooms, the drop was even more substantial—43 percent. The total charges for head-injured motorcyclists seen in San Diego County trauma centers fell from $9.8 million in 1991 to $5.5 million in 1992 and $5.4 million in 1993. A study of the effects of Nebraska's reinstated helmet use law on hospital costs found the total acute medical charges for injured motorcyclists declined 38 percent after the law was implemented.

Studies conducted in Nebraska, Washington, Massachusetts, and Texas indicate how injured motorcyclists burden taxpayers. Forty-one percent of motorcyclists injured in Nebraska from January 1988 to January 1990 lacked health insurance or received Medicaid or Medicare. In Seattle, 63 percent of trauma care for injured motorcyclists in 1985 was paid by public funds. In Sacramento, public funds paid 82 percent of the costs to treat orthopedic injuries sustained by motorcyclists in 1980-83. Forty-six percent of motorcyclists treated at Massachusetts General Hospital in 1982-83 were uninsured. At Brackenridge Hospital in Austin, Texas, 41 percent of injured motorcyclists who were unhelmeted had no insurance, compared with 27 percent of injured helmeted riders treated between February 1985 and January 1986.

Are helmet use laws applying to only young motorcyclists effective?

There's no evidence that weak helmet use laws (i.e., those that apply only to young riders) reduce deaths and injuries. In states that mandate helmet use for riders younger than 18, 3 percent of motorcyclists killed in crashes in 1994 were under 18, the same percentage killed in states without helmet laws. Helmet use rates for all riders remain low in states where restricted laws are in effect, and death rates from head injuries are twice as high in states with weak or no helmet laws, compared with rates in states with helmet laws applying to all riders.

How have courts resolved challenges to helmet use laws?

Courts have repeatedly upheld motorcycle helmet use laws under the U.S. Constitution. In 1972 a federal court in Massachusetts told a cyclist who objected to the law: "The public has an interest in minimizing the resources directly involved. From the moment of injury, society picks the person up off the highway; delivers him to a municipal hospital and municipal doctors; provides him with unemployment compensation if, after recovery, he cannot replace his lost job; and, if the injury causes permanent disability, may assume responsibility for his and his family's subsistence. We do not understand a state of mind that permits plaintiff to think that only he himself is concerned." This decision was affirmed by the U.S. Supreme Court.

Are motorcycle education/training courses a substitute for helmet laws?

There is no scientific evidence that motorcycle rider training reduces crash risk. "Numerous studies have shown that formal motorcycle education and training is not an effective loss reduction strategy," state authors of a 1989 Traffic Injury Research Foundation of Canada report. Some support for motorcycle training was found in a California study in which training was associated with reduced motorcycle crash risk. However, later research contradicted the results of this study, finding an increased crash risk associated with training. The most thorough analysis of motorcycle rider training was conducted in New York between 1981 and 1985 by the New York Department of Motor Vehicles. Motorcycle operator's license applicants were randomly assigned to one of three training programs or to New York's standard knowledge and driving test. Despite the fact that more riders were licensed sooner under New York's standard procedures, these riders had fewer motorcycle crashes in the subsequent two years than riders in the three experimental groups.

Do other countries have motorcycle helmet use laws?

Laws requiring motorcyclists to wear helmets are in effect in most countries outside the United States. Among them are Australia, Belgium, Canada, Czech Republic, Denmark, Finland, France, Germany, Hungary, India, Indonesia, Ireland, Italy, Japan, Luxembourg, Malaysia, Netherlands, New Zealand, Norway, Portugal, Singapore, South Africa, Spain, Sweden, Switzerland, Thailand, and the United Kingdom. Victoria, Australia had the first motorcycle helmet law in the world. It took effect January 1, 1961.

By the early 1970s, virtually all states had laws requiring motorcyclists of all ages to use helmets. However, Illinois repealed its helmet use law in 1970 and, by 1980, most states had abandoned or substantially limited theirs—usually restricting coverage to riders younger than 18. Legislators in some states later reinstated motorcycle helmet use laws, so that now all but three states require some or all cyclists to use helmets. (Colorado, Illinois, and Iowa don't have helmet laws.) These and other differences among helmet laws in the 50 states as of July 1995 are summarized below.

Alabama—all riders
Alaska—17 and younger[1]
Arizona—17 and younger
Arkansas—all riders
California—all riders
Colorado—
Connecticut—17 and younger[2]
Delaware—18 and younger[2]
Dist. of Columbia—all riders
Florida—all riders
Georgia—all riders
Hawaii—17 and younger
Idaho—17 and younger
Illinois—
Indiana—17 and younger[2]
Iowa—
Kansas—17 and younger
Kentucky—all riders
Louisiana—all riders
Maine—14 and younger[3]
Maryland—all riders
Massachusetts—all riders
Michigan—all riders
Minnesota—17 and younger[2]
Mississippi—all riders
Missouri—all riders
Montana—17 and younger
Nebraska—all riders
Nevada—all riders
New Hampshire—17 and younger
New Jersey—all riders
New Mexico—17 and younger
New York—all riders
North Carolina—all riders

North Dakota-17 and younger[4]
Ohio—17 and younger[5]
Oklahoma—17 and younger
Oregon—all riders
Pennsylvania—all riders
Rhode Island—20 and younger[6]
South Carolina—20 and younger
South Dakota—17 and younger
Tennessee—all riders
Texas—all riders
Utah—17 and younger
Vermont—all riders
Virginia—all riders
Washington—all riders
West Virginia—all riders
Wisconsin—17 and younger[2]
Wyoming—18 and younger

[1]Alaska's motorcycle helmet use law covers passengers of all ages, drivers younger than 18, and drivers with instructional permits.

[2]Motorcycle helmet laws in Connecticut, Delaware, Indiana, Minnesota, and Wisconsin also cover drivers with instructional/learner's permits.

[3]Maine's motorcycle helmet use law covers passengers 14 years and younger, drivers with learner's permits, and drivers plus their passengers during the first year of licensure.

[4]North Dakota's motorcycle helmet law covers all passengers traveling with drivers who are covered by the law.

[5]Ohio's motorcycle helmet use law covers all drivers during the first year of licensure and all passengers of drivers covered by the law.

[6]Rhode Island's motorcycle helmet use law covers all drivers during the first year of licensure.

Chapter 7

Advice from the U.S. Consumer Product Safety Commission

Falls from Shopping Carts Cause Head Injuries to Children: Safety Alert

Falls from shopping carts are among the leading causes of head injuries to young children treated in hospital emergency rooms. The U.S. Consumer Product Safety Commission estimated that in 1988 there were 12,000 hospital emergency room-treated head injuries to children under 5 years of age. These injuries were usually due to falls from shopping carts. About one-third of these head injuries were concussions, fractures, or internal injuries. Shopping cart-related injuries overall doubled from 1980 to 1986. These products are now often used in hardware stores, drugstores, toy stores, and grocery stores.

To prevent falls from shopping carts use seat-belts to restrain the child in the cart and watch the child closely while shopping.

Wear Helmets to Prevent Sports Related Head Injuries: Safety Alert

The U.S. Consumer Product Safety Commission estimates that about 3 million head injuries related to consumer products were treated in hospital emergency rooms in 1988. About 440,000 of these

This chapter contains text from U.S. Consumer Product Safety Commission, Safety Alert (Aug. 1991), Publication #93, and Documents 5075, 5044, and 5002.

were injuries such as concussions and skull fractures. Many of these accidents happened when helmets could have been worn.

The Commission's study of head injuries showed that these four products or activities had large numbers of hospital emergency room-treated head injuries related to them and high hospitalization rates for these injuries.

These findings also may be an indication of the potential for death from these injuries.

- Snow skiing . . . 10,000 head injuries (11 percent hospitalized).
- All terrain vehicles. . . 12,000 head injuries (14 percent hospitalized).
- Bicycles . . . 169,000 head injuries (6 percent hospitalized).
- Horseback riding . . . 8,000 head injuries (27 percent hospitalized).

Many people do not wear helmets. Fewer than 1 out of 10 bicyclists wear helmets. Three-fourths of ATV drivers with head injuries were not wearing helmets.

There are several nationally-recognized voluntary safety standards for helmets. These standards require helmets to absorb the energy of an impact to lessen or prevent head injuries. Crushable, expanded plastic foam can serve this purpose. Many helmets also have a hard outer shell to protect against collision with a sharp object.

To reduce head injuries, bicyclists, ATV riders, horseback riders, and skiers should wear the helmet appropriate for each activity.

Back to School Safety Alert: CPSC Urges Bicyclists to Wear Helmets

With many families "back-to-school" preparations well underway, the U.S. Consumer Product Safety Commission urges parents to include bicycle helmets on the list of items for those youngsters planning to bike to school.

Each year about 1,200 bicyclists are killed and more than half a million bicycle-related injuries are treated in hospital emergency rooms. About one-third of these deaths and two-thirds of the injuries involve school age children under the age of 15. Three out of four of the deaths are due to head trauma and about one-third of the injuries are to the head or face. It is estimated that helmets are now worn by fewer than one out of 10 bicyclists. Some of these deaths and injuries could have been prevented if the rider had been wearing a helmet.

The purpose of a helmet is to absorb the energy of an impact to minimize or prevent a head injury. Crushable, expanded polystyrene foam generally is used for this purpose. Many helmets also have a hard outer shell which can provide additional protection to the head in the event of a collision with a sharp object.

A bicycle helmet should have a snug but comfortable fit on the rider's head. Some helmets are available with several different thicknesses of internal padding to custom fit the helmet to the user. If a parent is buying a helmet for a child, the CPSC recommends that the child accompany the parent so that the helmet can be tested for a good fit.

For a helmet to provide protection during impact, it must have a chin strap and buckle that will stay securely fastened. No combination of twisting or pulling should remove the helmet from the head or loosen the buckle on the strap. Children should be instructed to always wear the helmet with the chin strap firmly buckled while bicycling.

There are two nationally recognized voluntary safety standards for bicycle helmets sold in the United States. Both of these safety standards contain requirements for the helmet features discussed above. When purchasing a helmet, consumers are urged to examine the helmet and accompanying instructions and safety literature carefully. The CPSC recommends that bicyclists consider wearing only those helmets that are labeled as conforming with the voluntary standards. The CPSC is currently evaluating bicycle helmet safety standards to determine if their effectiveness can be increased.

Safety Commission Warns about Hazards with In-Line Roller Skates

The U.S. Consumer Product Safety Commission (CPSC) warns that in-line roller skating—a popular new sport—can be hazardous if skaters do not wear helmets and other protective equipment or do not learn to skate and stop safely. As use of in-line roller skates has increased, it appears that the number of injuries also has increased.

CPSC recommends these safety tips to help prevent injuries with in-line roller skates:

- Wear a helmet, intended for use with skateboards or roller skates, along with knee pads, elbow pads, and gloves.

- Skate on smooth, paved surfaces without any traffic. Avoid skating on streets, driveways, or surfaces with water, sand, gravel, or dirt.

- Learn to stop safely using the brake pads at the heel of most in-line roller skates. With one foot somewhat in front of the other, raise the toes of the front foot and push down on the heel brake.

- Do not skate at night because of your difficulty in being seen and your difficulty seeing obstacles or other skaters.

Skateboards

According to the U.S. Consumer Product Safety Commission, approximately 26,000 persons are treated in hospital emergency rooms each year with skateboard related injuries. Sprains, fractures, contusions and abrasions are the most common types of injuries. Deaths due to collisions with cars and from falls also are reported.

Several factors—lack of protective equipment, poor board maintenance and irregular riding surfaces—are involved in these accidents. Skateboard riding requires good balance and body control, yet many young skateboarders have not developed the necessary balance and do not react quickly enough to prevent injury.

Who Gets Injured

Six out of every 10 skateboard injuries are to children under 15 years of age.

Skateboarders who have been skating for less than a week suffer one-third of the injuries; riders with a year or more of experience have the next highest number of injuries.

Injuries to first-time skateboarders are, for the most part, due to falls. Experienced riders mainly suffer injuries when they fall after their skateboards strike rocks and other irregularities in the riding surface or when they attempt difficult stunts.

Environmental Hazards

Irregular riding surfaces account for over half the skateboarding injuries due to falls.

Before riding, skateboarders should screen the area where they will be riding by checking for holes, bumps, rocks and any debris. Areas set aside especially for skateboarding generally have smoother riding surfaces.

Skateboarding in the street can result in collisions with cars causing serious injury and even death.

The Skateboard

There are boards with varying characteristics for different types of riding (i.e., slalom, freestyle, or speed). Some boards are rated as to the weight of the intended user.

Before using their boards, riders should check them for hazards, such as loose, broken, or cracked parts; sharp edges on metal boards; slippery top surface; and wheels with nicks and cracks.

Serious defects should be corrected by a qualified repairman.

Protective Gear

Protective gear, such as closed, slip-resistant shoes, helmets, and specially designed padding, may not fully protect skateboarders from fractures, but its use is recommended as such gear that can reduce the number and severity of injuries.

Padded jackets and shorts are available, as well as padding for hips, knees, elbows, wrist braces and special skateboarding gloves. All of this protective gear will help absorb the impact of a fall. With protective gear, it is important to look for comfort, design, and function. The gear should not interfere with the skater's movement, vision, or hearing.

The protective gear currently on the market is not subject to Federal performance standards, and, therefore, careful selection is necessary. In a helmet, for example, look for proper fit and a chin strap; make sure the helmet does not block the rider's vision and hearing. Body padding should fit comfortably. If padding is too tight, it could restrict circulation and reduce the skater's ability to move freely. Loose-fitting padding, on the other hand, could slip off or slide out of position.

Tips for Using a Skateboard

The U.S. Consumer Product Safety Commission offers the following suggestions for safe skateboarding:

- Never ride in the street.

- Don't take chances:
    - Complicated tricks require careful practice and a specially designed area.
    - Only one person per skateboard.
    - Never hitch a ride from a car, bus, truck, bicycle, etc.

- *Learning how to fall in case of an accident* may help reduce your chances of being seriously injured.
    - If you are losing your balance, crouch down on the skateboard so that you will not have so far to fall.
    - In a fall, try to land on the fleshy parts of your body.
    - If you fall, try to roll rather than absorb the force with your arms.
    - Even though it may be difficult, during a fall try to *relax* your body, rather than stiffen.

To Contact the Consumer Product Safety Commission

To report a dangerous product or a product-related injury and for information on CPSC's fax-on-demand service, call CPSC's hotline at (800) 638-2772 or CPSC's teletypewriter at (800) 638-8270. To order a press release through fax-on-demand, call 301-504-0051 from the handset of your fax machine and enter the release number. Consumers can obtain releases and recall information via Internet gopher services at cpsc.gov or report product hazards to info@cpsc.gov.

Chapter 8

Head Injuries Require Quick, Skilled Care

American deaths from head injury since 1977 exceed the total of war dead from all U.S. battles, including the Revolutionary War. Yearly, head injury creates 5,000 cases of seizure disorders, leaves up to 90,000 victims permanently disabled, puts 2,000 humans into a vegetative existence, and claims as many as 100,000 lives, including 10 of every 100,000 children.

And, in the 15 seconds it took to read those statistics, another head injury occurred.

Most likely it was a young man, for his risk is more than twice that of a woman. Most likely it was from a motor vehicle accident, for mishaps involving cars, motorcycles and other vehicles account for half of all head injuries.

The annual tally of head injuries is conservatively estimated to be over 2 million, with 500,000 requiring hospital admission.

Emergency!

In a 1986 report published by the National Head Injury Foundation (a nonprofit advocacy group), Thomas Kay, Ph.D., of New York University Medical Center defines moderate to severe head trauma as clearly serious, often life-threatening, with obvious disability and need for specialized treatment. In other words, an emergency.

FDA Consumer, September 1990.

"Head trauma? We put a neck collar on. We always suspect spinal injury," says Burton Conway, emergency medical technician on weekends in rural Virginia and medical physicist during the week at the Food and Drug Administration's Center for Devices and Radiological Health (CDRH).

It's a good idea for anyone to learn first-aid, including cardiopulmonary resuscitation. The American Heart Association and the Red Cross offer classes.

To someone at the scene of an accident involving a potentially serious head injury, particularly if that person is untrained, Conway cautions:

- Never risk spinal injury by moving the head-injured victim unless there's immediate danger, such as a fire.

- Never stem the flow of fluid from the nose or ears, which may be from the brain, as this can inflict damaging pressure on the brain.

- Never remove an object penetrating the skull, as this can cause massive bleeding.

"Get professional help right away," he says.

Emergency protocols vary from state to state. In the unique statewide Maryland Emergency Medical System, a 911 call reaches a "central alarm" communications center, one per county, that can dispatch ambulances from local fire departments and request a "medevac" helicopter. Maryland has eight helicopter bases and 11 trauma centers. Ambulances are staffed by emergency medical technicians, cardiac rescue technicians, or emergency medical technician paramedics, depending on the need. The helicopters carry paramedics able to provide the highest level of pre-hospital care.

Ameen Ramzy, M.D., who directs emergency medical services for Maryland, says the technicians arriving at the scene quickly assess injuries, determine where the patient should go, and begin radio communications with the receiving center. They start an intravenous line, administer fluids in case of shock, and may also apply medical anti-shock trousers to temporarily increase blood pressure.

"The emphasis," Ramzy says, "is rapid assessment, rapid evacuation, establishing and maintaining an airway—with a tube down the throat, if needed—and administering oxygen."

He stresses that severely injured patients should reach definitive care, not just the closest hospital, within an hour from injury—an interval some call the "golden hour."

The Trauma Center

"A young man we received today was injured in a car crash—an unbelted passenger," says Walker Robinson, M.D., acting chief of the University of Maryland's neurotrauma unit in Baltimore. "He's unconscious, unresponsive, and has rapid pulse. He's not moving his arms or legs and is gasping for breath. We've got shock, maybe from bleeding, problems with the chest, and a broken neck."

The first person who sees him, says Robinson, is a traumatologist, a surgeon experienced in treating accident injuries, who leads the trauma team in looking at the patient "to try to determine which bit and piece isn't working right."

Quickly, they measure vital signs such as heartbeat and blood pressure and place electrodes on the skin to attach lines to cardiac and other monitors. They set up life-support measures such as mechanical breathing (ventilation) and blood replacement to reduce the risk of imminent death. Seeing the young man has head injury, they consult the unit's neurosurgeon, Robinson.

A thorough physical examination follows. Systematic testing of reflexes determines the patient's level of consciousness—"the most important factor in evaluating a head-injured patient," says Robinson.

The computed axial tomography (CAT or CT) scan is the gold standard diagnostic radiological procedure (see also "What About Skull X-Rays?") for head injury because it depicts the critical soft tissue of the brain so well.

(CT scans produce mathematically computed cross-sectional images of the brain's soft tissue. CT uses an x-ray tube but provides much more information than ordinary x-rays. CDRH regulates the instruments as medical devices and as radiological equipment. For more on imaging techniques, see "A Primer on Medical Imaging, Parts I and II" in the April and May 1989 issues of *FDA Consumer*.)

Robinson looks to CT scans and other diagnostic tests to explain why the brain isn't working right. There may be a blood clot (hematoma) or a depressed fracture pushing on the brain, which requires surgery. Quite commonly, he says, "we don't find anything to operate on but see evidence of damage, such as contusion, or bruise, on the brain."

Early Diagnosis Essential

Early recognition of the extent of damage is vital to survival and to immediate appropriate care. Indeed, the risk of dying increases tenfold when there's more than a four-hour delay of needed brain surgery. Some studies indicate any delay is harmful, for injured neuron cells in the patient's brain are easily killed by lack of oxygen, and the brain cannot long endure shifting fluid or tissue.

Once the diagnosis is made, critical care may go on for weeks or months to prevent further damage.

"When there's evidence that a patient has increased intracranial pressure—pressure in the skull—it is critical that the pressure be brought down," says Russell Katz, M.D., deputy director, neuro-pharmacological drug division at FDA's Center for Drug Evaluation and Research. "One way to do that is to place the patient on a respirator and artificially hyperventilate the patient."

This rapid breathing reduces the blood carbon dioxide content, he says, causing vessels in the brain to constrict and become smaller. The resultant decreased volume of tissue in the skull can help mitigate the effects of a major unsolved problem caused by head trauma: brain swelling.

"The swelling brain presses harder and harder against the rigid skull, which causes dysfunction of the nerve cells," he says. "In a worst case, the brain begins to herniate down to the brain stem, at the top of the spinal column. The brain stem controls the vital functions, so when the brain starts pushing on it, the person may stop breathing, go into cardiac arrest, lose consciousness, and, if the herniation goes unchecked, die."

Management of Brain Swelling

Modern management of brain swelling often requires continuous monitoring of pressure inside the skull, says Robert Munzner, Ph.D., who heads CDRH review of neurological devices such as electronic brain pressure sensors. The sensor is placed on the surface of the brain through a small hole drilled in the skull.

"But the physician needs to know the cause of increased pressure," he says. "For instance, a hole may be drilled in the skull to drain the blood from a large hematoma causing excessive pressure on the brain surface. Or, a catheter may be inserted into the interior of the brain to drain excess fluid, providing a connection for use also in measuring the pressure."

Other methods to reduce brain swelling include elevating the head to encourage blood to drain and giving diuretic drugs such as mannitol or Lasix (furosemide) through a vein.

If those measures fail, in a practice that is not uncommon Robinson may administer the barbiturate pentobarbital to induce barbiturate coma. Though the physician labeling does not specifically list this use, it is a life-saving step that reduces pressure in about half the cases. It can cause liver damage and depress heart function, however, so it's only used in extreme cases, he says.

Early care includes follow-up CT scans as indicated to check for post-injury blood clots. Magnetic resonance imaging (MRI) may be used if it's available. MRI uses a large magnet and, like CT, produces computer-generated, cross-sectional pictures of the brain.

Anticonvulsant medication such as Dilantin (phenytoin) may be given to prevent seizures, and the body's chemical, fluid and nutritional balance is maintained. A plastic water-filled blanket can be temperature-regulated to heat or cool the patient, who may be left unclothed to provide total access and observation.

Thanks to increased knowledge about the brain, more accurate diagnosis, and earlier, aggressive care, 60 percent of head injury victims survive—compared with only 10 percent 25 years ago.

When patients become stable, they usually go to a regular bed in the hospital and then home or to a rehabilitation facility. About 1 percent require a chronic-care institution, says Robinson.

Coping with Coma

Rehabilitation should begin as early as possible to provide controlled stimulation and prevent further complications, even when the person is in coma, according to Beverly Whitlock, director of Head Injury Services in Gaithersburg, Md.

"There are many levels of coma, and nonresponsiveness is not always consistent and across the board," she says. "When impairment is primarily to the motor system, the person still mentally takes things in. Also, recovery from coma is a very slow process. It's not like on television where the hero wakes up before the end of the show and returns to his job as vice president of the firm. Rather, you may get nondirected motion, occasional response, some eye opening."

The survivors' cognitive (perceiving, thinking, remembering), behavioral, and physical disabilities can mean years of hopelessness and anguish, for neither medical science nor rehabilitation offers complete cure. The person is changed. Personality alteration, lack of inhibition, poor judgment, and impaired social perception can drive loved ones and their needed support from the patient, even to the point of family breakup—which is far more likely over a cognitive or behavioral handicap than a physical one. Financial ruin is not unusual.

Still, the brain continues healing for years, and medicine can support the body along the way while fine-tuned rehabilitation helps the person compensate for losses and accommodate the new self.

"The family should learn as much as possible about the problem," says Whitlock. "Otherwise they misunderstand some things that are going on and may begin to feel the person is having an emotional problem when it's really very organic."

She recommends getting in touch with the state head injury foundation or the National Head Injury Foundation for information and referral. Whitlock stresses that head injury rehabilitation requires professionals with special training in dealing with head injury patients. Since injuries vary, it's wise to keep close to the treatment team for specific advice, she says.

Head Injury Task Force

Responding to concern by Congress about head injury, the U.S. Department of Health and Human Services early in 1988 formed a federal task force of members from 13 agencies. Gordon Johnson, M.D., director of health affairs at CDRH, represents FDA.

"We were asked to identify gaps in all aspects of head injury," says Johnson, "and to make recommendations about how best to fill those gaps if funding were made available."

In February 1989, the group reported the need for research in every area: prevention, basic biology, treatment, rehabilitation, and community services. It recommended that the government institute a "traumatic brain injury" category in reporting systems, designate a lead federal agency and establish an advisory group, encourage state and local participation, create a national network of 15 head injury research centers, organize a treatment system tied into the centers, and study and document financial issues.

While the task force was developing its recommendations, the U.S. Department of Education's National Institute of Disability and

Rehabilitation Research was setting up five model research and demonstration systems for brain injury at: Baylor College of Medicine in Houston, Medical College of Virginia in Richmond. Mount Sinai Medical Center in New York City, Santa Clara Valley Medical Center in San Jose, Calif., and Wayne State University Medical Center in Detroit.

"At an annual cost of $1.5 million, the programs are now fully operational and provide rehabilitation research and comprehensive services from emergency care, through long-term rehabilitation, to re-entry into the community," says J. Paul Thomas, Ph.D., the institute's director of medical sciences and task force member.

Minor Head Injury

Older people are particularly susceptible to head injury that may go unnoticed, says Mark Schapiro, M.D., chief of the brain aging and dementia section of the National Institute on Aging. Not only are falls more likely because of failing eyesight, reduced agility, and degenerative disorders such as Parkinson's disease, but also the chance of brain injury from a fall increases in the elderly because the brain shrinks with age.

"The shrinking stretches the tiny blood vessels between the brain and skull," Schapiro says. "If one tears, blood collects, pressing on the brain. This happens in anyone, but to a greater degree in older people, especially the very old, because the vessels are already strained." Tearing can occur from a fall or when the brain jars back and forth against the inside of the hard skull, as in whiplash in a car accident.

Twenty years ago, Schapiro says, many elderly people with minor head injury went undiagnosed, though they probably had headaches and might even have seemed senile.

"Today, if we suspect a blood clot because an older person complains about a persistent headache, we can look for it with the CT scan," he says. "A good example is when former President Ronald Reagan fell from a horse last year. During a later medical checkup, a CT scan showed a collection of blood, which they drained, and he recovered."

In minor head injury, patients often spend little or no time in the hospital, make quick medical recovery, and are discharged without a perceived need for formal rehabilitation, according to New York researcher Kay.

But even though there may not be obvious problems, there may nevertheless be injury, such as widely scattered stretching or tearing of the brain's nerve fibers. This diffuse injury doesn't cause specific deficits such as language problems but results in a general disruption of the overall speed, efficiency, execution and integration of mental processes, Kay wrote.

"I'm convinced that everybody who gets hit on the head has some brain damage," says CDRH's Johnson. "Repeated injuries, such as a boxer receives, add up over time to cause some damage to some cells. This is true even if he's never knocked unconscious. But usually the damage is so small, microscopic or submicroscopic, there's no simple way to detect it."

To assess various kinds of damage, including minute damage not indicated by CT scans or MR imaging, researchers are investigating regional brain blood flow with nuclear scanning techniques: single photon emission computed tomography (SPECT) and positron emission tomography (PET), Johnson says.

(A radionuclide drug is given and tracked in blood through the brain by a scanner, which produces a cross-section or 3-D image. SPECT and PET are regulated by both CDRH and the Center for Drug Evaluation and Research, the latter taking the lead since it regulates the drugs.)

"If brain blood flow is less in one person than another, we don't really know what that means," Johnson says. "But if we measure a person one year, and then measure again at a later date and identify changes, that may be significant."

According to New York researcher Kay, the most effective handling of minor head injury is to educate the injured person and the family before discharge. He urged that patients be carefully evaluated and informed of the likely scenarios, not only for physical symptoms and recovery but also for cognitive, emotional and behavioral symptoms and recovery.

Dr. Judith Middleton of Tadworth's Court Children's Hospital in Surrey, U.K., wrote recently in *Journal of Child Psychology and Psychiatry* that when problems arise—whether behavioral, emotional or mental—"it might be salutary to ask routinely whether children have had a past blow to the head."

Prevention: The Sure Cure

"In a very real sense, head injury is a social disease," says Russell Katz, M.D., deputy director of FDA's division of neuropharmacological drugs. "People drive drunk, don't use seat belts, shoot each other, or don't protect themselves with headgear in high-risk activities. If the social disease were 'treated,' then the head injury—the medical problem—would largely be prevented."

Common-sense measures to reduce head injuries are:

- Wear a helmet when:

  Riding a motorcycle. Riders without helmets increase their risk of head injury two to four times and their risk of death three to nine times.

  Riding a bicycle. Bicyclists are at greater risk of head injury than motorcyclists—in part, because they tend to land on the head while motorcyclists usually hit another part of the body first. Head injury causes 75 percent of the approximately 1,000 bike-related deaths that occur each year, according to the May 1990 *Consumer Reports.* The report evaluated various brands of bike helmets, noting that helmets can prevent 85 percent of bicyclists' head injuries.

  Performing other high-risk activities, such as construction work, boxing, football, and rock climbing.

- Don't drink and drive.

- Use seat belts and approved infant and child restraint seats in automobiles.

- Keep infants and young children from open, unguarded windows.

- Don't leave youngsters unattended in highchairs, strollers, buggies, or walkers.

- Supervise children playing with projectile-type toys such as BB guns and archery sets.

- Pay close attention when using nailing machines and power staplers. The force can drive a nail or staple through a thin wall or board, making it a flying missile that could pierce the skull.

- Only use ladders in good condition. Match the length to the job, use stepladders opened, and prop straight or extension ladders against solid support. Face the ladder when using it.

- If you're an older person, make your environment as safe as possible. Remove scatter rugs, use a slip-proof tub mat, ensure stairways are well-lit, keep outdoor steps and walks safe from snow and ice, and hold onto handrails at stairways and in the tub or shower.

- Sidestep assault. If you jog in an isolated area, take along a partner. Keep the car doors locked. Instead of confronting a suspected burglar, leave the house and call the police from a neighbors.

Causes of Head Injuries

- Motor vehicle crashes 50%
- Falls 21%
- Assaults and violence 12%
- Sports and recreation 10%
- Other causes 7%

What about Skull X-Rays?

When it comes to diagnosing damage due to head injury, many physicians and most patients attach great importance to the detection of a skull fracture, says Philip M. McClean of FDA's Center for Devices and Radiological Health (CDRH).

"It's not unusual," he says, "for a physician to order an x-ray series because of pressure to do so by a parent or patient or because of fear of malpractice litigation."

But simple skull x-rays can't directly show intracranial injury because they don't depict the soft tissue. Further, McClean says, clinical studies show that without signs of nerve damage, discovery of a skull fracture usually doesn't affect treatment.

For these reasons, in 1979, CDRH convened a panel of experts representing family practice, pediatrics, neurological surgery, emergency medicine, and radiology to assess the value of skull x-rays following head injury and to develop a management strategy. McClean coordinated the study, which reviewed the records of more than 7,000 head injury patients. The findings were published in *The New England Journal of Medicine*, Jan. 8, 1987.

Among low-risk patients (those without symptoms or with only headache, dizziness, or a superficial scalp injury), the panel found that not a single intracranial injury had been discovered. They concluded that no such injury would have been missed by excluding skull x-rays for low-risk patients.

The panel recommended that low-risk patients be discharged under 48-hour observation by someone at home, as explained in a take-home instruction sheet. Typically, a "head" sheet lists symptoms requiring the patient's immediate return to the hospital, such as unusual drowsiness, confusion, persistent vomiting, blurred vision, neck stiffness, unrelenting headache, bleeding or fluid leakage from ears or nose, leg or arm weakness, convulsions, or unequal size of pupils.

The recommended strategy calls for withholding radiographic imaging unless additional symptoms develop. Should the physician deem the injury to be more than trivial despite the presence of solely low-risk criteria, the panel agreed patients may be reassigned as moderate risk or high risk, usually warranting computed tomography radiological examination, consultation with a neurosurgeon, and possibly supportive skull x-rays.

CDRH has made these criteria available to emergency departments throughout the country.

— by Dixie Farley

Dixie Farley is a staff writer for *FDA Consumer*.

Part Two

Types, Causes, and Consequences of Head Trauma

Chapter 9

Types and Consequences of Head Trauma

Driving home late at night from a high school graduation party, Frank lost control of his car. The car went off the road and struck a tree. Frank, only 18 years old, survived severe injuries—a fractured skull and a blood clot on the brain—but his life has never returned to normal.

Despite immediate surgery in the local hospital, Frank was comatose for 3 weeks. He then required hospital care for another 3 months. Now at home for more than 2 years, the left side of his body remains weak and he has such serious memory problems that he cannot hold a job or continue his schooling. He is quiet but occasionally gets angry and breaks things or threatens his family. His parents are having trouble coping with the heavy emotional and financial burden that has resulted from the accident. They do not know where to get help for him nor are they aware of support systems for the family.

Frank's story is a common one. According to one estimate, each year between 400,000 and 500,000 Americans suffer head injuries severe enough to cause death or admission to a hospital. Of course, many of these people do not experience head injuries as severe as Frank's. And not all are involved in car accidents. Some people receive head injuries while playing sports; others are hurt in falls; still others are victims of crime.

This chapter provides background and definitional information excerpted from NIH Pub. No. 84-2478 "Head Injury: Hope Through Research," August 1984. Current information on treatment, rehabilitation and research may be found in other chapters; please consult the table of contents or index.

But the most common cause of severe head injuries is motor vehicle accidents. The more serious the injury, the more likely it is to have been caused by a motor vehicle.

Victims of car accidents and other causes of serious head injury face years of disability and lost productivity. Like Frank, many of these patients struggle to regain memory and the ability to concentrate.

No Two Injuries Are Alike

The injuries that prevent head-trauma victims from participating fully in society are as varied as the functions of the brain.

Lying within the bony protection of the skull, and encased in a watery fluid, the brain works by means of signals that are passed from nerve cell to nerve cell through a network with billions of connections. Different regions of the brain are responsible for specific functions. One part of the brain controls speech; another regulates movement. The brain stem, at the base of the brain, controls heart rate, breathing, and blood pressure and regulates temperature.

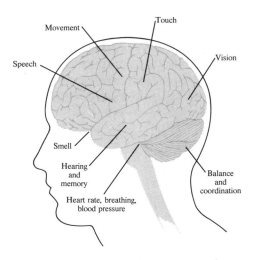

Figure 9.1. *Specific parts of the brain control specific functions, like the ability to see, to smell, to remember. The effect of a head injury is partly determined by the location of the bruise or wound. Damage to the left side of the brain, for example, may result in speech problems.*

Depending upon what areas of the brain are damaged, a head injury can produce losses in movement, sensation, intellect, and memory. There is no such thing as a typical brain injury. The effect of brain damage varies according to the location and the severity of the injury.

The outcome of a head injury is equally variable. Some victims die. Other people with serious head injuries become totally unresponsive for an indefinite time—a condition known as coma. Head-injured people may also suffer physical, emotional, intellectual, or psychological handicaps.

The more fortunate return to their regular employment and resume their social life with little or no disability.

Two Major Types of Injuries

Head injuries can be placed in two categories: penetrating injuries and closed head injuries.

Penetrating injuries occur when a penetrating object—a bullet, for example, or fragments of exploding shells—lacerates the scalp, fractures the skull, enters the brain, and rips the soft tissue in its path. The resulting stretching and tearing of nerve fibers, which kills many nerve cells in the damaged area, are the primary sources of harm in many penetrating head injuries. The severity of the injury depends on the type of object, its force, and its path through the brain.

Much of what we know about how penetrating injuries damage the brain and how the damage is best treated comes from studying the many thousands of soldiers who received head injuries during World War II, Korea, and Vietnam. Almost 1,000 men who were head injured during World War II participated in a Veterans Administration study designed to determine the long-term effects of head injuries. The study found that few men considered themselves "perfectly normal" years after the injury even though the results of their neurological examinations showed that they were normal. About 80 percent of these men still had injury related headaches 7 years after the trauma. In a similar collaborative study by the NINCDS, the Veterans Administration, and the Department of Defense, scientists are now evaluating the condition of head-injured Vietnam veterans 10 years after injury.

Penetrating injuries, however, are not limited to war. In any major hospital, surgeons are called upon to treat penetrating head injuries caused by objects such as a steak knife or an icepick.

Even do-it-yourself home repair may cause penetrating injuries. Great care must be taken when using stud guns and power staplers.

The force of the gun can easily drive a nail or screw through a thin wall or board, and the object may then become a dangerous flying missile that could pierce the head and cause a serious head injury.

Closed head injury is the most common type of head injury outside a war zone. In a closed head injury, damage is caused by the collision of the head with another surface such as a large stone. Although no object penetrates the brain, it may still be severely damaged.

A person's head hitting a car windshield is an example of closed head injury. When a person without a seat belt is thrown forward in a car that stops suddenly, the brain can be hurled against the inside of the skull. The soft brain collides with bone that is not only hard but has rough protrusions. This same kind of force can also squeeze and twist the brain in ways that are damaging.

In closed head injury, the blow may also injure the scalp and fracture the skull.

Where Is the Damage?

Regardless of the source of the head injury, the area of the brain damaged partly determines the resulting symptoms.

Focal Lesions

Focal lesions, injuries that affect a single, specific part of the brain, are of two types: *contusion*, which is like a bruise of a portion of the brain, and *hematoma*, which is a mass of blood resulting from bleeding in a confined space.

A contusion is a frequent result of severe head injury, occurring in almost 90 percent of cases. A contusion can occur at the point where an object strikes the head, or at a distant point where the jostled brain hits the hard surface of the skull.

The symptoms of a brain contusion vary according to the severity and location of the bruise. Some patients may be confused, restless, delirious, or even unconscious; others may develop severe headache, paralysis, or seizures which may lead to epilepsy.

A hematoma, which is generally considered a severe symptom of head injury, may accompany a contusion. Hematomas occur when a blood vessel is torn at the time of impact and blood leaks into the brain or its covering membrane (the dura). Intracerebral hematomas are formed within the brain tissue. Extracerebral hematomas occur between the brain and the skull—either below or above the dura. A

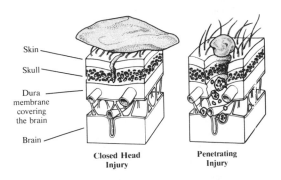

Skin

Skull

Dura membrane covering the brain

Brain

Closed Head Injury

Penetrating Injury

Figure 9.2. In this closed head injury (left) a large stone fractures the skull. But the skull helps absorb the blow, preventing the rock or bone fragments from entering the brain. In the penetrating injury (right), however, a small pellet fractures the skull sending bone fragments ripping into the brain.

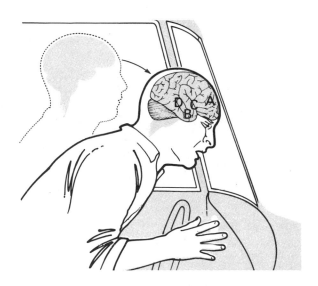

Figure 9.3. When the head smashes into a car windshield, momentum throws the brain against the inside of the skull. Brain damage often occurs in the frontal lobes (A) at the point of impact, the temporal lobes (B) as they jam against the skull, and at the junction of the frontal and temporal lobes (C) Large veins above the ear (D) may also tear, causing a subdural hematoma.

71

hematoma may be as small as a letter on this page or it may involve a large part of the brain.

Hematomas can result in increased pressure on the brain, causing further brain injury.

Diffuse Lesions

Focal lesions are confined to one brain site, but *diffuse* lesions are spread out and involve several areas of the brain. Billions of brain cells in these areas are distorted by the twisting, stretching, and compressing forces unleashed during the injury. This distortion can be temporary or can damage the nerve cells so severely that they die.

A physician describing the type of diffuse lesion suffered by a patient may use such terms as *mild concussion, concussion,* or *diffuse axonal injury.*

The least harmful form of diffuse lesion is the mild concussion, which occurs, for example, when a tall person bumps his or her head on the top of a low staircase and "sees stars." This sort of injury is reversible and probably leaves no ill effects.

In the mild concussion, a person experiences temporary neurological problems but does not lose consciousness. Mild concussions frequently occur in sports-related injuries. A blow to the head in a football game may cause confusion for a few seconds, and 5 to 10 minutes later the player may not remember the injury or events just before it. With more powerful blows, the player has longer periods of confusion and forgets events just after as well as just before the injury.

A person who has a full concussion loses consciousness for a period of time and also the memory of events just before and after the impact. Many people have no lasting ill effects from a concussion; however, some may show permanent subtle changes in personality or more prolonged memory loss.

In both the mild and severe concussions, the regions in the base of the brain involved in breathing and heart rate—called the brain stem—are temporarily disturbed. The parts of the brain that control memory are also affected.

Diffuse axonal injuries, the third type of diffuse lesion, involve a damaged brain stem as well as torn brain axons, the fiberlike projections from nerve cells that help transmit chemical "messages" from the brain to the body.

Diffuse axonal injuries range from mild to severe. All forms involve coma, a loss of consciousness triggered by brain stem damage. Recovery of consciousness is followed by confusion and memory lapses. Some patients recover to resume all normal activities, but others suffer intellectual, memory, and personality losses.

A severe diffuse axonal injury involves the tearing of many nerve fibers throughout the brain and brain stem. Patients with this type of injury remain deeply unconscious for a long time. They often have extensive loss of intellect, sensation, and movement. Some of them will die.

Coma

Brain damage caused by a head injury may cause a patient to lose consciousness for a prolonged period of time. Such a person is considered to be in a state of coma. Someone in a coma does not respond normally to stimulation. A comatose patient's eyes are closed, and he or she does not speak or move voluntarily. As one young man wrote about his brother who was in a coma after a car accident: "His body is whole, his brain is physically all there, but his mind, at least for now, is gone."

Coma can last from 6 to 24 hours or longer, depending on the severity of brain damage. Occasionally, a person remains unconscious for months or even years.

While in a coma, a patient must be given special care to survive. In an extended coma without intensive care, muscles will shrink and the body will become vulnerable to infection.

When patients first come out of a coma, they may follow people around the room with their eyes or blink in response to simple questions.

People often emerge from a coma with a combination of physical, intellectual, and psychological difficulties that need specialized attention. Recovery usually occurs gradually, with patients acquiring more and more ability to respond. Some patients never progress beyond very basic responses, but many recover full awareness.

A Threat to Survival

In addition to causing direct damage to the brain, a head injury may be complicated by pressure on the brain resulting from brain swelling or edema. These consequences of head injury can be life threatening.

Although poorly understood, brain swelling is thought to be partly the result of dangerously increased blood flow to the brain. The head injury disrupts the normal action of the brain's blood vessels, causing them to expand with blood and take up more space within the skull. Because the skull is a rigid container, this swelling may cause increased pressure on the brain. The brain is compressed and receives insufficient oxygen.

Swelling may occur immediately after injury, or be delayed by minutes or hours. The most common visible sign of brain swelling is a decrease in the patient's alertness. Some patients may lapse into unconsciousness. If the swelling can be controlled, it may not cause permanent damage. Uncontrolled, it may lead to the patient's death.

Scans, Surgery, and Drugs

Once initial care has been provided and the patient is not in immediate danger of death, the physician will turn to an array of tests and procedures to determine the extent of damage and restore function. Because the skull completely surrounds the brain, it is difficult to tell whether the brain has been injured and, if so, the type and extent of damage.

A technique called computerized tomography (CT) scanning has helped improve diagnosis and treatment of head-injury patients. The technique, perfected after years of research, creates a series of computerized x-ray images of the brain. After special x-rays are taken of the patient's head, a computer is used to reconstruct a cross-sectional view of the brain. With the CT scan, a neurosurgeon—a physician who specializes in surgery of the brain—can detect skull fractures and damage to the brain.

Rehabilitation: A Long-Term Goal

After receiving treatment in the hospital, the head-injury patient may be allowed to go home to complete the recovery process. Outpatient therapy may be provided at a rehabilitation center or in a hospital with a rehabilitation program.

People with more severe injuries, however, will live at a rehabilitation center for some time in order to participate in a more intensive program of physical and psychological therapy. These patients may make periodic visits home.

A number of specialists may be called upon to help rehabilitate the head-injury patient. Psychologists can help patients understand the consequences of their injury, cope with marital and sexual difficulties, and ask for assistance when they need it.

Other experts involved in the rehabilitation process include psychiatrists and speech, physical, and occupational therapists. Services offered to the patient include instruction in basic living skills such as bathing, dressing, cooking, and reading.

Some patients benefit from memory retraining therapy which helps them remember words by forming visual images. For example, they might picture Uncle Sam to remember "United States."

Another type of rehabilitation called cognitive therapy "opens the doors to understanding thinking processes," says a head-injury expert. Cognitive therapy may help people whose mental processes no longer interact in the normal, effective way. The training teaches patients to respond appropriately in a wide variety of situations, and improves attention span, self-awareness, and flexibility of thought. Techniques may include computer games, videotapes, and group role-playing sessions.

Rehabilitation may play a role even after mild head injuries, which can reduce a person's ability to process information. A patient who returns to work too soon after such an injury may not be able to succeed at ordinary tasks, especially at jobs requiring attention to several factors at once. A lawyer may not be able to follow court arguments; an insurance agent may find it hard to perform necessary calculations. Such difficulties can lead to tension, fatigue, irritability, anxiety, and depression—conditions that can only aggravate the cognitive or thought process.

Experimental occupational therapy tries to increase tolerance to fatigue and noise, thus improving work efficiency and ability to concentrate. The therapy program gives the patient increasingly abstract and complex activities to deal with—activities that are selected according to the patient's progress. The therapist also provides the patient with emotional support, while periodic tests measure patient improvement.

Occupational training and most other types of therapy are begun as soon as possible after the injury. Research has shown that this is the most effective way to approach the rehabilitation process. Exercise therapy, for example, is sometimes begun while the patient is still unconscious.

Physical Troubles Interfere

The patient's physical troubles often complicate the early stages of rehabilitation. The more severe the injury, the more lasting and serious will be the resulting physical problems.

Loss of muscle control and muscle weakness on one side of the body, interfering with leg and arm movement, can occur after head injury. Recurrent epileptic seizures may also be a problem. In fact, head injury is a leading cause of epilepsy. Fortunately, most seizures can be controlled with medicines.

Hematomas and skull fractures that press on the brain can cause facial paralysis, deafness, disorders in muscles controlling eye movement, and loss of the sense of smell.

Therapy for physical problems may restore old skills to damaged parts of the brain and teach new skills to brain areas that were spared by the injury.

Coping with Personality Changes

Just as important as the consequences of physical disabilities are the psychological and mental problems that are the most common result of head injury. Psychological difficulties include depression, anger, and behavior inappropriate to the situation.

Immediately following severe injury, most patients have impaired mental functions that can last for a long time. Some impairment may be permanent. Patients may have problems with abstract thinking, being unable to consider an idea in general terms without having a specific example in real life.

Patients may also have difficulty concentrating and they may find it hard to remember or to learn. Scientists have found that even a mild head injury such as a concussion impairs the brain's ability to handle new information for varying periods of time.

Children, like adults, may have persistent memory problems after head injuries. The ability to learn new things may be impaired, interfering with school progress. In NINCDS-funded research at the University of Texas Medical Branch in Galveston, investigators found similar patterns of memory problems in head-injured children, adolescents, and young adults. Among head-injured children, they found that nearly half later had trouble with the storage and retrieval functions of long-term memory. Those with the most severe head injuries suffered the greatest memory impairment.

Changes in personality, although harder to measure, seem to be more frequent than mental changes in head-injured patients, and are at least as disabling. One common personality change involves apathy—a reduced interest in life's activities and challenges.

Other patients may become overly optimistic—believing that things are better than they are. Or they may underestimate their disabilities.

A third common personality change is loss of social restraint and judgment. A person becomes tactless, talkative, and hurtful, and may have outbursts of rage in response to trivial frustrations. These rages occasionally become so violent that the patient may require hospitalization.

Patients may also react with psychiatric symptoms to the stress of mental disabilities and lifestyle readjustment. A law student might become depressed at having to change to a community college or a former accountant at having to take a menial job.

Regaining the Quality of Life

"Up until now," says one expert, "we've attended to the acute needs of the patient. But it is becoming apparent, as more and more head-injury patients are surviving, that we need to look at the quality of their lives. Many survive at least 40 years."

Generally, the greatest recovery occurs in most patients in the first year. Some people continue to improve for years. Therapists believe that patients who receive concentrated therapy soon after their injuries will continue to improve for a longer time. Long-term therapy can lead to a patient's continued improvement over a lifetime.

The Impact on the Family

When 16 year-old Lily found out that her younger sister, Fran, had been in a car accident and suffered a head injury, she felt "as if I had just been thrown into a make-believe world, one that I would just as soon not have known. I remember the endless trips to the hospital. I hated each and every one of them. My mother was there every day—all day. There was nothing else on her mind. I hated that too. In fact, I hated everything then. Fran was not the little sister I grew up with. She was a lifeless body—a part of machines and wires."

Whether it is a sister, brother, mother, or father who has been injured, the effect on the family can be dramatic. Relatives undergo tremendous emotional turmoil—from worrying whether the injured victim will survive to dealing with a mentally or physically handicapped person.

When a family member is injured, relatives need information about the condition of the patient and about the prospects for recovery. Later, they need to be taught to participate in rehabilitation and to plan for the patient's long-term care.

It is particularly difficult for a family to deal with a member who has trouble thinking, withdraws emotionally, and lacks initiative. Families need to be forewarned of ways in which the head-injury patient is likely to seem different, to experience difficulty, and to pose extra burdens. It is also important for the family to understand the reason for a patient's behavior. A person who recently awoke from a coma, for example, will probably experience confusion.

If a patient is disoriented and has visual, perceptual, and verbal problems, he or she can experience an overwhelming feeling of confusion and frustration. Not only does everything "look wrong," but the patient may be unable to talk about the unsettling after-effects of the injury. For that matter, the patient may have difficulty talking about anything if the part of the brain that controls speech and language is impaired. The patient's confusion and frustration can lead to a temporary state of agitation where he or she becomes verbally and physically abusive.

Although some patients remain combative, most people progress to a condition of greater control. Whatever the patient's disability, any denial of the problem by the family can subject the patient to more frustration and put pressure on the person to reassume responsibilities prematurely.

Even when a patient recovers, the rehabilitation process can be terrifying to relatives. Distressing effects of personality change and impaired intellectual function—no matter how temporary—can be overwhelming. One research study in Scotland found that an injured person's mental handicap tends to break up a family far more than does a physical handicap.

But many families learn to cope. "It's been 6 years since Fran's accident," writes her sister, Lily. "The waiting was worth it. Fran continues to improve; but mentally and physically she will never be the same. My sister is becoming a new person, a strong young woman whom I am growing to respect. It does no good to look for the Fran of yesterday—she is no more. There is only the Fran of today. I've learned to understand that the brain-damaged victims of head injury are new people with their own unique needs and desires. It is our responsibility to understand and accept."

Chapter 10

Fainting

Passing out is usually scary but not always serious.

You felt fine. Then with little warning, you found yourself lying on the floor with a circle of concerned faces peering down at you.

One in three people faints at least once in a lifetime, most often after age 65. Although frightening and maybe a bit embarrassing, fainting generally isn't a reason to panic.

When the Lights Go Out

Fainting, also called syncope (SING-kuh-pe), occurs when not enough oxygen-rich blood reaches your brain. Without adequate oxygen, brain metabolism slows, causing you to lose consciousness briefly.

You may have no warning. But usually you feel nauseated or lightheaded, become sweaty and pale, then experience a graying out of your vision. Within about a minute of lying flat, sufficient blood flow to your brain is restored and you regain consciousness.

A Symptom with Many Causes

About 25 percent of adults faint because of a heart condition (see "When fainting signals something serious"). In as many as 35 percent of people, the reason is unknown.

Reprinted from January 1996 *Mayo Clinic Health Letter* with permission of Mayo Foundation for Medical Education and Research, Rochester, MN 55905. For subscription information, call 1-800-333-9037.

In other cases, fainting may be due to a drop in blood pressure related to these factors:

Standing too quickly. When you stand, your sympathetic nervous system triggers release of the hormone adrenaline. This leads to an increase in your heart rate and blood pressure, preserving adequate blood flow to your brain.

With age, this cardiovascular response can slow. Standing too quickly may cause blood to pool in your legs, leading to a sudden drop in blood pressure.

Medications. High blood pressure drugs and antiarrhythmics that slow heart rate are typically associated with fainting.

These drugs can make you more susceptible to blood pressure changes. They also can keep your heart from beating fast enough to meet higher demands caused by a change in position or activity.

Anxiety. Emotional stress or sudden severe pain can trigger interplay between your neurologic and cardiovascular systems that results in stimulation of your vagus nerve. This signals your heart to slow and your arteries to dilate. When the changes occur too quickly, blood pressure drops suddenly.

Activity. Adequate sodium helps maintain blood pressure. Sodium lost through excessive sweat during strenuous activity, especially in heat and humidity, can lead to a drop in blood pressure.

Ways to Prevent Fainting

A few simple steps may keep you from fainting:

Lower your head. If you feel as though you're going to faint, lie down. Raise your legs above the level of your head to increase blood flow to your brain.

If you can't lie down, sit or bend forward with your head between your knees. Wait until the lightheadedness or nausea has subsided before trying to stand.

Stand slowly. This gives your blood pressure and heart rate more time to adjust to an upright position.

Check medications. If a new drug or change in prescription causes occasional lightheadedness, talk with your doctor. You may need an adjustment in your dosage.

If you take several medications, don't take them all at the same time unless your doctor advises otherwise. The combined effect may overwhelm your body's ability to maintain homeostasis.

Pace yourself. When working or exercising in heat and humidity, take frequent breaks and drink plenty of liquids.

Don't Minimize Fainting

If you have a chronic health condition such as cardiovascular disease, high blood pressure or diabetes coupled with recurrent fainting, have your doctor evaluate the problem. Contact your doctor about even a single fainting episode if you're more than 40 years old.

When Fainting Signals Something Serious

Serious causes of fainting typically involve problems with your heart or the blood vessels leading to your brain. An irregular rhythm, the most common heart condition, reduces blood pumped from your heart.

Severe narrowing of your aortic valve (aortic stenosis) or accumulation of plaque in your carotid arteries may cause fainting by limiting blood flow to your brain.

See your doctor right away if fainting occurs without warning, when you turn your head or extend your neck, or when accompanied by:

- Irregular heartbeat
- Chest pain
- Shortness of breath
- Blurred vision
- Confusion
- Trouble talking

Chapter 11

Minor Head Trauma

What is minor head trauma?

Minor head trauma is the temporary disruption of brain functioning due to an insult to the head. For our purposes, head trauma is called "minor" if the injury is not judged serious enough to require formal rehabilitation, and the patient is sent directly home from the hospital.

Is the head always struck in a minor head trauma?

No. Usually the head is struck, as in a car accident, fall, or blow to the head. But minor head trauma may occur as a result of sudden violent motion—such as a whiplash injury—without the head actually hitting anything.

Is there always loss of consciousness?

Usually, but not always. Brief loss of consciousness is common, but minor head trauma can occur even without loss of consciousness.

What happens during minor head trauma?

The damage during head injury occurs when the soft movable brain twists and collides with the rough interior surface of the skull during

"The Unseen Injury: Minor Head Trauma," Brain Injury Association, nd; Reprinted with permission.

violent motion to the head. Nerve fibers may be stretched and torn, and bruising may occur on the surface of the brain. (In more serious injuries, bleeding and swelling may occur within the brain.) Unconsciousness occurs if the activating system in the brain is temporarily "knocked out."

Why is minor head trauma called "The Unseen Injury"?

Because even though physical recovery may be complete, and the person may look fine, non-physical problems in the areas of thinking, behavior, and emotions may remain as a result of damage to nerve cells.

Does minor head trauma always result in permanent problems?

No. Most people who suffer minor bumps to the head will be OK. They will have temporary symptoms which will disappear with time. Only when enough nerve cells have been damaged—or if there are repeated minor injuries—will persons experience permanent changes in the way they think, feel, and act.

What is the normal course of recovery after minor head trauma?

Although recovery may differ between individuals, many people will experience headaches, dizziness, nausea, vomiting, confusion, disorientation, fatigue, and slowness immediately after their injury. Usually the events immediately preceding the accident, and for some time afterwards, are not remembered, even though the person may have been conscious for much of the time. For some time after the injury, persons may have problems with learning and memory, attention and concentration, a slower thinking process, and physical and mental fatigue. All these symptoms are common after a minor head injury, and mean that a person has suffered a "concussion." *Usually*, these symptoms will gradually disappear over a period of days, weeks, or sometimes even months, until the problems disappear or fade completely into the background.

When do more permanent problems occur?

When a sufficient number of nerve cells have been damaged, certain symptoms may remain and interfere with a person's life at home, in school, or on the job. Often these problems are not encountered until a person returns to the demands of work, school or home.

How will I recognize these problems?

You will notice that "something is off"; things just "aren't the same." Memory problems are common, not for things already known, but for new learning. You may be more forgetful of names, where you put things, appointments, etc. It may be harder to learn new information or routines. Your attention may be shorter, you may be easily distracted, or forget things or lose your place when you have to shift back and forth between two things. You may find it harder to concentrate for long periods of time, and become mentally fatigued, e.g., when reading.

You may find it harder to find the right word or express exactly what you are thinking. You may think and respond more slowly, and it may take more effort to do the things you used to do automatically. You may not have the same insights or spontaneous ideas as you did before.

Emotionally you may find yourself more irritable, quicker to get angry and more emotional. You may find yourself in conflict with your friends or co-workers, even when it doesn't seem like your fault. You may get depressed more easily, or laugh or cry when you don't expect to. Strong emotions may come and go very quickly. You may feel more argumentative. All these emotional reactions are a direct result of damage to nerve cells suffered as a result of your accident, and do not mean you are crazy or abnormal.

Finally, you may find it more difficult to make plans, get organized, and set and carry out realistic goals. You may feel like you are "spinning your wheels" and not able to accomplish anything. You may say and do things that others take offense at, that you wouldn't have done before. Your judgement may be off. You may miss the subtle cues that others give you that indicate how they're reacting to what you're doing. Often you will hear these observations from others who are concerned about you, rather than noticing them yourself. Your friends and family may comment that "you're not the same person" since your injury.

What do these changes mean?

When these changes persist for many months after your injury, it means that enough nerve cells were damaged to affect your thinking, emotions, and behavior. It also means you should seek help to learn to overcome or adapt to the changes that have occurred.

Will medical doctors find neurological damage if I have these problems?

Not necessarily. The nerve cell damage that occurs may be widespread and microscopic, so that it does not appear on x-rays, CAT scans, or on neurological exams. Also, your intelligence may still be measured in the average or above average. Your problems may be real and caused *by nerve cell damage* even if not medically obvious. Do not fall victim to being told you are malingering or imaging your symptoms.

Does this mean none of my problems are psychological?

No. When you cannot function the same as you used to, and do not understand why, it is natural to become frustrated, depressed, and to avoid situations where you might fail. If you are told you have no real problems and are just imagining things, it is easy to feel guilty, angry, frightened, or like you are going crazy. These feelings all complicate the problems you encounter because of the injury to nerve cells. It does not mean you are crazy or neurotic. It means you should seek proper help.

Of course, some persons who have pre-existing personality problems, or who are unconsciously tempted by the rewards of being incapacitated, may exaggerate or create their symptoms after a minor injury. However, this happens much less often than is commonly thought.

What should I do if I encounter these problems?

First, recontact the medical professional *you trust most* (regardless of his or her discipline). Explain your problems and ask for a referral for a *neuropsychological evaluation.*

A *neuropsychologist* is a psychologist who is specially trained to understand and treat the problems that occur following damage to the brain. While the evaluation is extensive, it is the best way for you to understand the nature of your problems, and to begin the process of adjusting and adapting.

Second, contact the National Head Injury Foundation (202-296-6443). They will provide you with information about head injury, tell you about local support groups, and refer you to local professionals who are active in treating persons with head trauma.

I have had a minor head injury. Should I be worried?

No. Most people recover after minor injuries, with time. Don't be so anxious that you start avoiding situations. Return slowly and gradually to your normal routine. But if your problems persist, seek help. Even when symptoms remain, early evaluation and treatment can head off many problems, and you will be able to lead a rich and productive life.

Chapter 12

Mild Head Injury:
Care of the Child at Home

Mild Head Injury

Your child has had a head injury. This is the most common injury for infants and young children. This booklet was written to give you information about head injuries, your child's return to school, and resources available for you and your child. The hospital team will meet with you to:

- talk about the specific type of head injury your child has and its treatment
- plan your child's care while in the hospital and at home.

Each child recovers differently from a head injury. Here are things to watch for in your child as recovery starts.

Your Child May:

- respond to your voice before someone else's
- respond to light and colors before words and pictures
- become fussy or irritable around new and strange smells and noises
- become calm around familiar music, touch, and people

- have changes in sleep patterns, for example, reversing night and day
- have bad dreams and trouble sleeping
- become very emotional or "act different"
- forget what happened right before and during the injury (amnesia, post-traumatic amnesia)
- have trouble paying attention and following directions
- become more dependent upon you and your family
- have problems with short term memory (who visited yesterday, food eaten for breakfast)

Mild Head Injury and "Post-Concussive Syndrome"

Mild head injury causes the brain to move around and hit the skull one or more times (coup-contracoup). This movement may bruise the brain. The child with a mild head injury may or may not lose consciousness at the time of injury.

As your child returns to regular activities, he or she may have a post-concussive syndrome, a collection of symptoms resulting from the brain injury (concussion or contusion). This syndrome usually lasts four to six weeks. Often these symptoms appear one or more days after leaving the hospital. Some of the symptoms your child may have with post-concussive syndrome are:

- loss of memory about the injury (amnesia)
- dull headaches that come and go
- feeling very tired, mostly at the end of the day
- mood changes and irritability
- disliking loud noises
- changes in sleep patterns
- short attention span
- trouble remembering and following directions
- trouble dealing with large groups of people
- greater need for individual attention
- greater need for supervision of safety behavior

Your child may have one or more of these symptoms. The symptoms should last no more than four to six weeks. After this time, your child should return to all normal activities and routines. Every child who has a head injury needs special help returning to home and school routines. How quickly your child recovers depends on the type and cause of the head injury.

To Help Your Child Recover:

- take extra time with him or her
- be patient
- give him or her the extra help needed to complete tasks
- provide quiet places for him or her to learn and work

Follow-Up Care

Call your doctors at the hospital to schedule the first follow up visit. If your child has problems after six weeks, make an appointment for him or her to see the head injury specialists. These specialists include:

- Neurosurgery
- Neuropsychology
- Speech and Language
- Rehabilitation Medicine
- Special Education

Returning to School After a Mild Head Injury

Your doctor will talk with you about when your child may return to school. Share the following information with your child's teacher. If you wish, the hospital staff will talk to your child's teacher also.

Each child recovers from a head injury in an individual pattern and time frame. In addition to dull headaches which come and go, the child may experience some common and usually temporary difficulties after a mild head injury.

Problems with Specific Learning Skills (cognition)

- Paying attention and concentrating
- Short term memory tasks
- Word finding and completing sentences
- Starting activities
- Completing assignments, especially timed work
- Judgment and complex problem solving
- Specific learning tasks
- Speed of language processing, memory tasks

Problems with Movement

- Coordination and speed, especially with walking (ataxia)
- Balance
- Fatigues quickly

Problems with Emotions

- Lack of awareness of other's feelings
- Recurrent dreams or nightmares of the event causing the head injury
- Frustration with difficult tasks
- Lack of impulse control
- Lack of knowledge of changes in self
- Easily angered at parents or peers

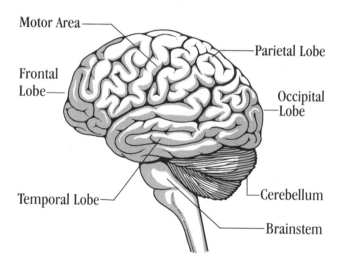

Figure 12.1. *Functions of Different Areas of the Brain.* Frontal lobe—*controls emotions, motivation, and social interaction, impulse control, voluntary movements, and organizing information;* Parietal lobe—*involved in sensation (feeling touch and pain), reading, and awareness of space;* Temporal lobe—*involved in memory, speech, and understanding language;* Occipital lobe—*involved in vision and understanding what is seen;* Cerebellum—*involved in the coordination of movement;* Brainstem—*controls consciousness, alertness, and the breathing and heart rates.*

Every child who has had a head injury needs special assistance as he or she returns to school. Most of these children will return to their normal activities and routines within four to six weeks. Teachers can help the recovery process by providing time, patience, extra assistance, and quiet situations in which the child can learn and work. Open communication with the child and parents is essential as the child returns to school and to a normal routine. The hospital staff is available to discuss any concerns with you.

References

Bowells, T.: *Minor Head Injury in Children*, Southboro, MA, National Head Injury Foundation, 1985.

Lehr, E., ed.: *Psychological Management of Traumatic Brain Injuries in Children and Adolescents*, Rockville, MD, Aspen Publishing Co., 1990.

Pediatric Head Trauma: A Guide for Families, New Kent, VA, Cumberland Hospital, Healthcare International, Inc. 1987. 1-800-737-7713.

Rosen, C., and Gerring, J., eds.: *Head Trauma: Educational Reintegration*, San Diego, College Hill Press, 1986.

Ylvisaker, M., ed.: *Head Injury Rehabilitation: Children and Adolescents*, San Diego, College Hill Press, 1985.

Chapter 13

Head Trauma:
Hearing Loss and Dizziness

Although the incidence of significant head injury in this country is unknown, the National Head Injury Foundation (now known as Brain Injury Association, Inc.) estimates that 2 million new cases of brain trauma occur every year. Of those 2 million, 500,000 require hospitalization, and 90,000 experience lifelong disability. Weisel et al. estimated that 10% of vehicle occupants in rear-end collisions will develop "whiplash syndrome," consisting of head and neck pain, neck stiffness, malaise, disequilibrium, and anxiety with depression.

The incidence of dizziness with even mild head injury ranges from 15% to 78%. This wide range is probably caused by different definitions of mild head trauma and by variations in the time of sampling after the injury. In one of the few long-term studies on untreated patients with mild head trauma injury, Berman and Frederickson showed vertigo persisting in 59% of the patients after 5 years of recovery. Initial complaints of vertigo in whiplash patients ranged from 40% to 80%. The symptoms were confirmed by objective electronystagmography (ENG) findings.

The incidence of hearing loss shortly after mild head trauma ranges from 7% to 50%. Some early hearing losses were conductive in nature and were quickly resolved, but interestingly, so were some sensorineural losses. One study by Feldman, however, warns of the possibility of late onset of hearing loss after trauma—even up to 18 years later.

The Journal of Trauma: Injury, Infection, and Critical Care Vol. 40, No. 3, March 1996 ©by Williams & Wilkins, reprinted with permission.

Dizziness can result from trauma through injuries to many different anatomic structures. Commonly, the maintenance of proper spatial orientation is held to involve the intricate interplay of three sensory modalities—vestibular, visual, and proprioceptive; central mixing and processing in the brain stem and the cerebellum; and final motor coordination by the central cortex, the spinal cord, and the peripheral muscles. "Dizziness" is defined as a disturbed sense of relationship to space—a sense of unsteadiness, with a feeling of movement within the head. More specific terms include "vertigo," an illusion of angular or linear movement; "ataxia," the failure of muscular coordination; and "disequilibrium," any derangement of proper balance. This study adheres to these definitions and interprets other studies accordingly.

Forces brought to bear on the central nervous system (CNS) during trauma are well understood, and the pathophysiology of traumatic brain injury also is well described. Magnetic resonance imaging (MRI) scanning of the head after trauma has supported the existence of brain contusion and hemorrhage in head injury patients with neurotologic symptoms. However, this study concentrates primarily on the peripheral sensory modalities of the vestibular and auditory systems, touching lightly on the subject of proprioceptive pathology (cervical vertigo).

For the sake of clarification, the term "trauma" includes both head blows and whiplash but not injuries severe enough to cause skull fractures or intracranial hemorrhage. No one doubts that head blows, even minor ones, can cause damage to the peripheral vestibular and auditory systems, but many physicians are suspicious of patients with hearing loss and dizziness resulting solely from a whiplash injury. Yet rear-end collisions at only 8 mph generate 5 g of force on the occupant's head. Such force has been shown experimentally to produce injury to the brain stem, cerebral concussion, and cranial nerve stretch in 50% of the monkeys and chimpanzees subjected to it. In reality, many rear-end collisions occur at far higher speeds than 8 mph, greatly increasing the possibility of damage to the CNS and to the peripheral auditory and vestibular structures.

The findings from the literature review and my own experiences concerning closed head injuries are presented below in two basic categories: first, those that produce dizziness; and second, those that produce hearing loss.

Injuries Producing Dizziness

Trauma and the Brain Stem—Eighth Nerve Complex

Many experimental and autopsy reports have described a shearing effect on the root entry zone of cranial nerves with head trauma. Even with mild trauma, this leads to petechial hemorrhages, often in the brain stem and especially in the area of the vestibular nuclei. Clinically, these patients experience acute signs of vertigo, leading to constant unsteadiness, which worsens in darkness and during fatigue, and to motion intolerance.

These patients experience a perpetually uncompensated vestibular disturbance for two reasons. First, the peripheral end organ input is probably only partially interrupted; and second, compensation in complete unilateral loss of peripheral vestibular input requires a *normally* functioning vestibular nucleus on the side of the acute loss. Because these patients have neither a total unilateral loss nor a healthy vestibular nucleus, they exhibit an unremitting vestibular dysfunction.

As mentioned previously, an MRI can reveal acute hemorrhage in these patients. Diagnostic vestibular testing shows a reduced vestibular response on caloric stimulation during an ENG battery, as well as an asymmetry of gain during low-frequency sinusoidal harmonic acceleration testing and an increased phase lag at low frequencies. With time, the asymmetry of gain would disappear, but the increased phase lag would remain indefinitely. Platform posturography using an Equi-Test profile (Neurocom International, Inc., Clackamas, Ore) would show poor function in tests 5 and 6. Some authors predict these patients to have a positive head-shaking nystagmus, but others have refuted this test's ability to detect a unilateral peripheral vestibular deficit. Finally, if the eighth nerve were, indeed, stretched, one might see an abnormality on standard diagnostic audiologic evaluations and auditory brain stem responses (ABR). Unfortunately, there is no known direct treatment for such an injury; vestibular rehabilitation might hold some hope, however, for these patients.

Trauma and the Semicircular Canals (Labyrinthine Concussion)

The pathophysiologic mechanism of trauma to the vestibular end organ is not fully understood. Excluding temporal bone fractures, with their obvious effect on the membranous inner ear, leaves us theoretical mechanisms of injury because the few autopsy studies available often show a paucity of pathology. One such study, however, found fibrous tissue and new bone formation typical of an inflammatory response to previous hemorrhage. Several indirect pathophysiologic mechanisms have been proposed. Brunner was the first to propose the idea that traumatic vasomotor changes in the inner ear (otitis interna vasomotorica) could affect the microcirculation to the sensory cells of the vestibular organ. Indeed, Axelsson and Hallen demonstrated small clots in the microcirculation of the inner ear after mechanical trauma. Other authors thought that there might be a physical disruption of the sensory epithelium by traumatic pressure waves transmitted from the intracranial cerebrospinal fluid to the fluids of the inner ear (commotio labyrinthi). Finally, Ilberg maintained that because of local hypoxia, biochemical alterations in the fluid of the inner ear could damage the sensory epithelium.

Whatever the exact nature of the pathophysiology, all accept the vulnerability of the semicircular canal epithelium to trauma. The vestibular end organ rarely has been entirely silenced by trauma, however, as evidenced by persisting caloric reactions on ENGs. Clinically, these patients present in exactly the same way as those with trauma to the brain stem—eighth nerve complex, described above. In fact; their diagnostic vestibular test results and long-term vestibular recovery are also identical. Only through the use of MRI, which is capable of finding hemorrhage in semicircular canals, can vestibular end organ injury be differentiated from a more proximal injury.

Why work so hard to make this distinction? The answer resides in the fact that surgery is available to provide relief from the long-term disability of an injured peripheral vestibular: end organ. The two options are either a labyrinthectomy or a selective vestibular nerve section. Labyrinthectomy has been used for decades to free patients of disabling peripheral vertigo when their hearing was not "serviceable" in the affected ear. When serviceable hearing remains, the vestibular nerve section will denervate the end organ and preserve the hearing.

Several factors must be considered before deciding whether a peripheral vestibular system should be ablated (through labyrinthectomy) or deafferented (through vestibular nerve section). First, common to both operations, is the assumption that the patient will undergo central adaptation when all unilateral peripheral vestibular information suddenly is removed. For reasonable assurance of this recovery within the usual 6 weeks, one must be very careful when the patient is more than 60 years of age. Although physiologic age and level of physical activity are probably more important than chronological age, this factor is one of the first to consider. In general, a patient functions better with *no* vestibular information from one inner ear, assuming the other inner ear is healthy, than with faulty and unpredictable information from a damaged organ. The CNS of injured patients can be compared with the pilot of a twin engine airplane with engine trouble. If one engine stops abruptly, there will be an immediate loss of control of the airplane, but with time, the pilot can bring the aircraft back in line and complete the flight. If the engine, however, continues to perform erratically, then the pilot is never able to resume control of the craft, and severe difficulties persist.

After surgery, whether an individual will compensate with time and therapy is often difficult to predict; certain circumstances, however, should raise a "red flag." A person who loses unilateral peripheral vestibular information, for example, must depend more heavily on the other two components of the sensory vestibular system—vision and proprioception. If there are deficits in these systems, as well, then recovery is less predictable but not necessarily unattainable. One difficult scenario would involve a diabetic patient who has both retinopathy and peripheral neuropathy, and then suffers trauma to the inner ear. In this particular case, one would proceed to surgery with extreme caution, if at all.

Another consideration is how soon after an injury a surgical intervention should be entertained. The prevailing opinion in the literature is that a patient with an isolated peripheral vestibular injury should reach maximal recovery 6 to 8 months after the injury, assuming the pathology of the inner ear is not progressive (for progressive conditions, see "Trauma and Ménière's Syndrome" and "Trauma and Perilymphatic Fistula"). Beyond consideration of age, other sensory deficiencies, and recovery time, other factors differ from one patient to another, including work, recreation, and general life activities. What a premorbid 75-year-old housebound patient can tolerate is not the same as what a 25-year-old individual with financial and parental obligations can endure. Taking all of these factors into account and remembering how disabling it is to have an erratically functioning inner ear (the *primary* balance system), the neurotologist finally must decide whether to recommend an operation to stop the peripheral vestibular input.

Once the decision is made to prevent this information from reaching the CNS, the next consideration is the hearing level of the affected ear. A labyrinthectomy produces total deafness in the ear that receives the operation. A vestibular nerve section preserves hearing at the preoperative level 95% of the time. Perceptions of what is serviceable hearing have changed over the last 10 years as cochlear implant candidates with minimal hearing are interviewed and tested. With this recent experience in mind, neurotologists are becoming less inclined to destroy inner ears with poor hearing. At one time, the 50/50 rule commonly was accepted. A pure-tone average exceeding 50 dB or a speech discrimination score worse than 50% indicated that an ear was "nonserviceable" and could be sacrificed. If, however, the better hearing ear were impaired or future hearing loss in the better hearing ear was a concern, then a hearing preservation operation—a vestibular nerve section—would be chosen. Physicians not familiar with these two operations rightly would ask: "Why not perform the hearing preservation operation routinely?" The answer is that the vestibular nerve section is a more complicated operation with higher risk levels than the traditional labyrinthectomy. So once again, the neurotologist must rely on published data and personal experience to counsel the patient with a vestibular disability properly. This counseling function must not be taken lightly or performed without adequate information because the wrong decision could consign a patient to a wheelchair or bed.

ENG is used routinely in these cases and should reveal a reduced vestibular response. An absent response without a temporal bone fracture is encountered only infrequently. An absent response even to stimulation with ice water, however, does not necessarily indicate an absence of residual vestibular function. One must always remember that caloric stimulation, as well as rotatory stimulation, tests only for *horizontal* canal function in standard testing protocols. Vestibular testing is also critically important in verifying the normal function of the contralateral ear on which the patient will rely for postoperative recovery. And finally, for ease of discussion, acute injury to the eighth nerve of the brain stem is separated from peripheral vestibular injury, although this separation is not so easy in the clinical situation. Sanna and Ylibosky caution that in cases of true vertigo, vestibular neurectomy was uniformly beneficial, even in patients with unsteadiness/positional vertigo and an accompanying hearing loss on the affected side. For unsteadiness/positional vertigo *without* hearing loss, even with a reduced vestibular response, however, nerve sectioning produced poor results, indicating a more proximal pathology or a combined central-peripheral injury.

Benign Paroxysmal Positional Vertigo

Positional vertigo after head trauma has been reported frequently. Considerable overlap and confusion exist in the nomenclature and diagnostic categories of positional vertigo. First, positional vertigo must be differentiated from postural vertigo. Postural vertigo, which occurs with changes from lying to sitting, lying to standing, or sitting to standing, is thought to be caused by transient hypotension seen in the elderly or in patients taking medication that affects the body's control of peripheral and central blood pressure. Usually, it is detected easily by monitoring the blood pressure during position changes specified above.

Positional vertigo (nystagmus) was subdivided into two types by Nylen in 1939: Type I, continuous and direction-changing (signifying CNS disease); and Type II, transient and direction-fixed (inner ear disease). Unfortunately, not all positional vertigo fits neatly into these two classifications. In 1952, Dix and Hallpike named a particular type of positional vertigo (first discovered by Barany in 1921), "positional nystagmus of the benign paroxysmal type," also known as benign paroxysmal positional vertigo (BPPV). They described a particular test for this condition, now generally referred to as the "Hallpike Maneuver" or "Dix-Hallpike Maneuver;" most ENG batteries, in fact, refer to a "Dix-Hallpike Maneuver" and to a separate group of tests called "positional or position tests." The difference is that the Dix-Hallpike Maneuver is not so much dependent on the final head position as the rapid *positioning* preceding it. Positional tests look for nystagmus produced when the head is in a certain position as the patient is moved into that position as slowly as possible. A positive positional nystagmus is regarded as a "nonlocalizing" sign, indicating a peripheral or central lesion, or both.

By definition, a positive "Classical" Dix-Hallpike Maneuver includes these characteristics:

1. A latent period of 3 to 10 seconds after the patient reaches the final position.
2. Transient rotatory nystagmus (clockwise with left ear down and counterclockwise with right ear down).
3. Severe subjective vertigo.
4. Fatigability—repeated maneuvers extinguish the response.

One exception is allowed for a nystagmus to fit the classical type: a latent period may be absent. Other characteristics are not essential but are often helpful in classifying responses as classical:

1. The response is usually unilateral.
2. The nystagmus is usually elicited with the affected ear undermost.
3. The caloric responses are usually normal.

That the pathophysiology of the Classical Dix-Hallpike Maneuver was a disorder of otoliths was suspected first by Barany and later supported in 1969 by Schuknecht, who proposed that loose otoliths would settle on the cupula of the posterior semicircular canal and coined the term "cupulolithiasis." Recent theories suggest that these dense particles accumulate in the endolymph of the posterior semicircular canal and would better explain the typical findings of a positive Classical Dix-Hallpike Maneuver. A more accurate term for this disorder would be "canalithiasis." Regardless, most authors agree that head trauma is one of the most frequent causes of BPPV. Clinically, the patient experiences severe vertigo when rolling in one particular direction in bed and, less frequently, also may report dizziness with quick head motion when up and around. For dizziness occurring at times other than in bed, cervical vertigo must be considered, especially in trauma cases.

After trauma, BPPV is commonly self-limited or intermittent in its expression. Many different treatments have been proposed. Initially, for those disabled by their symptoms, surgery to ablate the entire labyrinthine function of the affected ear was proposed. Gacek popularized a selective sectioning of the posterior ampullary nerve under the round window niche. This procedure became known as a "singular neurectomy," but because of the technical difficulty of identifying the singular nerve and the risk of damaging the cochlea in the process, the procedure was performed sparingly. McClure and Willett found antivertiginous medicine ineffective in controlling the disturbing symptoms. Brandt and Daroff described a specific exercise to disperse debris in the labyrinth. Toupet and Semont developed a rather violent maneuver called the "liberatory maneuver" to free the cupula of its supposed deposits. A technique I have used for the last 5 years with almost universal success has been found highly effective in alleviating the positional vertigo; Epley describes this maneuver, which he calls the "Canalith Repositioning Procedure."

Finally, most physicians dealing with patients who are dizzy after head trauma recognize BPPV and now treat it promptly and successfully as outlined above. Should a patient exhibit a positive nonclassical Dix-Hallpike Maneuver or a positive positional test, however, other causes must be sought in the peripheral or central vestibular system. A most exhaustive review of this literature is found in the work of Tuohimaa.

Trauma and Ménière's Syndrome—Vestibular Symptoms

Most physicians know that Ménière's disease produces hearing loss and dizziness. Typically, the dizziness involves episodic, whirling vertigo, often accompanied by nausea and vomiting. As the disorder progresses, the discrete attacks are often replaced by more constant unsteadiness, positional vertigo, and motion intolerance. Ménière's disease, which has endolymphatic hydrops as its pathologic substrate, is idiopathic by definition. When a definitive cause can be determined, it is then referred to as Ménière's *syndrome.* The symptoms of episodic vertigo—fluctuating hearing loss, tinnitus, and aural fullness—are exactly the same as those of Ménière's disease. Professor Ménière himself described patients who had a clear cause of trauma as the cause of their endolymphatic hydrops. Pulec found trauma as the cause in 3% of the 120 patients he followed. Animal studies have shown that disruption of the endolymphatic duct eventually leads to hydrops. Temporal bone fractures capable of interrupting the endolymphatic duct in humans have led to symptoms typical of Ménière's syndrome. Ylikoski et al., Nadol et al., and Paparella et al. provide clear examples of traumatically induced endolymphatic hydrops without temporal bone fractures. Characteristically, a symptom-free interval between the trauma and the onset of symptoms, often lasted as long as several years. The vestibular symptoms, rather than the auditory symptoms, seemed to predominate, and a reduced vestibular response on the ENG was more common than is usual in idiopathic Ménière's disease. The ENG, a test specific for endolymphatic hydrops, is very useful for confirming the diagnosis, although its sensitivity is thought to be only about 50%. In traumatic Ménière's syndrome, the auditory tests were often normal, thus fitting an older classification of "Vestibular Ménière's Syndrome."

Aside from hydrops resulting from disruption of the endolymphatic duct because of fractures, other theories explain the pathologic process, including those described earlier in this report involving hemorrhage into the fluids of the inner ear and displaced otoliths associated with head trauma. As the endolymph travels on a longitudinal path into the endolymphatic sac, where it is reabsorbed, blood and debris could block the flow and lead to obstructive hydrops. Debris could also accumulate in the endolymphatic sac, reducing the resorptive capacity of this delicate structure. After all, the volume of the entire endolymphatic space for a human inner ear is only 0.008 cc!

The same treatment as for idiopathic Ménière's disease—salt restriction, diuretic, and niacin—is used for 3 months. If medical treatment fails, an endolymphatic shunt, which has a long-term success rag of between 75% and 80%, is recommended. Failures of this conservative surgical procedure are rescued either through a labyrinthectomy or a vestibula nerve section, as described earlier, with a success rate in traumatic cases of 75% to 80%. The obvious reasons for the 20% to 25% failure rate include a concomitant CNS or bilateral disorder.

Trauma and Perilymphatic Fistula—Vestibular Symptoms

It has been known for decades that temporal bone fractures can result in perilymphatic fistulas (PLFs) and even cerebrospinal fluid (CSF) otorrhea. PLFs are ruptures that allow perilymph to leak into the middle ear. Assuming no fractures are present, these leaks occur through tears, either in the round window membrane or in the ligamentous attachment of the stapes footplate to the rim of the oval window. Fee, in 1968, was the first to describe traumatic PLFs clearly in the case of a patient who had been treated for traumatic Ménière's syndrome for 7 months, until an exploratory tympanotomy detected a perilymph leak, which was corrected successfully. This confusion over traumatic Ménière's syndrome and PLF will be a recurring theme and will require a detailed discussion. In the 25 years after Fee, more than 150 articles have chronicled the development of an understanding of the predisposition, causes, pathology, and treatment of PLFs. I have performed PLF operations in more than 350 cases, which will be the subject of a future article; a clear thread running through these cases, however, is some traumatic event, often whiplash or head trauma.

The pathophysiology of PLFs was clearly defined in 1971 by Victor Goodhill, who advanced the concept of two mechanisms for the round or oval window rupture—"explosive" and "implosive" routes. That the perilymphatic fluid pressure of the inner ear closely parallels the pressure of the intracranial CSF had long been known. Goodhill reasoned that a sudden increase in CSF pressure, often associated with head trauma, would be transmitted to the perilymph and could result in an explosive rupture of the round or oval window membranes. External pressure or trauma applied to the tympanic membrane (TM) would result in an implosive rupture.

With growing awareness of the disorder, it was only a matter of time until hundreds of cases of traumatic PLFs were reported. Unfortunately, these PLFs produced a confusing array of symptoms, and no diagnostic test 100% percent sensitive in determining the presence of a PLF is available yet. The history, therefore, remains the mainstay in the diagnosis of this disorder. In a monumental work, Strohm reviewed 232 cases of PLF and found that 25% occurred because of head or ear trauma. In the 350 cases my future article will review, 36% of the patients experienced direct head or ear trauma, often very mild in nature. I have reported on my own experiences with head trauma and PLF cases, many of which involved relatively minor head trauma. Grimm et al. published another landmark article, in which he defined the "PLF Syndrome" in mild head trauma and agreed with many others who have decried the use of the term "postconcussive syndrome." He presented information on 102 PLF patients, 33% of whom had incurred whiplash injuries only. The patients presented neurologic, perceptual, and cognitive deficits identical with those found in postconcussive syndrome, except that these symptoms uniformly *cleared* after the PLF was treated successfully, either through bed rest or surgical repair.

As noted by most who have written on the subject, PLF patients present myriad auditory and vestibular complaints. They may mimic traumatic Ménière's syndrome and, in fact, can involve a secondary component of endolymphatic hydrops brought about by the PLF. Most commonly, however, patients report constant disequilibrium and motion intolerance. They often report feeling worse in visually confusing environments, such as grocery stores or shopping malls. Some patients even report panic attacks and agoraphobia. If the patient also has aural pressure, unilateral tinnitus, or sensorineural hearing loss, the likelihood of PLF increases. The literature shows that PLF patients almost universally have positive tandem Romberg tests and fall to the side of the PLF. A simple office test, known as the "subjective fistula" or the "positive Hennebert's *symptom*" test, raises the likelihood of PLF to about 80% if positive, but the test's sensitivity is only 50%. This test is performed with the patient seated and instructed to fix vision on an object across the room. Using a pneumatic otoscope with an *airtight* seal to the external auditory canal, erratic pulses of pressure at approximately 120 mm Hg, are applied 8 to 10 times. The examiner then asks, "Did that bother you?" If the answer is "yes," indicating pain or pressure, then the result is negative. If, however, the patient reports that the object moved, feels nausea, or senses movement, then the result is positive. This test can be performed anywhere and takes only 1 to 2 minutes. It cannot be performed on patients with a perforated TM or an infected ear. A more sophisticated test, the platform pressure test, has been quite helpful in diagnosing this condition, with an amazing 80% reported specificity but only a 50% sensitivity in my experience. It provides information similar to that offered by the subjective fistula test. ENG testing may show a unilateral, reduced vestibular response or abnormal positional tests but rarely a positive Classical Dix-Hallpike Maneuver. ENG can aid in PLF diagnosis, however, as about 50% of PLF patients have a mildly abnormal summating potential/action potential (SP/AP) ratio. This abnormal ratio also has been observed by Gibson.

As mentioned previously, differentiation between a traumatic PLF and traumatic Ménière's syndrome often can be difficult. One distinguishing feature of a traumatic PLF is that its symptoms usually begin within 24 to 72 hours after injury, but traumatic Ménière's syndrome takes months or years to develop. A positive fistula test of any kind usually indicates a PLF but can sometimes also occur in Ménière's syndrome. On the ENG, Ménière's syndrome can be diagnosed with a moderately or markedly elevated SP/AP ratio.

Imaging, especially with MRI, has recently been shown to aid in diagnosing both PLF and Ménière's syndrome. An enhanced MRI can show hemorrhage in the inner ear after a round window PLF. Hemorrhages into the perilymph have been shown clearly in round window PLFs experimentally induced in animals. Gadolinium-enhanced MRIs can show segmental enhancement of the basal turn of the cochlea from traumatic inflammation after a PLF. My data indicate that the same technique sometimes reveals enhancement of the endolymphatic duct and sac, presumably presaging endolymphatic hydrops. Initial treatment of a traumatic PLF is bed rest for about 5 days. If the vestibular symptoms do not show clear signs of improvement, a simple middle ear operation is performed to place soft tissue patches over the oval window and round window membranes. This surgery has resolved the vestibular symptoms in approximately 95% of the traumatic cases, reviewed by Strohm.

Finally, traumatic PLFs may be one of the most underdiagnosed conditions known. Many mild head injury patients with PLFs are told to go home and await spontaneous improvement. The patients are not usually seen again until their conditions wear them down with frustration and exhaustion. The median duration of symptoms in my series was 3.5 years. Patients with severe head trauma and PLF have their auditory and vestibular symptoms overlooked while more serious problems are treated. Only with the knowledge that PLFs exist and that their symptoms can be obscured in a postconcussive syndrome package can these patients be rescued from years of unnecessary misery.

Cervical Vertigo

Cervical vertigo is a diagnosis/disorder that seems to be poorly understood. Relatively little has been written about this subject in the United States, and most of the world's literature on the subject comes from Japan and Europe. Ryan and Cope coined the term "cervical vertigo" in 1955 for this syndrome, which involves vertigo, in addition to tinnitus, hearing loss, and neck pain. The syndrome often results from trauma, such as a whiplash injury, but in one article on the subject, only 50% of the cervical vertigo patients in the group had experienced trauma. Macnah thought that the 575 patients he studied exhibited-little evidence of overt neck damage or of neurologic damage. He thought areas other than the neck itself, such as the brain, the brain stem, the cranial nerves, the cervical nerve roots, or the inner ear, might be responsible for the symptoms. Biesinger, on the other hand, proposed three possible origins: 1) a participant of the sympathetic nerve system, 2)vertebral vascular compromise, and 3) functional disorders of proprioceptive in segments C1-C2. He thought that some historical data was needed to support the theory that the neck was the source of the vertigo in 1) neck pain following trauma, 2) vertigo provoked by certain positioning or movements of the head, and 3) provoked vertigo of short duration.

The physical examination of such patients usually reveals some neck muscle spasm and limited neck mobility. Subjective dizziness is demonstrated best by rotational movements of the body, with the head stationary. Radiologic examination of the neck characteristically reveals excessive lordosis of the cervical spine.

Consistently, the ENGs of many patients have shown abnormalities. As early as 1907, Barany was investigating altered spinal proprioceptive afferents. Several investigators have shown nystagmus and disorientation when local anesthetics were injected into the neck muscles or when experimental animals underwent transection of cervical sensory roots. These alterations in the neck were signaled to the brain stem through spinovestibular pathways. In 1927, Klein and Nieuwenhuyse first demonstrated that simple rotation of the patient's neck, while the head was maintained fixed, caused vertigo and nystagmus. In 1976, Toglia reported objective ENG abnormalities in 57% of 309 patients with whiplash injuries. Wing and Hargrove-Wilson reported that 100% of their 80 patients showed nystagmus in ENG records with the head flexed, extended, or rotated to the right and left. Abnormal peripheral vestibular function was found using platform posturography in 90% of the 48 patients examined by Chester.

Treatment generally begins with conservative physiotherapy and antiinflammatory medications, once testing rules out an active inner ear disorder, such as a PLF. With time and therapy, most patients with abnormal ENGs end up having normal ENGs at follow-up testing. As for those patients who are thought to have vascular compromise, evaluation by a surgeon familiar with the diagnosis and management of this disorder is necessary.

Injuries Producing Hearing Loss

Trauma and the Brain

Few studies on the central auditory system after head injury exist. It is virtually impossible to have cortical injuries causing hearing loss in a conscious patient because the injury would have to be severe and bilateral. This type of injury would not be compatible with a conscious individual. Recently reported, however, was a bilateral midbrain injury after closed head trauma that resulted in total deafness in an otherwise alert individual. MRI scans showed that hemorrhagic lesions in inferior colliculi caused the deafness. This finding was regarded as a rare outcome of an isolated bilateral midbrain injury. These injuries are thought to result from contusion of the dorsal midbrain by the tentorium because of acceleration-deceleration forces. Other cases of such an injury typically include extensive hemorrhage causing coma and corticospinal tract signs. Hemorrhages of the brain stem also have been found in head injury patients and probably result from traction and shearing forces at the eighth nerve entry zone. Most patients with significant injuries to the brain stem are comatose and can be tested only with electro-physiologic tools, such as the ABR or the acoustic reflex. In 1970, acoustic reflex testing was shown to be abnormal in pontine lesions. In 1975, ABR became the dominant test for brain stem lesions. Peripheral auditory dysfunction in the cochlea and middle ear, however, can affect both tests. No treatment exists for the injuries described above.

Trauma and the Eighth Nerve

In general, it is virtually impossible to have isolated injuries to only the eighth nerve, unless a temporal bone fracture results in a severe crush injury or transection. Again, no treatment exists for this injury. Evaluation of the integrity of this nerve in traumatic cases of bilateral cochlear deafness is important, however, before cochlear implant surgery is undertaken. This evaluation is accomplished through a "promontory stimulation" test, in which a needle electrode is inserted against the promontory of the middle ear, electrically stimulating the cochlear afferent fibers, to look for a subjective auditory perception.

Trauma and Cochlear Concussion

The pathophysiology of cochlear concussion seems to be better understood than that of labyrinthine concussion. The principal theories include 1) disruption of the membranous portion of the cochlea by pressure waves transmitted from the intracranial CSF, 2) disturbance in the microcirculation of the cochlea, and 3) hemorrhage into the fluids of the cochlea.

Typically, damage to the hair cells of the cochlea is greatest in the region serving 4,000 to 8,000 Hz and mimics the changes observed in acoustic trauma. Most commonly, the hearing loss was noted immediately, with gradual recovery over the 6 months after the injury. If the hearing loss progresses or fluctuates, a diagnosis other than cochlea concussion must be entertained—PLF or traumatic Ménière's syndrome. Standard behavioral testing is often adequate to evaluate each ear individually. For years, as previously mentioned, site-of-lesion testing with the ABR and acoustic reflex was used to detect a retrocochlear lesion. In 1978, Kemp reported acoustic *emissions* detected in the human external ear canal after stimulation with clicks. These evoked otacoustic emissions are produced by contractile elements in the outer hair cells of the cochlea. They provide a unique opportunity to measure objectively the outer hair cell function of the cochlea and probably mirror the health of the entire cochlea. In the case of trauma resulting in deafness, evoked otacoustic emissions, if present, place the damage in a retrocochlear site and, if absent, tell us that the cochlea itself has been damaged. If there is damage to the cochlea, evoked otacoustic emissions will be absent with a loss of >30 to 40 dB in the 2,000 Hz range. As mentioned previously, MRI scanning would help detect a hemorrhage or an inflammatory reaction to hemorrhage in the cochlea.

Trauma and Ménière's Syndrome

As discussed previously, one of the hallmarks of traumatic Ménière's syndrome is the delayed onset of symptoms after the trauma. The hearing loss problems in traumatic Ménière's syndrome are less frequent than are the vestibular problems. The same diagnostic workup should be performed, as noted previously, and the same treatment should be applied, up to and including an endolymphatic shunt. In general, the control of fluctuating or progressive hearing loss in Ménière's disease with an endolymphatic shunt occurs in about 50% of the patients followed after surgery for up to 5 years. Labyrinthectomy and vestibular nerve section have no place in the treatment of the auditory component of traumatic Ménière's syndrome.

Trauma and Perilymphatic Fistula

As mentioned above, the incidence of hearing loss in PLFs in general seems to be less frequent than are the vestibular problems. Hearing loss after trauma can often be localized now, using the site-of-lesion auditory tests described above. These tests, combined with fistula tests, often aid significantly in the diagnosis of a PLF. The largest series of PLFs to date stresses that the speech scores on hearing tests seem disproportionately lower than the pure-tone scores, but this observation is not consistent with my experience. Another difference noted by most authors is that patients presenting only hearing loss symptoms because of a PLF more frequently have a round window fistula than an oval window fistula.

The surgical results in hearing loss problems because of a PLF are not as good as they are for control of vestibular symptoms. Most large studies have shown hearing improvement after surgical repair in the range of 30% to 40%. Hearing improvement has resulted in 43% of the PLFs I have repaired surgically (unpublished data). Although the success rate is not as high as that for the vestibular symptoms, these patients would not have experienced *any* improvement and, in fact, would have had progression of their hearing loss had they not undergone surgical repair.

Despite our best efforts, we struggle to differentiate traumatic Ménière's syndrome and traumatic PLF. When fistula tests are negative and the electrocochleography results are equivocal, I have followed the advice of previous writers in combining the PLF repair with an endolymphatic shunt when surgery is needed and a clear and separate diagnosis cannot be determined. In fact, it is my theory that *every* "active" PLF patient has some component of secondary endolymphatic hydrops, making a diagnostic differentiation an oxymoron.

Trauma and the Middle Ear

Because the middle ear structures contribute nothing to the vestibular system, trauma here can produce only hearing loss symptoms (excluding PLFs). In the 1950s, Hough sparked interest in middle ear injuries after head trauma. Until that time, little attention was directed toward traumatic hearing loss because it was assumed to be sensorineural and, thus, permanent and untreatable. Over the next 10 years, Hough diagnosed 33 cases of ossicular damage from head trauma. All of his patients had periods of unconsciousness and bleeding from the ear, signifying a severe head injury, including a temporal bone fracture. He coined the term "Traumatic Conductive Triad," meaning unconsciousness, bleeding from the ear, and hearing loss; thus, early on, we learned that head trauma alone had to be severe to disrupt the ossicular chain. Also, interestingly, none of his patients complained of "labyrinthine vertigo." Did the separation of the incudostapedial joint during the injury somehow protect the inner ear from developing an injury such as an implosive PLF? It is certainly food for thought. Hough's hearing results after surgery were excellent, with the ear closing the air-bone gap to 10 dB in 78% of the cases.

Conductive hearing loss after head injury is most often attributed to bleeding into the middle ear, sometimes because of a CSF leak associated with a temporal bone fracture. Because this report has avoided addressing the subject of skull fractures, we will only add that immediate testing of the auditory system in a patient with a head injury is rarely necessary, and a delay for 4 to 6 weeks after the injury allows the middle ear fluid to dissipate. If a TM perforation does not exist at the time the middle ear is aerated and a conductive loss is present, then an ossicular injury can be assumed. Standard middle ear reconstructive surgery, as pioneered by Hough and others, consistently provides excellent hearing improvement after surgery.

Conductive hearing loss secondary to head trauma without skull fracture does occur but is not common. In 84 head injury patients, Griffiths reported an incidence of 6% for a conductive hearing loss without skull fracture on conventional x-ray films (notorious for missing temporal bone fractures). All but one patient had spontaneous clearing of the conductive hearing loss 3 months after injury. Barber reported *no* conductive hearing loss in 56 head injury cases without fractures. Out of 307 such patients, Podoshin and Fradis found 15% with a conductive hearing loss, but again, only conventional skull x-ray films were examined to rule out temporal bone fractures. Perforation of the TM in head trauma is also rare unless direct force is applied to the external ear canal, producing a compression tear of the TM or a penetrating injury. Griffin reported his experience with 227 traumatic TM perforations, and only 5% resulted from head trauma (there was no mention of whether a temporal bone fracture was associated with the injury).

The treatment of a traumatic TM perforation varies from no treatment (because of the frequent spontaneous closure) to prompt surgical repair. The rationale for prompt surgical repair is the moderate incidence of an associated PLF, ossicular injury, or acquired cholesteatoma seen with trapped epithelium after spontaneous closure. I am aggressive when there are symptoms of a PLF (vestibular disturbance or sensorineural hearing loss); significantly large conductive hearing loss, indicating an ossicular dislocation; or a nearly total perforation. The edges of the TM perforation, otherwise, are everted in the office with an operating microscope, and a paper patch is applied over the perforation to assist in spontaneous healing. It must be remembered that fistula tests cannot be used when a TM perforation exists.

Discussion

This review was written to update the physicians caring for patients who have suffered closed head injuries. This care often falls to family practitioners, internists, neurologists, and physiatrists, especially when the injury has been mild and has not required hospitalization. Neurotologists and otoneurologists are trained to aid in the diagnosis and management of these patients. Before proper consultation can be obtained, the referring physician must have some knowledge of the causes and pathophysiology of closed head injuries with respect to neurotologic sequelae; otherwise, patients inadvertently are denied access to physicians who often can cure these vexing problems and provide long-term relief to frustrated and anxious patients. One final plea is made against assigning the wastebasket diagnosis of postconcussive syndrome to every head injury patient injury who complains of dizziness, hearing loss, and cognitive and perceptual problems. Physicians should look harder and seek consultation for their patients to maximize recovery from disabling and debilitating conditions.

— by Dennis C. Fitzgerald, MD

From the Department of Otology and Neurotology, Washington Hospital Center, Washington, D.C.

Chapter 14

Historic Studies Regarding the Incidence of Posttraumatic Epilepsy

An association between head injury and epilepsy has been suspected since Hippocratic times. Trauma to the head may be divided into A) closed or blunt and B) penetrating. In both, the key interest focuses on the potential brain damage caused by blows to the head. Early consequences of impact injury include focal cerebral injury such as in contusion or hemorrhage, raised intracranial pressure, reduced cerebral perfusion, cerebral edema, and epileptic seizures. The late or delayed effects of severe brain injury also include posttraumatic epilepsy. Such epilepsy depends upon the extent of cortical damage and on the inherent susceptibility of the individual patient. Both the amount of localized cortical damage as well as the extent of diffuse damage (reflected in the duration of posttraumatic amnesia) may contribute to producing a potential epileptogenic lesion.

Severe head injuries have been studied extensively in the war injured. Posttraumatic epilepsy has been reported to occur in up to 45% of this group of patients. A study regarding Vietnam veterans has indicated that 53% of patients with penetrating head injury have posttraumatic epilepsy and approximately half of these patients continue to have seizures after 15 years.

This chapter contains excerpts from a 1986 Brain Injury Association fact sheet developed by Kevin H. Ruggles, MD. It provides statistical information about the incidence and risk factors for epilepsy following head trauma. For more information about epilepsy and current treatment options, contact the Epilepsy Foundation of America: (800) EFA-1000.

Factors other than penetrating brain injury which have been associated with a heightened risk of posttraumatic epilepsy include loss of consciousness, or posttraumatic amnesia for more than 24 hours, focal neurologic signs, and early seizures (those that occur within one week of injury). Depressed skull fractures, intracranial hematoma, and dural lacerations are other risk factors. When two or more of these factors are associated the risk is still higher.

Nonmissile, or blunt head trauma, as it relates to epilepsy has been studied most extensively by Dr. Bryan Jennett (Jennett, W.B. *Epilepsy After Non-Missile Head Injuries*, Ed. 2, London, Heineman Medical Books, 1975). He has attempted to answer questions relating to early and late posttraumatic seizures and their prognosis. Answers to these questions are important so that appropriate treatment can be instituted as early as possible or treatment may be withheld if unnecessary. Secondly, answers to these questions are needed to address medicolegal issues and to advise patients in terms of restricting their activities, such as driving, if they are at risk for seizures.

Early seizures occurring soon after injury are often given a different significance than those seizures occurring later. Jennett found that epilepsy occurs more frequently in the first week after injury than in any of the next seven weeks. Furthermore, seizures which occur within one week of injury are significantly less likely to recur than seizures beginning in the next few weeks. A seizure was never the only or first sign of a developing intracranial hematoma. Less than 2% of patients who had early seizures proved to be developing an epidural hematoma at the time of the first seizure. Late epilepsy, or remote posttraumatic seizures, occurred significantly more often when there had been early seizures.

The overall risk of late epilepsy in unselected blunt head trauma patients in Jennett's study was about 5%. Risk was increased by three factors—acute hematoma (31%), early seizures (25%), and depressed skull fracture (15%). Without these risk factors, late epilepsy was around 1%.

After depressed skull fracture the incidence of late epilepsy varied from 4-50%, depending upon other factors. Depressed skull fracture in a patient less than age 16 had less risk. Depressed fracture plus posttraumatic amnesia of greater than 24 hours increased the risk to 33%. Addition of early seizures increased the risk to 66%.

In more than 50% of cases of late epilepsy, the seizure onset was less than one year after trauma. One patient in five had seizure onset more than four years following injury. Patients who had early as well as late epilepsy less often had the onset of late epilepsy after four years.

In 1980 a population study done at the Mayo Clinic involved 2,747 patients followed for 28,176 person years. Injuries were defined as severe (contusion, intracranial hematoma, or posttraumatic amnesia greater than 24 hours), moderate (skull fracture, or 30 minutes to 24 hours of posttraumatic amnesia), and mild (briefer posttraumatic amnesia). The risk of posttraumatic seizures was 7.1% within one year and 11.5% in five years in the severe group; 0.7% and 1.6% in the moderate group; and 0.1% and 0.6% in the mild group. The incidence of late posttraumatic epilepsy in the mild head injury group was not significantly different from the general population.

This study has varied from many previous studies in that all cases with loss of consciousness were studied whereas many other studies had looked only at patients who had actually been admitted to a hospital or examined by a neurosurgeon. Thus, other studies may have excluded many of the mildly injured patients. Some other studies have also included patients who had preexisting epilepsy. Yet other studies included many patients who presented with sequelae of head trauma such as seizures thus being biased toward a higher incidence of posttraumatic epilepsy. In Jennett's study, only 100 of 896 patients had mild head injury. The overall risk of 5% in that study may reflect more severely injured patients. Most other studies have revealed lower rates: 0.14-2.7%.

In addition to clinical neurological evaluation and consideration of epidemiological information, what can be done in an individual patient to more clearly define that patient's risk for seizures? EEG, which is helpful in diagnosis of epilepsy in general, has been disappointing in detecting those at risk for posttraumatic epilepsy. Jennett and van de Sande studied 722 patients with high risk of late epilepsy (43% did develop epilepsy). Although abnormal records were more common in patients who developed epilepsy, this reflected more severe brain injury which was already clinically evident. Twenty percent of patients with late epilepsy had at least one normal EEG in the first three months following injury. Some patients with persistent or newly developing EEG abnormalities never had a seizure. Jennett and van de Sande as well as Walton (1963), Courjon (1969), and Terespolsky (1972) have all concluded that EEG is not helpful in predicting posttraumatic epilepsy.

More recently, computerized axial tomography (CT) as it relates to posttraumatic epilepsy has been studied. D'Alessandro, et al., studied 233 head injured patients. Forty-nine had at least one risk factor for posttraumatic epilepsy and 10 cases studied with CT scan developed late seizures. All 10 of these patients had CT scan abnormalities. Twenty-one patients, however, had focal CT abnormalities and did not develop late seizures during the three to five year follow-up period. These authors concluded that an early CT scan abnormality is a risk factor for posttraumatic epilepsy and it may be possible to select patients for prophylactic anticonvulsant therapy on the basis of CT scan alone.

Riesner, et al., found that combined clinical neurologic evaluation, CT scan and EEG yielded an abnormality in all but 3 of 64 patients with posttraumatic epilepsy. CT scan was normal, however, in 22% and EEG was normal in 19%.

Some data from animal as well as human studies suggests benefit from prophylactic administration of anticonvulsants. Clinical studies thus far present conflicting results.

Salazar, et al., in a report of the Vietnam head injury study (Salazar, A.M. et al., "Epilepsy After Penetrating Head Injury. I. Clinical Correlates: A Report of the Vietnam Head Injury Study," *Neurology* 35:1406-1414, 1985) have looked at data regarding 421 patients with penetrating brain wounds. Treatment with Phenytoin in the first year following injury did not prevent later seizures. Young, et al., reported results of a randomized double blind placebo controlled study of 41 patients (Young, B., et al., "Failure of Prophylactically Administered Phenytoin to Prevent Posttraumatic Seizures in Children," *Child's Brain* 10:185-192, 1983). Phenytoin was instituted within 24 hours following trauma. Only patients estimated to have greater than 10% probability of late seizures were included. There was no significant difference in the incidence of late posttraumatic epilepsy between the treatment and placebo groups.

McQueen, et al., looked at 164 patients with severe head injury. They concluded that because of the low incidence of posttraumatic epilepsy, at least six times the number of patients that they studied would be required to draw valid conclusions (McQueen, J.K., et al., "Low Risk of Late Posttraumatic Seizures Following Severe Injury: Implications for Clinical Trials of Prophylaxis," *J.N.N.P.* 46:899-904, 1983).

In summary, head trauma in general places patients at an increased risk for developing epilepsy. Severe penetrating head trauma results in a 45-53% incidence of posttraumatic seizures. Severe blunt head trauma with an acute hematoma, prolonged posttraumatic amnesia, early epilepsy and depressed skull fracture have a risk of late epilepsy which varies between 15 and 35%. When two of these factors occur in combination the risk is greater. Mild head trauma carries at most a minimal increased risk of epilepsy.

—by Kevin H. Ruggles, MD

Chapter 15

Aphasia

The breakdown of communication ability in an adult resulting from brain damage is usually called aphasia—an impaired ability to understand and/or express language. Individuals with aphasia differ not only in the severity of communication problems but also in the forms the disorder takes. A single area of language can be affected, such as a slight difficulty in recalling words in conversation, or there may be almost total loss of language communication. Some aphasic people talk a lot; others speak very little. Some speak fluently; others struggle to get each syllable out. Some understand better than they speak; for others, the reverse is true.

Who is aphasic? The National Aphasia Association (NAA) reports that one out of every 275 adults in the United States has some type of aphasia. There are over one million aphasic persons in the United States. Strokes result in aphasia for some 80,000 persons annually. Others acquire aphasia as a result of head injuries, often resulting from car and motorcycle accidents. According to Glazer, an aphasia specialist from New Zealand, strokes and head injuries are the most common causes of aphasia in young adults. Aphasia can also result from tumors, neurological illnesses, or other trauma to the brain. As aphasia specialists Rosenbek and colleagues have noted, aphasia does *not* result from dementia, schizophrenia, sensory or memory loss, or institutionalization.

Rehab BRIEF, Vol. XIII. No. 5 (1991) National Institute on Disability and Rehabilitation Research (NIDRR), Office of Special Education and Rehabilitation Services, Department of Education; prepared by PSI International, Inc.

This chapter provides an overview of clinical perspectives on aphasia. It includes a discussion of changing views of the nature of aphasia and implications for clinical practice. The reference drawn upon is "Aphasia Rehabilitation, An Approach to Diagnosis and Treatment of Language Production Disorders" by Mitchum and Berndt in Eisenberg and Grzesiak's *Advances in Clinical Rehabilitation, Volume 2*.

Many concerns about service delivery in aphasia management are international in scope. Observations from specialists in the Pacific Basin have been collected by Sarno and Woods and provide insight into similar problems in the United States. The main sources for this discussion are Walsh's "Aphasia Rehabilitation in New Zealand and Australia" and the monograph edited by Sarno and Woods, *Aphasia Rehabilitation in Asia and the Pacific Region: Japan, China, India, Australia, and New Zealand*. In Sarno and Woods' monograph, Ferguson provided observations on aphasia rehabilitation for Australia, Glazer for New Zealand, Karanth for India, Sasanuma for Japan, and Wang for China. Additional information for the United States was drawn from Rosenbek, LaPointe, and Wertz's *Aphasia: A Clinical Approach*.

The Nature of Aphasia and Its Management

Traditional treatment of aphasia incorporates a medically oriented, hospital-based model, with services provided by speech-language pathologists. Diagnosis and intervention are completed in the hospital setting, with center-based outpatient rehabilitation services after release. Aphasia affects four major modalities: auditory comprehension, spoken language, reading, and writing. Standardized tests for each modality form the backbone of assessment.

Recovery from aphasia is most rapid during the first days and weeks after onset. Rosenbek et al. (p. 106) cite evidence from a variety of studies that spontaneous recovery from aphasia continues for up to six months after onset. Additional evidence suggests that beginning therapy immediately after onset enhances its efficacy.

In intervention, modality-specific tasks are used to help improve abilities in deficit areas, for example, in auditory comprehension, the naming of objects, or the identification of pictures on flash cards. Since the activities have little resemblance to real-world ones, therapy also addresses functional skills—the use of language in naturally occurring, everyday situations. It may also involve the development of alternative communication strategies.

Changing Views on the Nature of Aphasia and Its Management

Mitchum and Berndt describe recent findings that suggest a review of our basic understanding of aphasia. This evidence challenges traditional assumptions about modality-specific impairments in aphasia and the effectiveness of rehabilitation for persons with chronic aphasia. They describe language and aphasia not only in terms of modalities but also in terms of the underlying processing components of language. Impairment in the processes underlying any one of these may result in aphasia.

Mitchum and Berndt review recent research evidence in a discussion of word-finding problems, which are very common for people with aphasia. These occur when an individual cannot recall a word needed to communicate a specific meaning—similar to the "tip of the tongue" phenomenon most of us experience from time to time. Recent evidence cited by Mitchum and Berndt suggests that these problems may not be due to a simple loss of the word from the individual's vocabulary or memory but may represent a more complex problem—or a variety of problems.

For example, difficulty in correctly identifying a pictured object could result from a general disruption in overall ability to recall words into memory. Alternatively, the person may have trouble distinguishing the word of interest from words in similar categories, that is, distinguishing difference in meaning between *nail* and *screw*, a comparatively fine level distinction, or between *nail* and *hammer*, a broader distinction. An additional difficulty that might underlie a word-finding problem is with phonological analysis—a difficulty in connecting the word or concept with the pattern of speech sounds used to represent that concept. Finally, failure on such tasks may be due to problems unrelated to the suspected language disorder. A person with a visual perceptual impairment may call a *noose a balloon* for reasons that have nothing to do with a language disorder.

Clinical application of such findings will require understanding of both the underlying processes involved in the naming process and the treatment techniques most likely to be effective for different types of naming deficits. No single therapeutic approach is likely to work with all persons with word-finding problems.

While word finding is necessary for language, it is, by itself, not enough. The speaker must also organize these words into grammatically well-formed sentences. The process by which unimpaired speakers create sentences is not well understood. We can convey a given piece of information in different ways, for example, *John gave Mary the cat*; or *Mary was given the cat by John*. However, slight differences between sentences can profoundly change the meaning, for example, *John can go to school*; and *John can't go to school*.

As with word finding, difficulty with several different processes are hypothesized to underlie aphasic people's problems with language at the sentence level. Some potential difficulties lie with word-finding problems, some with difficulties with the structural elements used to form sentences, and others are failures to integrate structural elements with semantic (word meaning) information. Again, as with processing at the word-finding level, there is evidence that information about the nature of the processes underlying a problem helps to develop intervention strategies to improve sentence-level processing. Since little is known about normal processes in structural formation of sentences, remediation techniques directed at improving these structural aspects remain relatively uncommon.

Findings challenge the notion that rehabilitation is ineffective with the chronic aphasic. Rehabilitation that is directed to the disruption of underlying processes can benefit even individuals with long-standing aphasia.

Mitchum and Berndt note that conventional aphasia intervention categorizes the nature of the individual's communication problems and works categorically with the overt symptoms of the problem. They conclude that the traditional stopping point in diagnosis of language deficits should best be viewed as only a starting point. In the future, identifying the process-related difficulties that underlie aphasia may help clinicians establish more individualized therapies specifically tailored toward improving functioning of these underlying processes. Moreover, therapies may be devised for aphasic populations not routinely served, such as those resistant to present techniques or chronic aphasics who have ceased responding to present therapeutic methods.

Meeting Needs in Service Delivery for Aphasic People

After the individual is discharged from active treatment, rehabilitation services and formal support may be limited or available for only a brief period of time. The resources of people with disabilities, their families, and the availability of community resources will determine how those with aphasia manage their disabilities and become reintegrated into the community.

Issues in the Pacific Basin

In reviewing reports on aphasia management from the Pacific Basin region, several common concerns are apparent. As Sarno has noted, most of these are reported by aphasia specialists from around the world.

Support for people. People with aphasia needing services and their families can soon become discouraged by the slowness of the rehabilitation process. While families are experiencing these frustrations, their traditional outside social supports may be dwindling. Professional services in other areas—such as physical or occupational therapy—may be terminated. It can become increasingly difficult to persevere when day-to-day communication is poor and progress is slow. A homemaker who is now also caregiver for her aphasic husband no longer has her own social sphere—just as he has lost his. Friends and acquaintances may not persevere in conversation. Casual conversation in public may be labored, embarrassing, or impossible. Occasions that used to be pleasurable can become frustrating.

Personnel. Observers in Japan, China, India, Australia, and New Zealand have noted the need for more specialized personnel such as speech-language pathologists to work with aphasic people. This concern is shared by observers in the United States (Rosenbek et al., p. 131), who note that speech-language pathologists in this country often have a generalist background in working with a broad range of disorders and not in-depth training in meeting the needs of the aphasic person.

Service delivery in urban and rural areas. In countries with large rural areas—such as India, China, and Australia—service delivery is complicated by the fact that speech-language pathologists tend to be concentrated in large urban centers. Center-based services then require families to travel long distances, while home-based services may be infrequent or unavailable. The large geographical distances found in some areas of the United States may present similar difficulties.

Cultural and linguistic diversity. Multilingualism can affect services to aphasic persons in several ways. As Ferguson has noted for Australia, aphasics from linguistic minority groups may have no

language in common with the speech-language pathologist, complicating assessment and remediation. In India, with a population of 800
million people and literally hundreds of languages, it is not uncommon for an individual to speak one language at home, another at work,
and use a third for reading and writing. For such an individual—or
any bilingual person—the effects of aphasia may vary across languages or modalities. Formulating adequate assessment or remediation strategies may be complicated not only by the aphasia and
multilingualism itself but also by client or family preference and
service availability. Sarno expresses concern about the need for qualified clinicians to work with linguistic minority aphasic people in the
language-of-choice.

Responding to Needs in Service Delivery

Only recently have programs been developed to meet needs. Aphasia peer circles, organizing and operating primarily at the local level,
have evolved to ease social readjustment. In the United States, the
recently formed National Aphasia Association is working to organize
national support of aphasic people and their families.

New Zealand's Counterstroke Program. Both Glazer and
Walsh have described a program of national scope developed in New
Zealand in 1981. Counterstroke New Zealand, Inc., was organized by
professionals but is staffed by volunteers trained to help people with
aphasia after they have left the hospital. It includes home-based,
volunteer-centered programs. Counterstroke helps meet the need for
providing quality speech and language intervention services in spite
of shortages of professional personnel. Community services of
Counterstroke include liaison between families and available community resources and organization of stroke clubs, which provide social
activities, therapy, and spouse support groups. Its goal is to unite those
connected in stroke care, rehabilitation, and prevention and to fill
political and advocacy roles for families. Its volunteer Scheme for Com-
munication-Impaired Stroke People is a network of speech-language
pathologists and volunteers.

Speech-language professionals provide extensive training for volunteers about aphasia and in ways to stimulate communication for
aphasic people and oversee language activities at stroke clubs. This
allows limited resources to reach many more aphasic persons. Volunteers meet with their aphasic partners on a weekly basis in their

126

homes. They might hold general conversation, complete specific speech-language activities, go on outings, or enjoy activities in the home.

Activities are pursued that focus on helping the aphasic individual regain communication function. These may include simple friendship and companionship; naming objects and their uses; simple reading activities, such as matching words to pictures; writing activities, such as copying, solving simple crossword puzzles, or letter writing; initiating and maintaining conversations on enjoyable topics; playing word or board games; and practicing functional language tasks, such as making shopping lists or using the telephone. The goal is to encourage any form of communication, verbal or nonverbal, with the assistance carried out in a friendly, tolerant atmosphere.

Excerpts from a Survey by the National Aphasia Association

- Approximately 50 percent of aphasics have had aphasia therapy for over a year.

- 72 percent of aphasics are unable to work.

- 70 percent of aphasics feel people avoid contact with them because of their communication difficulties.

- Almost 90 percent of aphasic persons surveyed felt more information about aphasia was needed for the public—and for themselves.

Discussion and Conclusion

While speech-language pathologists are gaining new insight into aphasia and effective aphasia management, advocacy and support groups, such as those discussed above, have emerged to offer aphasic people—even those with significant long-lasting language deficits—better opportunities for renewed participation in career and community.

At the diagnostic-therapeutic level, according to Mitchum and Berndt, the communication problems aphasic people experience are not accurately characterized by conventional modality-specific approaches alone. Rather, speech-language pathologists are finding it necessary to look beyond the modality of concern to basic processes that underlie it. The identification of process-specific disabilities, in turn, appears to promote development of treatments that focus on these processes. Efficacy of aphasia therapy should improve as speech-language pathologists are better able to offer treatments that are increasingly individualized to the patterns of deficit of the aphasic individual. Moreover, by applying a new process-oriented focus in aphasia assessment and remediation, intervention may offer even chronic aphasics enhanced function.

The model for support of aphasic people and their families described by Glazer and by Walsh emerged from personnel shortages and the need for support and advocacy for families common in many countries. It also appears to hold potential for alleviating some of the other difficulties that have been inherent in aphasia management, while enabling more effective response to individual needs. Programs such as New Zealand's Counterstroke, Inc., can accommodate the need for services of people in rural areas. While not specifically addressed by Walsh or by Glazer, Counterstroke-type programs and nonprofessional volunteers hold potential for responding to needs of individuals from minority linguistic and cultural groups or for aphasic people with long-standing language deficits. There is an important role for volunteers in the aphasia rehabilitation process which needs to be developed. Speech-language pathologists working with aphasic patients need experience with the many ways in which volunteers can help enhance their work, especially in providing social supports.

A common thread binds the work reported by Mitchum and Berndt and the areas of concern identified for the Pacific Basin in the delivery of services to aphasic persons. There appears to be a need for increasing individualization of services to effectively meet the needs of the aphasic individual. The work discussed here describes both clinically oriented and community-based strategies from widely varied perspectives that are working to meet these needs.

Sources

Mitchum, C.C., & Berndt, R.S. (1988). Aphasia rehabilitation: An approach to diagnosis and treatment of language production disorders. In M.G. Eisenberg & R.C. Grzesiak (Eds) *Advances in clinical rehabilitation, Volume 2*. New York: Springer Publishing Company.

Sarno, M.T., & Woods, D.E. (Eds). (1989). *Aphasia rehabilitation in Asia and the Pacific region: Japan, China, India, Australia, and New Zealand*. World Rehabilitation Fund.

Walsh, P. (undated). *Aphasia rehabilitation in New Zealand and Australia*. Unpublished manuscript.

Additional References

Aphasia: National Aphasia Association Newsletter. (Spring 1989) 1:1.

Aphasia: National Aphasia Association Newsletter. (Spring 1989) 1:2.

Rosenbek, J.C., LaPointe, L.L., & Wertz, R.T. (1989). *Aphasia: A clinical approach*. Boston, MA: College Hill Press.

For More Information

National Aphasia Association
P.O. Box 1887
Murray Hill Station
New York, NY 10156-0611

Information about family and peer support for aphasic persons, stroke clubs, and support groups can also be obtained through your local chapter of the American Heart Association or Easter Seal Society.

Chapter 16

Severity and Outcome of Traumatic Brain Injury: A Review of Methods of Measurement

In the past two decades, a means to measure virtually every aspect of traumatic brain injury has been developed. The purpose of this paper is to describe those which are most commonly used in order to provide a basic understanding of each. It is hoped that these explanations will help the reader to be more informed about the strengths, limitations, and uses of such scales. It should be noted, however, that the measurement of traumatic brain injury using scales such as those described below offers only one of many, many factors which are considered when an individual's prognosis and potential for progress are determined.

Severity of Injury

Measurement of severity of injury requires consideration of many factors including the type, nature, and location of the brain injury, duration of coma or loss of consciousness, findings on clinical tests such as computerized axial tomography (CT) scans or magnetic resonance imaging (MRI) to name a few. There are however, some standard ways in which severity of injury is measured which one might encounter. The most widely used is the Abbreviated Injury Scale (AIS).

Abbreviated Injury Scale

The Abbreviated Injury Scale (AIS) was designed to provide *crash investigators* with a simple numerical way to rank and compare injuries by severity and to standardize the terminology used to describe injuries. The AIS results in a single score for each injury an individual sustains by body region. The AIS measures injuries, not the impairments or disabilities (outcome) which result from injury. One of its primary uses today is to assist in assessing the efficacy of motor vehicle design changes.

Individual injuries are classified by body region using a six-point scale which ranges from AIS 1 (minor) to AIS 6 (maximum or currently untreatable). The single highest AIS code in an individual with multiple injuries is known as the Maximum AIS or MAIS.

While the AIS is of greatest value to researchers at present, two important aspects should be noted. First, the Brain section of the AIS 90 (as the 1990 revision is referred to) has been significantly expanded. Second, the Association for the Advancement of Automotive Medicine which developed the AIS, is currently working on development of a companion scale which would measure impairment or disability.

Coma

Individuals with severe traumatic brain injury are frequently in coma. Coma is defined as the inability to open the eyes, utter words, or obey commands (Jennett and Teasdale, 1974). Coma (also referred to as loss of consciousness) represents a life-threatening complication of brain injury. The duration of coma has been found to be an indicator of the severity of injury and to have a strong association with the outcome of injury. While there are several measures of coma, the most widely used is the Glasgow Coma Scale (GCS).

Glasgow Coma Scale

Eye Opening	**Verbal Response**	**Best Motor Response**
4 = spontaneous	5 = orientated	6 = obeys commands
3 = to speech	4 = confused conversation	5 = localizes
2 = to pain	3 = inappropriate words	4 = withdraws
1 = nil	2=incomprehensible sounds	3 = abnormal flexion
	1 = nil	2 = extensor
		1 = nil

(Teasdale and Jennett, 1974)

In order to determine a score in each area, each response is tested and scored separately and a total score is determined by adding the best eye opening, verbal and motor responses. The highest possible score is 15, and represents an individual who is awake, oriented, and following commands. The lowest score is three (3), which represents an individual who is deeply unconscious with flaccid limbs. Scores of eight (8) or lower have generally been accepted as indicative of severe brain injury (Cooper, 1987).

The following are examples of the tests used, individual's response, and the corresponding score.

Modality/Test	*Response*	*Score*
Eye opening		
speech	opens eyes when asked to in a loud voice	3
pain	does not open eyes	1
Best motor		
commands	follows simple commands	6
pain	pulls body part away when pinched	4
pain	no motor response when pinched	1
Verbal		
speech	carries on conversation correctly, oriented to person, place and time	5
speech	talks so examiner can understand but makes no sense	3
speech	makes no noise	1

(Teasdale and Jennett, 1974)

In instances when a particular modality cannot be tested (for example, when an individual is intubated and verbal response cannot be tested), the best motor response is used. This has been found to only slightly decrease the predictive power of the GCS in comparison to the sum of the scores (Eisenberg, 1985).

Some individuals come out of coma within minutes, while others may take hours or days. Still others remain in coma for weeks, months, and longer. An individual's emergence from coma occurs gradually.

Frequently characterized by confusion, agitation, emotional lability, inappropriate speech, inability to attend and recall ongoing events, this period of time is known as post-traumatic amnesia (PTA).

Post-Traumatic Amnesia

Post-traumatic amnesia (PTA) is the duration of time from the point of injury until continuous memory occurs. This includes the duration of coma. The length of time after injury until return to work and the occurrence of late traumatic epilepsy have been related to PTA duration. The length of post-traumatic amnesia has also been found to generally relate to the severity of injury as follows:

PTA Duration	Severity of injury
1 hour or less	mild
1 to 24 hours	moderate
1 day to 1 week	severe
more than 1 week	very to extremely severe

(Rosenthal, Griffith, Bond, and Miller, 1983)

While long periods of PTA are difficult to estimate accurately, there is less need for a precise estimate of lengthy PTA. An expanded scale for minor injuries has been devised because it is possible to more precisely estimate brief durations of PTA. Thus:

PTA Duration	Severity of injury
0-10 minutes	very mild
10-60 minutes	mild
1-24 hours	moderate

(Rosenthal, Griffith, Bond, and Miller, 1990)

The end of PTA does not occur merely when an individual appears awake and can speak, since many individuals begin to speak before they are able to retain information from one day to the next. Similarly, the apparent return of normal memory function may not indicate the end of PTA because it is common for memory to return temporarily. This may then be followed by another period of PTA. This temporary return of memory is referred to as an "island" of memory. It is quite common for individuals to recall some, but not all (or even to recall none) of the events which occurred during PTA. In order to more accurately assess the end of PTA, orientation and memory are usually monitored daily. The Galveston Orientation and Amnesia Test (GOAT) is frequently used for this purpose.

Galveston Orientation and Amnesia Test

The Galveston Orientation and Amnesia Test (GOAT) is a ten item test which provides a global index of amnesia and orientation. It also estimates both anterograde amnesia (the time *after* injury during which memory is lost) and retrograde amnesia (the time *prior* to the injury during which memory is lost). The GOAT is reliable and may be administered quickly and easily at an individual's bedside.

Individuals are asked a series of questions which include:

- What is your name?
- When were you born?
- Where do you live?
- What is the first event you can remember after injury?
- What time is it now?
- Can you describe the last event you recall before the accident?

(Levin, Benton & Grossman, 1982)

Responses are scored, with those less than 66 indicating impairment, from 66 to 75 borderline, and 76-100 normal. Serial GOAT scores are graphed to offer a clear record of recovery from PTA. Serial scores have been found to relate to the severity of acute cerebral disturbance after a brain injury. In addition, they have been found to relate to Glasgow Coma Scale scores and the findings on CT scan (computerized axial tomography, which is an indicator of the severity of brain injury) and outcome. (Mysiw, Corrigan, Carpenter, and Chock, 1990)

While the GOAT offers a reliable and quick way to assess PTA, it has been criticized because it permits individuals to learn the correct, desired response. Another way PTA is often assessed is through the Orientation Group Monitoring System (OGMS).

Orientation Group Monitoring System

The Orientation Group Monitoring System (OGMS) is administered in a group setting rather than individually. During the course of a daily orientation group, behavioral observations of individuals are conducted in seven areas: orientation to time, to place, to self and other group members, attention span, semantic memory (for facts, often learned through repetition) and episodic memory (for ongoing events), and the use of planning and scheduling aids. While the tasks performed daily in the group vary, the objectives of the group remain the same. Scoring is done as follows:

1 = failure to respond correctly
2 = attempted to respond but the accuracy of the response was unclear
3 = correctly performed the desired behavior

(Jackson, Mysiw, and Corrigan, 1989)

Average scores in each of the seven areas are collected weekly. The average of these scores then determines the weekly OGMS score. An OGMS score of 2.75 over a two week period is indicative of the resolution of PTA. The OGMS has been found to assess subtle changes in behavioral and cognitive deficits. A decline in the OGMS has been found to be one of the earliest indicators of adverse drug effects, hydrocephalus, and expanding chronic subdural hematoma.

Comparison: the GOAT and the OGMS

The GOAT may be administered easily at bedside. Its results typically reflect a shorter period of PTA than the OGMS. In comparison, the OGMS requires more time, staff, and a group setting. It offers the advantage of being a more conservative instrument, and is intended to remediate the deficits of PTA while monitoring PTA duration. Both the GOAT and the OGMS have been found to monitor PTA reliably and effectively.

Rehabilitation usually begins during PTA and continues after it has resolved. The focus of measurement then turns to what is referred to as outcome. This is a general term which reflects the return to previous capabilities an individual attains. There are several methods used to describe outcome.

Outcome

It is important to note that the following outcome scales do not ordinarily offer a clear picture of the actual functional abilities and impairments of an *individual* because they result in a single score which represents abilities in many areas. Rather, they are best able to predict the outcome of a group of individuals. The most commonly used outcome scales are the Glasgow Outcome Scale (GOS), the Rancho Los Amigos Levels of Cognitive Functioning (RLA), and the Disability Rating Scale (DRS).

Glasgow Outcome Scale

The Glasgow Outcome Scale (GOS) offers a general method for assessing the degree of recovery achieved. The categories it contains are composites of cognitive, physical, and social functioning. Originally, the scale offered only four categories. Today, it is more commonly used in either a five or eight category form. Descriptors in the five category scale are:

Good Recovery (GR). Individuals have the capacity to resume normal occupational and social activities despite minor physical or cognitive impairments.

Moderate Disability (MD). Individuals are "independent but disabled." While able to take care of themselves, to get out and to use public transportation independently, they are unable to return to some prior social or work activities as a result of physical or cognitive deficits.

Severe Disability (SD). Individuals are conscious but require the assistance of another person for some activities of daily living (ADL's). This is a wide group ranging from individuals who are totally dependent on others to individuals who require assistance for only one activity.

Persistent Vegetative State (PVS). Restricted to individuals who show no evidence of meaningful response. Individuals who obey commands or speak even one word are assigned to the severe disability group. In PVS, individuals breathe spontaneously, have periods of spontaneous eye opening and may track objects, show reflex responses, and swallow food placed in their mouths.

Persistent Vegetative State (PVS) is a term used to describe those individuals who never regain any degree of consciousness in the sense of cortical function. Individuals neither speak nor follow commands but do regain their alerting mechanism which includes eye opening and sleep-wake cycles. It **does not** mean "vegetable."

Death. Resulting either as a direct result of brain injury or due to secondary complications.

(Jennett and Bond, 1975)

The eight category scale is more sensitive since good recovery, moderate disability and severe disability are each subdivided into a best and worse category. While the GOS sacrifices detail for simplicity, it has been found to be reliable and valid.

Rancho Los Amigos Levels of Cognitive Functioning

The Rancho Los Amigos Levels of Cognitive Functioning (RLA) were designed to measure and track an individual's progress early in the recovery period. They have been used as a means to develop "level-specific" treatment interventions and strategies designed to facilitate movement from one level to another. A RLA level is determined based on behavioral observations. The RLA scale designates eight levels of function:

I. No Response. The individual appears to be in deep sleep and is completely unresponsive to any stimuli.

II. Generalized Response. The individual reacts inconsistently and nonpurposefully to stimuli. Responses are limited in nature and often the same regardless of the stimuli presented. Responses may include gross motor movements, vocalization, and physiologic changes. Response time is likely to be delayed. Deep pain evokes the earliest response.

III. Localized Response. The individual responds specifically but inconsistently to stimulus. Responses are directly related to the type of stimuli presented. For example, an individual's head will turn toward a sound or his/her eyes will focus on an object when presented. The individual may follow simple commands and may respond better to some people (i.e., family and friends) than others.

IV. Confused-Agitated. The individual is in a heightened state of activity with severely decreased ability to process information. Behavior is nonpurposeful relative to the immediate environment. Attempts to climb out of bed, remove restraints, and hostility are common. The individual requires maximum assistance to perform self-care activities. An individual may sit, reach, or walk, but will not necessarily perform these activities upon request.

V. Confused-Inappropriate. The individual appears alert and responds to simple commands fairly consistently. Agitation which is out of proportion (but directly related) to stimuli may be evident. Lack of external structure results in random or nonpurposeful responses. Inappropriate verbalizations and high distractibility are common. Memory is severely impaired, but the individual may self-feed with supervision and requires only assistance for self-care activities.

VI. Confused-Appropriate. The individual shows goal oriented behavior, but is dependent upon external input for direction. Response to discomfort is appropriate. Responses are incorrect due to memory problems, but are appropriate to the situation. Simple commands are followed consistently and carry-over for relearned activities is evident. Orientation is inconsistent but awareness of self, family, and basic needs is increased.

VII. Automatic-Appropriate. The individual appears appropriate within hospital and home settings, goes through daily routine automatically but is robot-like, with shallow recall of activities performed. Has absent-to-minimal confusion and lacks insight. The individual frequently demonstrates poor judgment and problem solving and expresses unrealistic future plans. With structure, the individual is able to initiate tasks or social and recreational activities.

VIII. Purposeful-Appropriate. The individual is alert and oriented, able to recall and integrate past and recent events and is aware of and responsive to the environment. Independence in the home and community has returned. Carry-over for new learning is present, and the need for supervision is absent once activities have been learned. Social, emotional and cognitive abilities may still be decreased.

(Hagen, Malkmus, and Durham, 1980)

The RLA scale is quite popular and is widely used, particularly within rehabilitation facilities. It has not however, been subjected to critical peer review which is generally viewed as desirable for an evaluation instrument.

Disability Rating Scale

The Disability Rating Scale (DRS) (Rappaport and Hall, 1982) was designed to chart an individual's progress (or the lack of progress) between early arousal from coma and early sensory awareness and functioning. It consists of eight items in four categories. A score of 0 is indicative of no disability.

1. Arousal and Awareness—(a modified Glasgow Coma Scale):
    a. Eye Opening (rated 0-3)
    b. Verbal Output (rated 0-4)
    c. Motor Activities (rated 0-4)

2. Cognitive ability to know *how and when* to perform self-care activities:
    a. feed self (rated 0-3)
    b. use the bathroom (rated 0-4)
    c. groom self (rated 0-3)
    The physical ability to perform these functions is not rated in this category.

3. Physical dependence upon others (rated 0-5):
    Rates the individual's need for physical assistance from others. Ratings include completely independent (0), mildly dependent—requires limited assistance from a non-residential helper (2), and completely dependent (5).

4. Psychosocial adaptability (0-3):
    Rates "employability" for age-related work responsibilities (such as student, housewife, or employee). This area measures both physical and cognitive abilities to perform work functions. Scoring includes not restricted (0), able to perform selected competitive jobs (1) and not employable (3).

Each area is scored separately. The totals are then added to determine the DRS score. Total DRS scores and their corresponding level of disability are:

DRS Score	Level of Disability
0	None
1	Mild
2-3	Partial
4-6	Moderate
7-11	Moderately Severe
12-16	Severe
17-21	Extremely Severe
22-24	Vegetative State
25-29	Extremely Vegetative State
30	Death

In contrast to all other scales discussed thus far, the DRS ratings are based on level of **dis**ability. Thus, a low score is reflective of a low level of disability, and a higher score reflective of a more significant disability.

The DRS has been found to be more sensitive in measuring progress than the GOS. A change of even one point on the DRS represents a significant change in clinical status. In one study, the DRS has been found to surpass the RLA in both reliability and validity. However, it is not as widely used as either the GOS or the RLA scale.

Conclusion

As one can see, measuring traumatic brain injury by using the above scales is not precise. Each has strengths and limitations. None are universally used. However, these and other scales are particularly useful in research because they provide a means to compare and contrast groups of individuals with traumatic brain injuries. In this way, they have contributed to the advancement of knowledge about what types of treatments and services are most likely to be beneficial to individuals with traumatic brain injuries.

Despite the tremendous advances in knowledge about traumatic brain injuries, it is difficult to say with certainty how much improvement in what time frame an individual may make. Therefore, it is vital that the determination of a particular individual's prognosis and ability to progress be made by an individual's physician(s) and treatment team (including the family) based upon many factors. Included among these are the type and nature of brain injury, other bodily and systemic injuries, medical complications, and age.

Bibliography

Adamovich, B.B., Henderson, J.A., & Auerbach, S. (1985). *Cognitive Rehabilitation of Closed Head Injured Patients*, San Diego: College-Hill Press.

Association for Advancement of Automotive Medicine. (1990). *The Abbreviated Injury Scale, 1990 Revision*. Des Plains, IL.

Bleiberg, J., Cope, D.N., & Spector, J. Cognitive assessment and therapy in traumatic brain injury. (1989). In Horn, L.J., & Cope, D.N. *Physical Medicine and Rehabilitation: State of the Art Reviews*. (pp. 95-121) Philadelphia: Hanley & Belfus, Inc. 1989.

Corrigan, J.D., & Mysiw, W.J. (1988). Agitation following traumatic head injury: Equivocal evidence for a discrete stage of cognitive recovery. *Archives of Physical Medicine and Rehabilitation*; 69(7):487-492.

Eisenberg, H.M. (1985). Outcome after head injury: General considerations and neurobehavioral recovery Part I: General considerations. In Becker, D.P., & Povlishock, J.T. (Eds.), *Central Nervous System Trauma Status Report* (pp. 271-280), U.S. Government Printing Office: 1988-520-149/00 028.

Freeman, E.A. (Ed.) (1987) *The Catastrophe of Coma: A Way Back*. Australia: David Bateman, Ltd.

Giannotta, S.L., Weiner, J.M., & Karnaze, D. 1987. Prognosis and outcome in severe head injury. In P.R. Cooper (Ed.), *Head Injury*, (2nd ed., pp. 464-487) Baltimore: Williams & Wilkins.

Gouvier, W.D., Blanton, P.D., Kittle LaPorte, K., & Nepomuceno, C. (1987). Reliability and validity of the disability rating scale and the levels of cognitive functioning scale in monitoring recovery from severe head injury. *Archives of Physical Medicine and Rehabilitation*; 68:94-97.

Hagen, C., Malkmus, D., & Durham, P. (1979). Levels of cognitive functioning. In *Rehabilitation of Head Injured Adult: Comprehensive Physical Management*. Downey, CA: Professional Staff Association of Rancho Los Amigos Hospital, Inc.

Hall, K., Cope, D.N., & Rappaport, M. (1985). Glasgow outcome scale and disability rating scale: Comparative usefulness in following recovery in traumatic head injury. *Archives of Physical Medicine and Rehabilitation*; 66(1):35-37.

Heiden, J.S., Small, R., Caton, W., Weiss, M., & Kurze, T. (1983). Severe head injury. *Physical Therapy*; 63(12) 1946-1951.

Jackson, R.D., Mysiw, W.J., & Corrigan, J.D. (1989). Orientation group monitoring system: An indicator for reversible impairments in cognition during posttraumatic amnesia. *Archives of Physical Medicine and Rehabilitation*; 70(1):33-36

Jennett, B., & Bond, M. (1975). Assessment of outcome after severe brain damage: A practical scale. *Lancet*, 1:480-484.

Jennett, B., Snoek, J., Bond, M.R., & Brooks, N. (1981). Disability after severe head injury: Observations on the use of the Glasgow outcome scale. *Journal of Neurology, Neurosurgery, and Psychiatry*; 44:285-293.

Jennett, B., & Teasdale, G. (1974). Assessment of coma and impaired consciousness. *Lancet*; 2:81-84.

Jennett, B., Teasdale, G., Galbraith, S., Pickard, J., Grant, H., Braakman, R., Avezaat, C., Maas, A., Minderhoud, J., Vecht, C.J., Heiden, J., Small, R., Caton, W., & Kurze, T. (1977). Severe head injuries in three countries. *Journal of Neurology, Neurosurgery, and Psychiatry*: 40:291-298.

Levin, H.S. Neurobehavioral sequelae of head injury. (1987). In P.R. Cooper Ed., *Head Injury*. (2nd ed., pp. 442-463). Baltimore: Williams & Wilkins.

Levin, H.S., Benton, A.L., & Grossman, R.G.(1982). *Neurobehavioral Consequences of Closed Head Injury*. New York: Oxford University Press.

Mysiw, W.J., Corrigan, J.D., Carpenter, D., & Chock, S.K.L. (1990). Prospective assessment of posttraumatic amnesia: A comparison of the GOAT and the OGMS. *Journal of Head Trauma Rehabilitation*; 5(1):65-70.

Rappaport, M., & Hall, K. (November, 1982). *Severe Head Trauma: A Comprehensive Medical Approach. Project 13-P-59156/9.* Report to the National Institute for Handicapped Research.

Rappaport, M., Hall, K.M., Hopkins, K., Belleza, T., & Cope, D.N. (1981). Disability rating scale for severe head trauma: Coma to community. *Archives of Physical Medicine and Rehabilitation*; 63:118-123. 1981.

Rosenthal, M., Griffith, E.R., Bond, M.R., & Miller, J.D. (1983). *Rehabilitation of the Head Injured Adult.* Philadelphia: F.A. Davis Company.

Rosenthal, M., Griffith, E.R., Bond, M.R., & Miller, J.D. (1990). *Rehabilitation of the Adult and Child with Traumatic Brain Injury* (2nd ed.), Philadelphia: F.A. Davis Company.

—by Mary S. Reitter, MS

Chapter 17

Outcome After Severe Traumatic Brain Injury: Coma, the Vegetative State, and the Minimally Responsive State

The estimated annual incidence of severe traumatic brain injury (TBI) in the United States is 20 cases per 100,000 persons. Extrapolating from these figures, the number of severe brain injuries per 1 million people is approximately 200. Assuming a 15% mortality rate, the number of survivors admitted to hospitals with severe TBI is approximately 170 per 1 million persons per year. This number inflates to 44,200 when the total population of the United States is considered (based on 1994 data from the US Census Bureau).

Rehabilitation costs associated with care and treatment of the patient with severe TBI range from $35,000 to $85,000. Projecting an average expense of $60,000 per patient, the cost of rehabilitation is approximately $265,000,000 annually. Although these figures are meant to represent only a gross estimate of the costs associated with severe TBI, they clearly illustrate the scope and enormity of the problem.

The purpose of this article is to discuss the "state of the art" in assessment, treatment, and research related to outcome after severe traumatic brain injury. The discussion focuses on three distinct subgroups within the population of survivors of severe brain injury. These three subgroups comprise patients who are comatose, vegetative, and minimally responsive. The specific intent is to describe and critique the available literature regarding pertinent nomenclature, assessment methods, outcome prediction, and treatment interventions used with

Excerpted from *Journal of Head Trauma Rehabilitation*, 10(1):40-56, February 1995 © Aspen Publishers, Inc.; reprinted with permission.

this population. Controversial issues are highlighted, and recommendations for advancing the state of the art are suggested.

The Importance of Outcome Prediction

Determining a reliable prognosis after brain injury presents unique problems for the clinician, patient, family, and payer. For the clinician, recommendations regarding the nature, intensity, and duration of treatment typically rest on the prognosis. A number of recent studies have shown that patient management is directly influenced by the prognosis in terms of the number and type of treatments recommended. For this reason, it is imperative that the patient's clinical status be monitored across the recovery course so that the diagnosis and appropriateness of the corresponding treatment plan can be confirmed. Outcome monitoring also allows the clinician to assess the effectiveness of the prescribed interventions.

Outcome prediction and diagnostic accuracy primarily affect the patient as the direct recipient of the contingent treatment decisions. Recovery of neurological, cognitive, and functional abilities depends, to varying degrees, on the type and duration of treatment provided. A patient mistakenly diagnosed to be in a "persistent vegetative state" (PVS) at 3 weeks after injury, for example, may have less chance of being referred for the same rehabilitative services as a second patient with the same clinical presentation who does not carry the diagnosis of PVS.

Family members are affected by prognostic information insofar as the adjustment process is concerned. For the family to be able to develop realistic expectations for recovery, specific information must be provided that addresses the degree of improvement anticipated, the long-term needs of the patient (e.g., medical, physical, cognitive), and the chances of achieving functional and vocational independence. Misinformation can complicate the already arduous process of emotional adjustment faced by all members of the primary support network.

Finally, resource allocation is often determined on the basis of predictions about the potential level of functional recovery that is deemed attainable. For this reason, third party payers typically request prognostic information early in the acute period. Subsequent decisions regarding the allocation of funds tend to be premised on early outcome predictions, which may influence provision of services throughout the recovery course.

Nomenclature

One of the major problems faced by clinicians in the field of neurotrauma care has been the lack of a consistent nomenclature germane to low-level neurological states after severe brain injury, both traumatic and nontraumatic. Another major issue has been the relative lack of understanding of the existing nomenclature and a tendency toward inappropriate diagnoses and subsequently incorrect conclusions regarding neurological and functional prognoses and necessary treatment. Ultimately, clinicians must have a universally agreed on nomenclature and must understand the clinical implications of such a system relative to diagnosis, prognosis, and treatment.

The bedside assessment of the patient with severe TBI requires that adequate time be taken to conduct a thorough neurobehavioral assessment, given the normal expected fluctuations in arousal and responsiveness levels. In addition, the examiner must understand what clinical findings are consistent with cortical versus subcortical neurobehavioral responses, as well as what factors, neurological as well as medical, may confound the neurobehavioral assessment.

The major diagnostic neurobehavioral terms that are germane to a discussion of nomenclature in persons with severe alterations in consciousness are *coma, vegetative state, persistent vegetative state, akinetic mutism, locked-in syndrome,* and *minimally responsive state.* These six terms describe the scope of neurobehavioral presentations for persons after severe brain injury who typically present at Rancho Los Amigos Cognitive Levels I to IV based on apparent outward "neurobehavioral appearance." Although there is no direct relationship between Rancho level and the six conditions discussed, patients in coma typically fall between Rancho levels I and II; those in the vegetative state, within Rancho level II; and minimally responsive patients, within Rancho levels III and IV. Patients with akinetic mutism usually fall within Rancho level III, although the degree of responsiveness may be highly variable depending on the nature and intensity of stimulation provided. Patients with locked-in syndrome typically fall within Rancho levels V through VIII, as cognitive functions are relatively well preserved. The locked-in syndrome is included in this discussion because these patients are often misdiagnosed as comatose or vegetative. To the clinician who has become sensitized to the importance of careful neurobehavioral assessment, there are discernible differences among these subgroups that must be recognized.

Coma is a state of unarousable neurobehavioral unresponsiveness. Neurobehaviorally, these patients typically present with eyes closed without evidence of eye opening either spontaneously or in response to external stimulation; they do not follow commands, do not demonstrate goal-directed or volitional behavior, do not verbalize or mouth words, and cannot sustain visual pursuit movements beyond a 45° arc. Neurobehavioral signs and symptoms of "coma" secondary to pharmacological treatment with agents such as paralytic or sedative drugs must be excluded.

Patients in the vegetative state (VS) demonstrate arousal without behavioral evidence of the capacity to interact with the environment. Neurobehaviorally, there are periods of eye opening, either spontaneously or in response to stimulation; subcortical responses to external stimulation, including generalized physiological responses to pain such as posturing, tachycardia, and diaphoresis, as well as subcortical motor responses such as a grasp reflex; return of so-called vegetative (autonomic) functions, including sleep-wake cycles, and normalization of respiratory and digestive system functions; and there may be roving eye movements without concomitant visual tracking ability. The presence of subcortical responses should not be considered as pathognomonic of VS, as these findings may also be seen in patients who demonstrate neurobehavioral evidence of environmental awareness (i.e., minimally responsive). In addition, there is no way that we are aware of to clinically assess "internal awareness" in a patient who is otherwise unable to express awareness relative to external environmental stimuli. Thus, it is theoretically possible that some patients who are indeed conscious at some level are incorrectly labeled as being in a VS. Practitioners should also understand that there is no neurodiagnostic or laboratory test that allows the clinician to diagnose VS per se, the diagnosis is only made by serial neurobehavioral assessment.

Considerable confusion and controversy surrounds the term PVS. Although there are no differences in the neurobehavioral criteria required for PVS relative to VS, the label "PVS" conveys prognostic information, as opposed to the diagnostic term, VS. Recently, the Multi-Society Task Force on PVS (sponsored by the American Academy of Neurology) adopted the position that the term PVS can be utilized at one month post-injury and that the VS can be considered permanent after 3 and 12 months following non-traumatic and traumatic injuries, respectively. Contrary to the AAN position, we do not believe that the descriptors "persistent" and "permanent" clarify either the diagnosis or prognosis of the patient in the VS. Choi and others found that 52% of 71 patients who were vegetative at 3 months recovered consciousness by 12 months post-injury which suggests that one month is too early to apply the term "persistent." We also do not believe that the VS can be reliably termed permanent at 1 year after injury, as this implies no potential for further improvement and the literature contains a number of well-documented cases of recovery that exceed this time frame. Furthermore, smallpox, tuberculosis, bubonic plague, and spinal cord injury were all once thought to be "permanent." Introduction of the term *permanent vegetative state* serves only to create a self-prophesizing environment that surely does not encourage clinicians and scientists to pursue treatments that may ameliorate if not cure the condition (W. Young, personal communication, 1994).

Minimally responsive (MR) patients are those who are no longer in coma or VS but demonstrate primitive neurobehavioral responses (e.g., grasp reflex), as well as basic cognitively mediated responses (e.g., inconsistent command following). MR patients are able to demonstrate, albeit intermittently and possibly incompletely, some level of awareness to environmental stimulation consistent with the presence of cortical function. The examining clinician must take into consideration both the frequency and the context of the behavioral response to interpret the meaningfulness or purposefulness of a given behavior.

Akinetic mutism (AM) is a neurobehavioral condition marked by severe disturbances in behavioral drive. In actuality, it is a neurobehavioral subset of the MR subgroup. Generally, a minimal degree of movement (kinesis) and speech is elicitable. As opposed to most other low-level neurobehavioral disorders, AM is associated with damage to dopaminergic pathways, including the mesoceruleal, diencephalospinal, or mesocorticolimbic pathways. Patients with frontal AM tend to be more vigilant than those with midbrain AM and may even demonstrate episodic agitation. Patients with AM typically demonstrate eye opening with visual tracking; little or no spontaneous speech; and infrequent as well as incomplete command following. AM is distinct from the MR state in that the low frequency of movement and speech cannot be attributed to neuromuscular disturbance (e.g., hypotonus) or decreased wakefulness as is typically noted in the minimally responsive patient.

Locked-in syndrome (LIS) is a relatively rare, albeit important, neurobehavioral condition that is distinct from the previously discussed conditions in that cognition and conscious awareness remain relatively well preserved. Clinically, patients with LIS present with anarthria and quadriplegia in the "classic" form of the condition. The causative lesion disrupts corticospinal and corticobulbar pathways in the ventral pons, sparing rostral and dorsal pontine function and thereby preserving cognitive functions and arousal. Although there is significant lower cranial nerve and sleep-wake cycle dysfunction, vertical eye movements and blinking are typically preserved and can be used to communicate and operate environmental control devices.

Methods of Assessment

Standardized Procedures

The number of assessment methods designed specifically for use with the severely brain-injured patient has increased significantly over the past 5 years. Most have been developed to supersede the Glasgow Coma Scale (GCS) and the Disability Rating Scale (DRS), which are of limited utility for monitoring recovery in this population during rehabilitation. The GCS and DRS consist largely of items that tend to lose their predictive utility subsequent to the acute period and are relatively insensitive to subtle changes in neurological responsiveness over time. Characteristically, these recently developed specialized assessment instruments employ standardized methods and behaviorally defined response scoring systems. Table 17.1 compares four of the most widely used assessment procedures. Giacino et al, for example, have shown that determining the rate of recovery across the first month of rehabilitation, measured by the change in total score on the Coma Recovery Scale, enhanced outcome prediction relative to GCS and DRS scores. Although these measures have been shown to be capable of detecting subtle changes in responsiveness, there is relatively little information available regarding their ability to predict long-term outcome.

Nonstandardized Procedures

Before publication of the GCS, clinicians relied exclusively on nonstandardized strategies for evaluation of the comatose, vegetative, and MR patient. Nonstandardized approaches continue to be widely used. The "pathological sign" approach, for example, relies on analysis of the pattern of neurologic abnormalities observed. The pattern

	Coma/Near-Coma Scale[18]	Coma Recovery Scale[19]	Sensory Stimulation Assessment Measure (SSAM)[20]	Western Neurosensory Stimulation Profile[21]
Target population	DRS=21–29	DRS=17–29 RLA Levels II–IV	RLA levels II–V	RLA levels II–V
Content	11 items; 8 subscales: Auditory Command Visual Threat Olfactory Tactile Pain Vocal	25 items; 6 subscales: Auditory Visual Motor Verbal Communication Arousal/attention	5 response scales: Visual Auditory Tactile Gustatory Olfactory	33 items; 6 subscales: Arousal/attention Auditory comprehension Visual comprehension Visual tracking Object manipulation Expressive communication
Scoring system	Ordinal; 3 severity grades based on quality of response; yields 5 levels of "awareness or responsivity"	Ordinal; items scored for presence/absence of a criterion-referenced response to standard stimuli	Ordinal; points assigned based on type of stimulus applied and change in eye, verbal, and motor response	Ordinal; scores based on nature of stimulus, nature of response, response latency, need for cueing
Interrater reliability	r=0.97	r=0.83	r=0.89	r=0.70
Validity	DRS: r=0.97	DRS: r=–0.93 GCS: r=0.90	DRS: r=–0.61 GCS: r=0.70 RLA: r=0.68	RLA: r=0.73
Research findings	Patients with scores in near-coma range (<2 or below) most likely to improve	Rate of improvement in CRS score over first 4 wk of rehabilitation predictive of outcome at discharge	No evidence for efficacy of sensory stimulation based on changes in SSAM score over 4 mo	Specific items capable of predicting rehabilitation readiness and recovery rate

Table 17.1. Summary of specialized assessment methods RLA = Rancho Los Amigos

of abnormal neurological signs elicited on examination suggest a particular location or region of brain injury, which is then associated with a prognosis. The methods used to elicit the neurological signs and the criteria for judging their integrity vary among examiners and consequently may be unreliable.

More recently, a nonstandardized approach has been formulated based on principles of single-subject research design. This procedure, developed by Whyte et al. and referred to as *Individualized Quantitative Assessment*, allows the assessment procedures to be tailored to a specific clinical question. It provides as much flexibility as is required to define and investigate the target question (e.g., "Is there evidence of command following?"). The results are then subjected to statistical analysis so that conclusions can be drawn. The reliability and validity of this approach have not yet been made available.

Comprehensive assessment of the patient with severe TBI should include both standardized and nonstandardized strategies. This furnishes the clinician with the advantages of standardization (e.g., comparability across subjects) while concurrently avoiding the disadvantages (e.g., inability to answer case-specific questions).

Prediction of Outcome: Factors Influencing Accuracy

There have been numerous investigations, most in the neurosurgical literature, on predicting outcome in the severely brain-injured population. Although the majority of studies conclude that it is possible to predict outcome after brain injury, the variability inherent in prediction makes it difficult to apply findings from these studies to decisions pertinent to individual patients. Despite the level of complexity involved, single-case outcome prediction is possible when prognostic statements are well formulated and relevant decision-making guidelines are adhered to.

Nature of Outcome Predicted

The precision with which outcome predictions can be made varies according to how outcome is defined and which domains are of interest. Outcome can be broken down into five domains: mortality; recovery of consciousness; and neuropsychological, psychosocial, and vocational domains.

Mortality is concerned with the likelihood of survival. Studies have consistently identified a number of variables associated with death after severe TBI (e.g., GCS score <5, bilateral nonreactive pupils, hypotension, advanced age). Although there is some evidence that mortality can be predicted during the acute period after severe TBI, it is necessary to bear in mind that the level of predictability deemed acceptable varies according to the individual considering the consequences of the prediction. For example, the neurosurgeon may be inclined to forego aggressive intervention when there is an 80% chance of death based on the clinical parameters. The patient's family, on the other hand, may be more likely to proceed according to the 20% chance of survival.

The remaining four outcome domains concern morbidity (i.e., extent of disability). Recovery of consciousness pertains to whether the patient regains environmental and self-awareness (i.e., capacity to interact meaningfully with the environment). Although numerous studies have successfully identified factors that predict outcome according to global ratings of function (e.g., Glasgow Outcome Scale [GOS], DRS), few studies have addressed recovery of consciousness per se as an outcome. This is due in part to the difficulties involved in defining consciousness. Studies that have addressed this question have not found consistent indicators of recovery of consciousness. Prediction of neuropsychological outcome is concerned with the degree of residual cognitive dysfunction expected to persist after the period of spontaneous recovery. A linear relationship appears to exist between severity of injury and neuropsychological outcome, with greater impairment associated with more severe injuries. Psychosocial (or functional) outcome relates to the patient's capacity to socially reintegrate and function independently. There is growing consensus that the most disabling residua of TBI are the psychosocial consequences. Finally, there is the question of vocational outcome. This domain concerns the probability of return to work and the eventual level of work reentry anticipated. Although injury characteristics (e.g., coma duration length of posttraumatic amnesia) and cognitive variables have been shown to be related to vocational outcome, more recent studies suggest an association with patient variables such as awareness and acceptance of deficits.

Etiology of Injury

Differences exist relative to comparative prognosis across different groups of patients with brain injury from an etiologic standpoint, assuming all other factors (e.g., injury severity) are constant. Hypoxic-ischemic brain injury has a much poorer neurological and functional prognosis than "pure" traumatic brain injury, regardless of the type of primary brain injury incurred (i.e., diffuse versus focal injury, or both, at any given time after injury). Clinicians should avoid making clinical and prognostic decisions based on literature garnered from studying TBI populations in cases of hypoxic-ischemic brain injury.

Type of Prognostic Indicator

Prognostic indicators commonly used to predict outcome during rehabilitation generally fall into one of six categories: demographic variables, severity indices, neurological signs, neuroimaging studies, neuromedical markers, and psychosocial ratings.

Of the demographic measures, the relationship between age and outcome has been investigated most heavily. Age is more closely related to survival than to morbidity. More specifically, outcomes tend to contrast sharply at the outer limits of the continuum with a higher percentage of younger patients (age <20) attaining good outcomes and a higher percentage of older patients (age ≥60) achieving poorer outcomes.

Injury severity and neurological signs have been studied extensively in the neurosurgical literature on outcome prediction. Interestingly, recent literature suggests that the duration of VS, in and of itself, may be one of the strongest, if not the strongest, predictor of long-term neurological and functional outcome after severe TBI (assuming no concurrent complicating neuromedical issues exist). Further analysis of outcome studies suggests that a number of conclusions can be drawn. Severity indices and neurological signs are most useful when they are used during the first 2 weeks after injury. In the acute period, the major predictors of poor outcome are the following:

- GCS ≤5 (with motor score most highly predictive of outcome),
- prolonged posttraumatic amnesia,
- abnormal brainstem findings, and
- elevated intracranial pressure (i.e., >40 mm Hg).

However, low initial GCS scores (3 to 5) and coma of relatively short duration (<2 weeks) are not reliable predictors of long-term outcome in that they characterize patients whose eventual functional status on the Glasgow Outcome Scale (GOS) range from mild to severe. In contrast, abnormal oculomotor findings are powerful predictors of persistent cognitive disability. In general, injury factors are capable of predicting functional outcome, but with low specificity, and they generally are not highly predictive of late (>6 months) functional or neuropsychological outcome. They do, however, appear to be useful for early identification of patients who will require intensive medical and rehabilitative treatment.

Multiple electrophysiological measures have been examined in an attempt to provide further prognostic information pertaining to severe TBI outcome. The potential applications of electroencephalography (EEG) in a variety of formats have been studied in coma, VS, PVS, and MR patients. Some patients show normalization of their EEG with time, even in PVS. Certain coma EEG patterns may aid in prediction of outcome (e.g., alpha coma versus theta coma and burst suppression patterns, which are commonly seen in cases of severe hypoxic brain injury). Overall, late, low-voltage, nonreactive EEGs, although not precluding neurorecovery, are generally not harbingers of good neurological and functional recovery. Emergence from VS may be accompanied by EEG changes consisting of diminution of theta and delta activity and appearance of a reactive alpha rhythm, but these findings are not, per se, predictive of the extent of future functional improvements. Early data using compressed spectral array analysis EEG suggest that patients with changeable spectrograms and desynchronization eventually emerge from VS. Other researchers have concluded that changeable spectrograms alone correlate more strongly with survival and not necessarily with emergence from VS.

Evoked potentials have also been studied in great depth relative to their predictive relevance after severe TBI. Of the three commonly used evoked potential (EP) modalities—somatosensory, visual, and brainstem—the somatosensory EPs (SEPs) are the most sensitive and reliable relative to outcome prediction, particularly in the acute postinjury period. Most of the research to date has centered on acute and subacute (i.e., during the first 2 weeks) use of EP data relative to predictive utility for short-term complications (morbidity and mortality), as well as long-term functional outcome. Bilateral absence of early SEPs strongly correlates with death or VS outcome. Bilateral absence of the N-20 response, as opposed to prolongation or presence of an N-20 response, correlates best with a poor outcome (that is, the presence of an N-20 response does not necessarily imply a good outcome). Multimodal EP analysis significantly increases predictive validity. Some researchers have also begun to look at the predictive utility of intermediate and early long-latency cortical potentials relative to long-term functional disability in the post-acute setting. Work is also in the very early stages relative to cognitive evoked potentials (so called P-300s) and their possible utility in outcome prediction after severe TBI.

The role of static neuroimaging computed tomography (CT) and magnetic resonance imaging (MRI) relative to long-term functional outcome prediction after severe TBI remains vague. There is no question that early static imaging correlates strongly with short-term morbidity and mortality. Risk factors in the acute period include high-volume lesions (>4,100 mm³), subdural hematoma, subarachnoid hemorrhage, midline shift, perimesencephalic cistern obliteration, and evidence of diffuse axonal injury. In the postacute period, static imaging may still be helpful. Specifically, significant atrophy—particularly with evidence of a very wide third ventricle, generalized atrophy, or both—as well as clinical suspicion of communicating hydrocephalus may be associated with poorer outcome from VS. Given the greater sensitivity of MRI for diffuse axonal injury (DAI) detection in this methodology remains the static imaging test of choice in the postacute period. Clinicians should understand, however, that numerous articles question the predictive utility of static imaging in TBI relative to long-term functional outcome or recovery from VS.

Functional imaging, including single photon emission computed tomography (SPECT) and positron emission tomography (PET), to assess cerebral blood flow and cerebral metabolism are just beginning to be explored as methods to add to the clinician's armamentarium of "predictive tools." SPECT is currently used as an adjuvant tool for brain death diagnosis; however, use of the technique for prognosis is premature, because the current database is too sparse to make predictions with any degree of medical probability. Early data suggest that functional imaging may offer practitioners additional information regarding the extent of brain dysfunction, rather than simply representing structural disintegrity as a static image. Clinicians should realize that the science does not exist to state that certain functional imaging patterns are consistent or inconsistent with cognition or pain perception.

Many attempts have been made to correlate a variety of laboratory measures with outcome after severe traumatic brain injury. Typically, these factors have been shown to be most significant relative to prognostic value when used in combination with other predictive factors in multiple regression analyses. The following laboratory measures have been found to be correlated with less favorable outcomes: acute hyperglycemia (>250 mg/dL), leukocytosis, hyperkalemia, hypercortisolemia, significant blood alcohol levels, elevated catecholamine levels (especially norepinephrine) in both plasma and cerebrospinal fluid (CSF), elevated serum myelin basic proteins, elevated CSF creatine kinase (BB type), as well as elevated ventricular lactate and pyruvate levels. The exact methodology by which these measures should be taken into consideration when making outcome predictions has yet to be definitely clarified.

Various neuromedical factors have been correlated, both early and late after injury, with a poorer overall neurological and functional outcome, in addition to a decreased likelihood of emergence from VS. Acute and subacute secondary medical complications have been associated with poorer long-term outcome. These include, but are not limited to, systolic hypertension, acidosis, impaired autoregulation, secondary hypoxemia, and disseminated intravascular coagulation. In the early posttraumatic phase of recovery (first week), Sazbon and Groswasser noted that certain parameters were associated with nonemergence from VS: central fever, diffuse diaphoresis, antidiuretic hormone (ADH) disturbances, abnormal motor reactivity, respiratory disturbances, and diffuse nonneurologic injuries. Contrary to this, in the subacute phase of care (after the first week), studies have shown that posttraumatic epilepsy (PIE) and communicating hydrocephalus (CH) were negative prognostic indicators for recovery from VS. Finally, of all the known neuromedical factors, duration of VS may in and of itself be the strongest predictor of the chance or lack thereof for emergence from VS.

The method used to analyze the prognostic indicators is perhaps the most important factor influencing the specificity of outcome prediction. There are two major methodological determinants. The first concerns whether unidimensional or multidimensional procedures are relied on for analyzing the prognostic indicators. There is conclusive evidence that more confident outcome predictions can be made when predictions are based on a combination of prognostic indicators. This is due to the inherent interactions between predictors (e.g., GCS score and CT findings). For example, Narayan and colleagues demonstrated that outcome, measured by a two-category collapsed version of the GOS, could be predicted with more than 90% confidence in approximately 65% of 133 severe TBI patients using a combination of GCS score, pupillary responses, intracranial pressure (ICP) data, multimodal evoked potential data, and age. The percentage of outcomes predicted with more than 90% confidence fell to 25% when the GCS score was used alone.

The second methodological consideration concerns the degree to which predictions are based on static versus serial assessment ratings.

Serial assessment allows the clinician to generate an index of change from which the rate of recovery can be estimated. There is increasing evidence that change indices are superior to static ratings in predicting outcome. This suggests that outcome predictions should also take into account the rate of change in prognostic markers over time.

Although numerous associations have been shown to exist between predictors (individual as well as combined) and outcome, a reliable "predictive formula" has not been derived. Although it is incumbent on the clinician to be well versed in the existing knowledgebase regarding prognostic indicators, empiricism continues to significantly influence how that knowledge is used. For this reason, outcome prediction remains as much an art as a science and should be routinely accompanied by skepticism.

—by Joseph T. Giacino PhD and
Nathan D. Zasler, MD, FAAPM&R, FAADEP

Joseph T. Giacino, PhD is Associate Director of Neuropsychology, JFK Johnson Rehabilitation Institute, Center for Head Injuries, Edison, New Jersey, Assistant Professor, Seton Hall University, School of Graduate Medical Education, Department of Neurology, South Orange, New Jersey.

Nathan D. Zasler, MD, FAAPM&R, FAADEP is Executive Medical Director, National NeuroRehabilitation Consortium, Inc., Medical Director, Concussion Care Center of Virginia, Richmond, Virginia.

Part Three

Rehabilitation and Research

Chapter 18

Life After Brain Injury: Who Am I?

Introduction

This book is written for you—the head injured patient. It is not for your family, not for your therapists, not for your employer, not for your attorney, and not for your rehabilitation nurse. It is very important that all these people understand what has happened to you and why you are who you are today. They are very welcome to read this booklet, but it was developed with only you in mind.

You have experienced an accident or medical complication that has changed your life. The changes may be mild or they may be far-reaching. In any event, you are not the exact same person you were before the injury. Damage to the brain, however mild, results in various circuits being either destroyed or at least short-circuited. Some circuits can be repaired, some can be detoured to other pathways, and others are permanently destroyed.

Most head injured individuals become aware at some point that changes have occurred and they are different or that they at least are perceived differently by others. This may occur when one of your friends tells you that "you are not the person I knew before" or when your boss demotes you, saying "you are not able to handle your previous job responsibilities." You may believe these statements are true or you may feel that others are imagining problems or acting unfairly. No matter what you believe is true, the reality remains that all insults to the brain lead to some changes in lifestyle, family structure, employability and social interactions.

As you recover and are involved in an appropriate rehabilitation program, cognitive deficits resulting from this damage begin to resolve fairly quickly. However, resolving some of the higher level problem-solving and social interaction deficits may take much time, therapy and hard work on your part. In some cases these skills may not completely return to the pre-injury level.

Behavioral and Emotional Reactions

We are all brought up to equate "bad behavior" with a "bad person." If you had a friend who was always getting into trouble, it was either because he was mean or his family never taught him right from wrong. If you had a friend who was highly emotional, such as depressed or anxious, it was because he had psychological problems. These very simple explanations for behavioral and emotional reactions do not provide an adequate picture now for you and your head injured peers.

During the injury to your head, various parts of your brain that deal with your emotions and your behavior were damaged. In the hospital you probably acted and felt very differently than you did before the accident. Gradually, these behaviors that may have been uncharacteristic for you will have decreased somewhat. Over time you begin to return to your old self or at least close to your old self. However, some people continue to experience personality changes many years past injury.

Please do not feel that you can now blame all of your undesirable behavior on your head injury. Yes, you may have lost some behavioral control. Yes, you may have been placed in a position such as loss of job or income which would justify an emotional reaction. But no, you cannot say that all your actions are not your fault.

This next section lists many reactions that are common consequences of head injury. They may not all apply to you, but it would be good to read each one so that you can have an understanding of all the possibilities. Remember, you are in control of your life. You must work to help yourself.

Denial

We have chosen denial as the first behavioral area to address since it has such a large impact on how you view your entire existence. From the time you can remember (since the injury), therapists have been talking to you about your problem areas and they have been setting goals for you to accomplish in therapy. Some of these problems you totally agree exist and others you have probably rejected. Physical weakness, speech misarticulations or slurring, slowed reactions and vision problems are those areas that are readily recognized by you and your head injury peers. However, cognitive problems are not as easily perceived by the one who is experiencing them.

This is not a psychological problem. You are not crazy. Instead, the neurological damage you received prevents you from completely recognizing all your difficulties. Moreover, it is natural for you to avoid those things that are hard for you. When you avoid them, you do not have to see that you have a problem. If you do not see the problem, then it does not exist. Right? Wrong.

This is not a problem area that can be resolved easily by reading this book. The best advice that we can give is to have an open mind. Listen to what others are saying. They are not being mean or enjoying themselves by listing all your weaknesses. They truly want to help. Let them help you.

Overoptimism

Overoptimism is a symptom of holding on to your denial. You may have expected that once you were out of the hospital you could start to make plans for becoming "normal" again. You may have set arbitrary goals such as "I'll be back to work by Thanksgiving" or "I'll be driving by Christmas." When you did not meet these goals you probably felt defeated, angry, or at least frustrated. This is a very common occurrence with those who have had an injury to the head.

One of the reasons for overoptimism with head injury is that you often look so good physically that you and your loved ones expect too much too soon. "Getting well" is mostly associated with physical recovery such as the healing of a broken leg. Healing of the brain needs much more time than you might expect or your friends and family might expect from just looking at you or talking to you.

Impatience

Head injured individuals are notoriously impatient and our guess is that you are no exception. There are three factors that appear to explain this condition. First, the areas of the brain that help you to control your emotions have, in all likelihood, been damaged—thus, the ability to control frustration and anger is affected. Second, head injury often leads to self-centered behavior which will be described in greater detail under egocentrism. Because you are tending to look at all issues from your viewpoint, you have a hard time understanding the other person's reasons for being delayed or late in responding to your wishes. Last, because of possible cognitive difficulties, such as problem solving or abstract reasoning, you may misinterpret a situation and find yourself very impatient for what other people think are illogical reasons.

Irritability

Almost all head injured patients go through a period of time where they are easily agitated. Some remain what might be termed as "grouchy" for the rest of their lives. You may be well aware of your increased irritability or you may not recognize it. If your family and loved ones tell you that you are overly sensitive, believe them; it is probably true.

This increased irritability is due to organic problems which have changed your ability to: 1) completely understand a situation accurately; 2) perform simple tasks that used to be second nature to you; 3) filter out unimportant information or noise. Any one or a combination of these three problems can cause you to be more annoyed by trivial matters.

Even though you have a decent excuse for acting this way, you will not be accepted by peers, employers or even family if you continue to let every little thing put you in a bad mood. No one freely chooses to spend time with a grouch when they can be somewhere else.

Verbal Outbursts

At first, when you were in the hospital, you may have said things to people that you either do not remember or would like to forget. You did not become a mean and ugly person overnight. Instead, when your brain was damaged, your filtering system was affected. This means that the areas that keep you from saying things that you would normally think but never say out loud are dysfunctional.

It would be very easy for you to say, "Well, this is the way I am and I can't help it." But this would be a cop-out. In order to fit back into society, you must identify and attempt to change the head injury characteristics that set you apart from others. Your desire to say the first thing that comes to your mind can be controlled. You are the only person who can do this—it is your job. If you feel you need assistance, ask a family member or close friend to help you.

Temper Outbursts

Temper outbursts are the physical manifestation of the same problem that leads to verbal outbursts described in the preceding section. Here you act before you think rather than speak before you think. Again, the underlying problem is primarily organic. Again, you cannot continue to use this as an excuse. No one wants to live or be around for any extended period of time with a person who resorts to physical displays of anger or frustration.

Family Abuse

In the area of head injury rehabilitation, we often say that the family is as "damaged" as the patient. We are not trying to minimize your suffering; however, after watching hundreds of families from ICU (Intensive Care) for two or more years post injury, it is quite evident that they have also been traumatized.

Although you may not fit into the usual pattern, many head injured individuals make life for their families almost unbearable. At first you may not have been aware of your actions—they were out of your control. Later, you may have realized that you were being difficult, but you figured your family understood your frustrations and would be willing to put up with you. For the most part, you are right. Your family will accept much more inappropriate and ungrateful behavior from you than will therapists, teachers, friends or employers. Nevertheless, is this how you want to treat the people who are most likely to stick by you for the rest of your life?

Why risk the possibility that those who care the most about you will gradually be soured by your harsh words or insensitive actions? Manners begin at home. When the chips are down, who will be there for you? Act to make sure it will be your family.

Egocentrism

It is natural for someone who has gone through a traumatic illness to focus primarily upon himself. We all do this. You are not acting in a self-centered manner. You are like the three or four year-old who thinks that the world revolves around him. Eventually, you have to grow up and realize that the feelings and desires of others are also important.

Sometimes head injured individuals continue to focus almost entirely on themselves. You may have had family members or friends who have accused you of being selfish. You may not have taken their accusations seriously. Now that you are on your way to recovery, you need to take a good look at your life and see if you are thinking about others—not just yourself.

Impulsivity

Do you find yourself acting or talking before you think? If so, you are probably engaging in impulsive behavior. Why? The part of your brain that deals with attention and concentration has probably been affected so that you act without clearly thinking about what would be the best response. Your filtering system or the device that applies some control over your behavior is not working up to par.

Undoubtedly, you have gotten yourself into trouble by doing things that others feel are not appropriate for the circumstance. This is undoubtedly very frustrating as well as aggravating for you. Families too can become very put out with you. It is to everyone's advantage for you to slow down, think, and then act.

Suspiciousness

At times you may think that other people are doing things to you or talking about you behind your back. Even when they assure you that they are not, you may not believe them. This is a common feeling with head injured patients. It does not mean that you are crazy. Instead, this behavior is a result of your difficulty sizing up a situation and drawing accurate conclusions about what is going on. Some cognitive deficits are affecting your ability to think clearly. You may be misinterpreting certain cues and then blowing things out of proportion.

Moreover, since your head injury many people have been involved in your life telling you what to do and what not to do. You may be feeling that too many people are too concerned about your life. Why don't they worry about their own lives? Remember, they are concerned or they would not be involved. Look on the positive side—there could be nobody around to care.

Depression

Depression is a very common emotional consequence that usually comes after you have progressed in your rehabilitation program. At first you do not feel down or depressed because you really do not understand or comprehend all the changes that are taking place in your life. As you become more and more aware of the possibility that things will not return to normal immediately, you may begin to react with frustration and depression.

You may be saying, "I'm not depressed," and, in fact, you may not be, but—consider it a possibility if you find that you have one or more of the following symptoms: 1) lack of interest in life in general; 2) excessive sleeping; 3) loss of ability to feel happy or excited about anything; 4) lack of motivation; 5) loss of desire to be with any of your friends; 6) constant TV watching.

Lack of Motivation

Has your "get up and go got up and went?" Do you feel like nothing is of any real importance? Early in your recovery process this lack of motivation was the result of injury to the brain. You were fatigued, confused and unable to make plans and follow through with them. All thoughts of goal-setting were overwhelming. Now that you are better, you still feel this inertia or lack of movement.

The continuation of this general lack of interest is often related to the previously described behavioral reaction—depression. Another possibility is that you have tried to do things and failed miserably. Now it is easier and less threatening to remain stagnant, still, unmotivated.

Inappropriate Social Behavior

As you grew up, you gradually became socialized under the direction of your parents, teachers or guardians. It was a long, drawn out process probably involving a lot of trial and error as well as punishment here and there. When your head was injured, particularly if it was a severe injury, you probably became very childlike in your behavior. Thus, it was necessary for nurses and therapists to reteach you the social graces.

It is possible that you have been resentful of people telling you what to do and what not to do. You may not even feel that you are doing anything wrong. Instead, people are just trying to give you a hard time. It is important to remember, however, that many people who have experienced head trauma behave in ways that would have been unthinkable prior to their injury. Appropriate social behavior, like other forms of conduct, must be relearned.

Dependency

Over the past few days, months, or even years of your rehabilitation process you have had to rely heavily on other people to help you accomplish many things you could not do on your own. You have come to rely on certain people, especially those who were there for you at all times.

Now it is time to break away and become more self-sufficient. You may be very anxious to do this or you may be very hesitant. In any event, it is important for you as well as your primary support system that you gradually become more and more independent. This is a sign of "getting well" and reintegrating yourself back into the community.

Increased or Decreased Sexual Interest

A large majority of head injured patients find that their outlook on sexual matters may have been altered. You may find that you shy away from any sexual encounters, thinking that you are no longer attractive to the opposite sex. You may have tried and been shot down, leading you to be very reluctant to venture out again.

On the other hand, you may have discovered that you are extremely interested in talking about sex as well as participating in it. You may be much more open with your feelings and have fewer inhibitions. Reactions to your newfound interest may vary from people laughing and joking with you to others completely avoiding being in your presence.

You must remember that sex and discussions or jokes about sex are viewed very differently by those around you. You must learn to determine when this subject is appropriate and when it is not. Head injured individuals who have not been able to make these discriminations have lost jobs, friends and spouses over this issue. Making sexual innuendoes may be fun and enjoyable, but it is not worth damaging your future.

Excessive Talking

Excessive talking indicates a loss of control or a display of outward anxiety. You may not realize this, but head injured patients often discuss the same topic over and over. You do this for a number of reasons: 1) You may have difficulty remembering that you have already had many previous discussions of this topic; 2) You are using your numerous talks with others to come to some conclusions about your problem; 3) You are not able to stop yourself from bringing up the same topic many times.

This habit may be very frustrating to your family and friends. It may make you feel better, but it may not endear you to other people. If you are concerned about what others are thinking, you will need to first recognize the problem and then take steps to bring it under control. Ask someone who really cares about you to help you with this.

Loss of Control

Many head injured individuals express the feeling that their lives are really out of their control. You may have felt that you no longer have the freedom to work wherever you want, live wherever you like, or make the major decisions in your life. Your future seems to be out of your hands.

Psychosocial Problems

After a head injury, you may find yourself thinking, feeling and acting in ways that are different from how you thought, felt and acted before your injury. Cognitive and behavioral problems can create another set of problems for you called psychosocial problems. Psychosocial problems are problems adjusting to everyday living. Do you feel out of place or different? Are your relationships with family members strained? Have you lost all your friends and do you have difficulty making new ones? Are you experiencing difficulty returning to work or school? Have you lost your job or your career? Is your life less enjoyable and more unsatisfactory? If you answered yes to any of these questions, you may be experiencing psychosocial problems.

Others with head injuries have faced the same problems you are going through now. Your awareness of psychosocial problems will increase. This is very important because an awareness of any problem is the crucial first step toward its solution. Recognizing your psychosocial problems and realizing that other persons with head injuries are having the same problems do not solve your problems. To solve, reduce or cope with your psychosocial problems, you need to do something about them. You must take some type of action if you want to make your everyday life better. You cannot expect some type of pill or medical procedure to cure your psychosocial problems. It's your life so you must accept the responsibility for dealing with it. Others—parents, spouse, therapists and friends—can help you help yourself, but ultimately it is you who must do it. That's the bottom line.

Sometimes it is hard and lonely, but at other times it can be gratifying when you overcome a seemingly impossible obstacle. You know this already because you already are a survivor. You probably cheated death and successfully overcame many physical and medical problems. Maybe you have already overcome some cognitive and behavioral problems. Congratulations! But you can't stop there. You have to channel the motivation and desire you used in your physical and cognitive rehabilitation into the rehabilitation of your everyday living. It won't be easy and it won't be quick, but it will be well worth it. The payoffs are increased productivity, greater human intimacy and more enjoyment of life.

Chapter 19

Background Information about the Rehabilitation of People with Traumatic Brain Injury

Traumatic brain injury (TBI) is defined as brain damage from some externally inflicted trauma to the head that results in significant impairment to an individual's physical, psychological, and/or cognitive functional abilities. It is characterized by altered consciousness (coma and/or posttrauma amnesia) during the acute phase after injury, the duration of which varies greatly among individuals, usually depending on the severity of the injury.

Myths of Recovery vs. Factors in Improvement

Rehabilitation of brain-injured clients is certainly feasible and can be successful, but client, family, friends, and even rehabilitation practitioners must be constantly aware that TBI brings *permanent* damage that causes *permanent* limitations. The Twelfth Institute on Rehabilitation Issues (IRI) Prime Study Group working under a grant from the National Institute of Handicapped Research (NIHR) reports:

Almost never does a patient 'recover.' ...The continual expectation of recovery can lead clients and families into denial, frustration,

Background information on rehabilitation principles excerpted from Rehab BRIEF, Vol. IX, No. 4, 1986(?), National Institute of Handicapped Research, Office of Special Education and Rehabilitative Services, Department of Education, Washington, DC 20202; prepared by PSI International, Inc. For information on obtaining the complete document, see the Brain Injury Association's current Catalog of Educational Materials, #CEM 86-007. The Brain Injury Association, Inc. may be reached at (800) 444-6443 or (202) 296-6443.

171

disappointment, and ... extremely unrealistic expectations... We prefer to speak in terms of hope for as much *improvement* as possible.

There are several commonly held "myths" that rehabilitation practitioners may meet, or even hold themselves.

Recovery Occurs in a Year. It used to be traditional for doctors to tell people that whatever recovery will occur will happen in the first 12 months. While this may be the case *neurologically*, it is not the case functionally. Severe injuries may improve more slowly. This myth often causes people to believe that the client's level of performance at one year is what everyone is stuck with. The FACT is that while the major brain healing may have occurred, *true rehabilitation may be just beginning*.

The Plateau. This concept holds that "recovery" begins after coma, continues at an upward pace, and then slows down and levels off. Families despair at this plateau, and some therapists may terminate clients when they appear to stop progressing. The FACT is that head-injured people are notoriously inconsistent in their progress. They may take one step forward, two back, do nothing for a while, then unexpectedly make a series of gains. A "plateau" is by no means evidence that functional improvement is arrested.

The Lourdes Phenomenon. Many families, unwilling to accept less than a return to "normal," believe that a miracle of recovery will occur if *only* they find the right doctor or program. "Doctor and program hopping" are not unusual. It is true that significant gains are most likely with competent therapists, and there is always need to improve rehabilitation programs. However, the FACT is, that a solution lies not in finding a "cure" but in working toward improvements, accepting limitations, and developing new, realistic expectations and goals.

Normal IQ. Too often, psychologists naive to TBI are persuaded to administer batteries of intelligence tests to TBI clients. When the IQ scores are in the average range, they may pronounce the clients "cognitively recovered" or "capable of functioning intellectually in the average range." This myth can seriously misrepresent the clients' deficits and create unrealistic expectations. "Average IQ" is largely irrelevant to the assessment of brain-injured persons. The FACT is, traditional intelligence test interpretations bear little relationship to the mental processes required for everyday functioning. Head-injured people may perform very well on brief, structured, artificial tasks, yet have such immense deficits in learning, memory, and executive functions that they are unable to cope in the real world.

The Need for Psychotherapy. Many people who enter traditional psychotherapy do so because they are dissatisfied with their lives; their goals are unclear; their relationships are failing; they cannot accomplish what they want; they are angry, fearful, or depressed. While these may be the traits of a TBI client, the *causes* may be organic, *not* psychological. The FACT is, the disorder in a TBI client's life may not reflect underlying psychological conflict so much as the cognitive and executive dysfunctions of damaged brain cells. Psychological conflicts may exist in addition to the injury, but traditional psychodynamic approaches seldom offer head-injured people relief from their particular sorts of disordered lives.

Debunking such common myths is not meant to imply that improvement is impossible. To the contrary, it is programs like those represented in the IRI Study Group that believe most strongly in the possibilities for improvement.

Improvement after TBI needs to be considered from two points of view:

- *Neurological / Neuropsychological*—the amount of nerve tissue that returns to functioning and the extent to which this results in restored physical and cognitive ability; and

- *Functional*—the ability to carry out tasks of day-to-day living effectively.

Vocational Rehabilitation Intervention

Referral to a vocational rehabilitation counselor may come early after injury or at some later time. Early referral may not be appropriate if the client is not yet in a position to face vocational issues. Although some medical stability may have been achieved, it must be determined if *functional* stability is sufficient to begin addressing vocational concerns. The IRI Study Group sets out four factors for the vocational rehabilitation professional to consider.

Client's Ability to Participate. The client must be awake, alert, oriented, out of posttrauma amnesia (i.e., able to remember ongoing events from day to day), able to understand what happened to him or her, and prepare to take an active part in realistically planning for the future.

Stage of Improvement. The first 6 to 12 months after injury are often characterized by steady, spontaneous improvement. Physical, cognitive, and behavioral changes are so rapid that evaluation is often useless for determining eventual vocational potential. Wait until this early phase of marked change is complete before attempting to evaluate the client for indications of ultimate potential. Keep close to the client, monitoring progress, but defer evaluation until the rate of change slows.

Appropriateness of Services. The vocational rehabilitation counselor is often asked to purchase services that are not directly related to *vocational* concerns. If intervention begins too early, services that are more medical in nature may be requested. The practitioner needs to evaluate the appropriateness of such requests.

Alternate Sources of Funding. The astute vocational rehabilitation counselor will become aware of alternate funding sources to recommend when requests for services do not seem specific to the process of vocational rehabilitation.

Developing a Rehabilitation Plan

Developing an Individualized Written Rehabilitation Plan (IWRP) may present unique problems. TBI clients typically present a wider range of cognitive, social, physical, and self-care deficits than do other client groups; and a team of specialists may be involved, requiring creative, flexible scheduling. Some appropriate services may include:

- **Cognitive Rehabilitation.** Systematic, goal-oriented therapeutic intervention designed to improve cognitive abilities (attention, perception, planning and organization, memory, control of impulsiveness, making judgements) may be needed.

- **Behavioral Management.** Identifying specific maladaptive behaviors and modifying them or replacing them with more adaptive behaviors may help. For TBI clients, such behavioral problems as failure to organize daily life, argumentiveness, and lack of emotional control can interfere with social and vocational improvement.

- **Psychosocial Rehabilitation.** Social isolation or social inappropriateness can be a serious problem for TBI clients. Programs that use group training methods may enable clients to relearn social skills to form and maintain relationships.

- **Physical Therapy.** Neuromuscular and orthopedic problems may require therapy to develop muscle tone, range of movement, balance, and coordination.

- **Occupational Therapy.** Skills related to activities of daily living such as dressing, eating, and caring for personal hygiene may need improvement.

- **Speech and Language Therapy.** A number of communication disorders typically occur after TBI, including dysarthria, aphasia, and apraxia.

- **Neuropsychology.** Assessment of the cognitive and emotional functioning of the client or treatment in emotional/behavioral or cognitive skill areas may be needed.

- **Counseling Services.** While it will not cure behavioral and attitudinal problems that are organically based, counseling can provide emotional support in facing disability.

- **Recreational Therapy.** This service can help the client make productive use of leisure time.

- **Vocational Services.** While traditional job-seeking training may prove ineffective for clients with organically based planning, organization, and follow-through deficits, supported work or job trial situations can be helpful in establishing positive work behaviors.

  Vocational placement may rest heavily on job modification and restructuring. Training of work supervisors and coworkers may be essential. Consultation may be required about aids and services to make accommodation more likely. Follow-up with the client at work may be crucial to successful vocational rehabilitation.

Chapter 20

Selecting and Monitoring Head Injury Rehabilitation Services

The Health Care System In Brief

The 1980's brought radical changes to the health care industry in the United States. At the same time, the availability of specialized head injury rehabilitation programs and services grew dramatically. Competition became a hallmark of the health care industry as first the federal government, and then private insurance carriers began to rethink the way they paid for health care services. Competition for consumers has perhaps been strongest among head injury rehabilitation programs and services, in large part as a result of the proliferation of proprietary programs.

Models of Rehabilitation

In the past, rehabilitation programs for people with head injury were largely provided in a "medical model." Although this model is still predominant, the trend today is toward more community-based rehabilitation models. And, more community-based programs and services serving people with head injury are becoming available all the time. Restrictive insurance policies tend to favor the medical model. However, many carriers are becoming more willing to negotiate both types and settings of services they will pay for. In some states, this is also true of Medicaid.

An Informed Consumer Makes the Best Customer

The purpose of this guide is to enable you to make well-informed decisions about the services you or your family member receives. Through general guiding principals and specific questions, it provides a framework for the collection and evaluation of information regarding head injury rehabilitation programs and services. Contact your Brain Injury Association, Inc. state association if you have questions or need additional assistance.

—Mary S. Reitter
Deputy Director,
Brain Injury Association, Inc.

Guiding Principles

1. **You Know Your Needs Best.** People with head injury and their families know themselves and their needs best. Rehabilitation professionals can help provide the information you need to make informed choices, but *you* have to live with the decision you make.

2. **Be Curious.** Ask questions. Learn about the program, its staff and rehabilitation philosophy and methodology. If you don't understand something, insist that someone take time to explain it in the detail you need. Rehabilitation is as much an "art" as a "science."

3. **Learn from Others.** When researching available programs, talk with *at least three* individuals who have participated in each program you are considering. You can benefit from listening to their experiences with the program.

4. **Explore More Than One Program.** There are hundreds of rehabilitation programs and services to choose from. The closest one, or the one that offers the most services, is not necessarily the one which will best meet your needs.

5. **Listen to Your Instincts.** Make decisions when you are ready. If you are unsure or uncomfortable, find someone who

has no stake in the decision to help you sort things out. Be wary of anyone who tries to pressure you. If you feel pressured, report this to the program's corporate office, licensing agencies and accrediting organizations.

6. **Get It in Writing.** This cannot be emphasized enough! Keep a log of who you spoke to, the date, the time, and a summary of your conversation. Keep copies of all correspondence. During this emotional time, it is easy to forget information. You may wish to tape record your conversations so you can refer to them later. The person you are speaking with should readily agree to be taped. Get any commitments for services (the types and quantities to be provided as well as costs) in writing *before* you choose program.

7. **Looks Aren't Everything.** The quality of rehabilitation services cannot be judged by how nice the facilities or marketing materials look.

8. **The Ultimate Goal is Take Charge.** Rehabilitation programs should promote self-determination to the extent possible and maximize integration into the community. Self-determination can be achieved by taking charge of the decision-making process—for example, deciding how you wish to use your own time and energy and money.

9. **Know Your Financial Situation.** Talk with your insurance carrier or other health care provider to find out how much they will pay and for what. Get a copy of your policy and read it. Find out the extent of your financial obligations (i.e., co-payments). Get regular (at least monthly) updates about where you stand financially with the carrier and program. Find out what other public or private benefits you may be eligible for and apply promptly.

10. **Be Involved.** Distance is no excuse for poor communication. Participate in team meetings. Establish regular verbal contact with key people in the program. Voice your opinions, questions, and concerns promptly. You should be welcome to visit, to observe, or to participate at any time.

11. **The Customer is Always Right.** As a customer of head injury rehabilitation services, *you* are the customer. While someone else may pay the bills, *you* are the one who must be satisfied with the services provided. If you are not satisfied, work with the program and funding source to remedy the situation promptly.

In these difficult times, choosing head injury rehabilitation programs and services may be the single most important decision you make—emotionally, financially, and in terms of outcome. Take time to make good decisions. And, once you are receiving services, stay on top of what is being provided, why, and what other options exist. Be an informed consumer.

Specific Questions You Might Ask

The following questions may not apply to all programs in all settings. We encourage you to select those questions which make sense for your particular situation, and, there may be others you feel are important as well. Add them. Write down the responses you get. Ask the same questions of each program you are considering, and then compare the responses. If you need more information, or something isn't clear, don't hesitate to call the program and ask again.

Please don't be concerned about the amount of time it may take you to ask the questions you have selected. Selecting a program which meets the needs you have is important.

Monitoring services once they have begun is important, too. Refer to this guide from time to time and reflect on how well the program staff is doing what they said they would do. Ask questions you didn't consider during the selection process but which are important as rehabilitation progresses. Remember, information is power.

Discharge Planning

Planning for discharge must begin at admission. It is imperative to have an understanding of what the next step is after discharge and what kinds of services might be needed, and their availability. Be clear about your intent to be involved in discharge decisions. As with other information, it is important to get discharge planning commitments in writing. It is virtually impossible for anyone to tell you the particular level of recovery which will be achieved. They can, however, commit to what they will do to achieve *maximum* recovery.

1. What are all the possible options after discharge?

2. What is the role of the person with head injury and their family in decisions about discharge?

3. Where do you think the person will go after discharge?

4. How and who decides when the individual is ready for discharge? What would make the program extend or shorten the anticipated discharge date? If this is done, how much notice is given, and what is the role of the individual and their family in this decision?

5. What if a person decides to leave the program with or without advance notice?

6. How does the program help research discharge options? Who does this?

7. What kinds of follow-up after discharge are provided to the person with head injury? What kinds of follow-up are offered to the family? Why is follow-up offered? How long is follow-up offered? What are the charges for this service?

8. What is the average length of stay?

9. How do I get a complete set of records for my files upon discharge? Is there a charge for this? How much and who pays?

10. Where are the people with head injury the program served in the past?

11. What happens if the place the person is expected to go after discharge falls through?

12. What happens if it appears the person has no discharge options except with family, and the family is unable to provide

the care or supervision needed, or for any other reason they feel they are not a viable discharge option?

13.   What does the program do to locate affordable community housing with a package of supports provided by a variety of state and community agencies to afford the individual the opportunity to live independently (i.e., transportation, recreation, vocational, educational, and personal assistance)?

Financial Responsibilities/Arrangements

People with head injuries have had to leave programs before they are ready because their funding has been exhausted. Large unexpected bills for rehabilitation services have surprised many people and dramatically changed their financial stability and status. The best way to prevent these occurrences is to stay informed about your continuing financial status both with the program and your funding source.

1.   Regarding costs...

A.   What is the daily cost of the program?
B.   What does this include (room & board, medications, physician services, therapy, transportation, etc.)?
C.   What is billed extra (i.e., telephone, laundry)?
D.   How are charges calculated (i.e., per diem, per unit)?

2.   What agreement does the program have with my funding source?

3.   What do I need to do to get copies of all correspondence (including bills submitted and payments rendered) between the program and my funding source?

4.   Who is billed for services my funding source won't pay for? What happens if the second source doesn't pay?

5.   Am I (or is my insurance) billed for services which are planned or scheduled but not provided (i.e., if a therapy session is missed)?

6.   What sources of funding does the program accept?

7. How do home visits or other leaves of absence effect payment? Is there a bed hold charge? If so, who is expected to pay if insurance won't?

8. What assistance does the program offer to determine which other public or private insurance and financial benefits the individual may be eligible for? How will they help you apply and follow the application in process for these?

Admission Planning

1. What are the rights and responsibilities of people participating in this program? How does the program inform the individual of these? Can I have a copy?

2. How do you make decisions about who to admit into the program?

3. How will you get previous medical and other important (i.e., school) records and other information you may need in order to decide?

4. I would like a proposed service or treatment plan before I decide. How can I get this?

5. How do you involve the program or service I am in now in the admission and transition process?

6. If I choose this program, what do you need to do prior to admission? How long will that take? What do you need me to do?

7. How can I arrange to spend a half-day or day observing the program?

8. What is your understanding of the role my funding source has in the decision-making process about the program I select?

9. What forms or contracts am I expected to sign prior to admission?

10. How can I get a copy of each to read thoroughly before I sign?

Involvement of Family & Friends

The active involvement of family members and friends throughout the rehabilitation process is a key component to achieve maximum success.

1. How does your program involve family members and friends?

2. How are family members and friends involved in team meetings? How will we be informed enough in advance so we can plan to participate?

3. What do I need to do to get copies of written reports regularly? Who is responsible for sending me these?

4. How will you schedule regular conference calls for me to speak with the team if I cannot get there to be at the meeting?

5. If I have a question about a particular area (i.e., physical therapy), what do I need to do to speak with the therapist directly?

6. What kind of family training, support groups and therapy is offered? Is there a charge for participation?

7. Since I live far away, what overnight arrangements are made for me to visit for a few days? How about for the person's friends?

8. What arrangements are made for staff to explain services and reports to me in non-technical terms?

9. What is your policy about visitors?

10. What are your policies which would affect friendships the person being served makes with other people served by your program? What provisions are made for them to spend time together as they might choose?

11. What arrangements are made if we wish to have conjugal visits?

Legal Considerations

1. How does a legal settlement affect the program's expectation about payment?

2. Has the program ever recommended guardianship, conservatorship or representative payees for people being served? Has the program ever recommended that these are no longer needed? If yes, what assistance is provided to the individual, family members or friends who can choose to pursue the recommendation?

3. Is the program licensed? By whom? How can I contact them to learn more about what they require for licensing? Can I see the license?

4. When was the last state or local inspection and what were the results?

5. Is the program CARF brain injury accredited? Any other CARF accreditation? When was the last survey?

6. Is the program accredited by JCAHO? At what level (1 year, 3 year, type 1)? When was the last survey?

7. What recourse does the person being served have if they question or disagree with the quality or necessity of services received?

8. What recourse do family members or friends have if they question or disagree with the quality or necessity of services received?

9. What provisions are made for personal banking services? Where do you keep money which belongs to people being served in your program? How/who accounts for money which is put into your program's care?

About the Program

Every component of every program is not addressed here. For example, specific questions about physical therapy are not included. The components below are those which tend to have broad implications, that is, to touch more than one specific discipline, often simultaneously. You will also wish to ask questions about the philosophy and methodology used in specific disciplines which are central to the services needed in your individual situation.

A. Observations to make about aesthetics:

1. Are the facilities clean?

2. Are people being served clean and dressed in a manner you are comfortable with? Do they appear to be well cared for?

3. Do staff seem attentive, to know people being served by name, and to care genuinely about people in the program (i.e., do they stop in the hall to say hello or joke)?

4. Is the food appealing? How does the program accommodate special diets, personal preferences, and requests for a different meal schedule? Any charge for this?

5. Do people being served seem comfortable with the way they are being treated? It helps to ask them.

B. Experience with people with head injuries:

1. How many people with head injuries has the program worked with in the past year? How many total individuals have they served?

2. What is the average staff turnover rate? Do they recruit people who have experience serving people with head injury? What staff training is provided?

3. How long has the program been in existence? When did it begin to serve people with head injury? Why was it established?

C. Program administration and organization:

1. Who is responsible for the overall supervision of the services rendered to people served? How often are they at the program?

How much direct contact do they have with individual people served?

2. What types of people are part of the team? What are the training and licensure requirements in the state for staff? Does the staff meet these standards?

3. How does the program integrate the individual's expressed desires and goals in service planning? For example, if an individual dislikes to cook and will not be expected to cook at home, is cooking an expected program component? If it will take a person three hours to feed themselves, and they decide this wastes energy they'd prefer to use in another manner, how will the program support them in this decision and what assistance will be provided to find ways to have feeding done by someone else—both at the program and at home?

4. Is there a consistent schedule for an individual's day? What involvement does the person have in directing the schedule and selecting the program components?

5. What do people generally do during unscheduled times?

6. What is the evening schedule?

7. What is the weekend schedule?

8. How is the need for specialized adaptive equipment identified? How is the equipment provided and paid for?

9. What access do people being served and their families have to their records? If I wanted to see my record now, what would I have to do? What recourse do I have if I disagree with something in the record?

D. Medical services/medications:

1. Who is responsible for providing the medical services? What is their background? Is the same person available at different times, or are multiple medical practitioners used?

2. How is my personal physician included in providing medical services while I'm in the program?

3. How does the program handle medical emergencies?

4. How are routine medical issues (i.e., regular dental and ophthalmological services) provided?

5. How would the program manage the special medical needs which have resulted from the injury?

6. I've heard that people can have trouble with bedsores. How does the program here avoid or prevent these?

7. What is the policy for the use of psychotropic or other mood-altering medications? What role does the individual have in these decisions? What does the program do if the person declines medical advice?

8. Who monitors medications and medication interactions? How often is this reviewed? What steps are taken to assure that therapeutic levels of medications are maintained and not exceeded?

Program Components:

Cognitive Services

1. What approaches does the program use to address cognitive strengths and limitations?

2. Is neuropsychological testing done? How much emphasis is placed in test reports on recommendations to build on an individual's cognitive strengths? How much emphasis is placed on reporting test scores and the person's limitations? When is retesting conducted?

3. If a "cognitive therapist" or "cognitive remediation specialist" is a member of the team, what particular qualifications do they have?

4. How is the effectiveness of cognitive services measured?

Behavioral Interventions

1. What approaches does the program use to address behavioral concerns? What role do the individual and his family play in determining the types of behavioral interventions used?

2. What steps does the program take to assure that behavioral interventions are clearly understood by all staff the person has contact with and that the plan is being implemented consistently by all staff (even at 3:00 in the morning)?

3. How is the effectiveness of behavioral interventions measured?

4. What role does medication play in "behavior management?"

5. Are physical restraints used? In what circumstances? What policies or protocols exist for the use of physical restraints? Can I see a copy of these?

6. Is a "secure" or locked unit available? When does the program recommend the use of these? Who decides when a person is ready for an open unit after being on a secure unit? How?

7. At what point is an individual's behavior deemed unacceptable to the program? How much notice does the program give the individual and his family? What efforts are made by the program to assist in locating another comparable program which can better meet the needs of the person?

Vocational Services

1. What is the extent of vocational services provided by the program?

2. How are situational vocational evaluations conducted? How are job trials, training, or placement provided? How are job coaches used? For how long?

3. What interface is there between the program and state vocational rehabilitation services?

Educational Services

1. What educational services are offered? To children? To college students? To adults?

2. Does the program have a teacher on staff with expertise in educating children with head injury?

3. What is the interface between the program and the person's school?

Community Re-entry

1. What components of the program take place in the community? How frequently is the individual in the community?

2. How are the person's ability to get around and to use community services and resources evaluated and addressed?

3. What local resources are used by the program to address the needs of the individual?

4. How does the program accommodate an individual's request to participate in community activities (i.e., AA or league bowling)?

5. What outreach does the program do to help educate the community about head injury and its consequences?

6. What does the program do to learn about the individual's home community and to identify resources and contacts there? What linkages are made with these resources and contacts prior to discharge?

7. What efforts are made to work with the person in their home, even if the program is "facility-based"? How often can this be expected—once for evaluation only, or multiple times to prepare the person for the return home?

8. What is the interface between the program and the local Independent Living Center?

Recreation

1. How does the program accommodate the individual's continued involvement in recreational interests and activities? Are modifications of activities or equipment suggested, and opportunity for situational exploration of the effectiveness of modifications included?

2. What does the program do to support the individual's desires to become active in new recreational pursuits?

3. How does the program help the individual identify ways to participate in recreation and social opportunities in their community?

4. What interface does the program have with the local recreation department? With community therapeutic recreation services? With social support and activity groups?

Chapter 21

Memory Rehabilitation

Some of the psychological approaches to memory rehabilitation are listed below. They include techniques that emphasize imagery and rehearsal, behavioral approaches to learning, and the use of computer technology and external memory aids in the rehabilitation of persons with brain injuries.

Imagery As a Therapeutic Mnemonic

Many investigations have shown that memory capacity can be increased dramatically when to-be-remembered verbal items are linked with a visual image. Perhaps the earliest description of the use of imagery comes from the ancient Greeks. Allegedly, the poet Simonides was called upon to identify the unrecognizable bodies of banquet guests who had been killed when a building caved in upon them. Simonides, who had performed at the banquet earlier that day, relied upon his memory of the banquet's seating arrangement in order to identify the victims.

Many researchers have explored the uses of imagery as a potential therapy technique for patients with memory disorders. For instance, patients may be taught to think of a visual image to link a person's name with their face (e.g., they might imagine "Joe Smith"

Excerpted from *Brain Injury Rehabilitation: Management of Memory Disorders* by Amy Weinstein, copyright 1995 by HDI Publishers. P.O. Box 131401, Houston, TX 77219; reprinted with permission. To order the complete booklet or to obtain a free catalogue of available materials call (800) 321-7037.

actively engaged in work as a blacksmith). In general, this strategy facilitates subsequent recall. However, studies with brain injured subjects have been controversial, with some demonstrating remarkable improvement and others showing only limited efficacy.

Perhaps the greatest drawback of imagery is that it requires vigilance and planning during the initial encoding stage of memory. Individuals with normal memory functions rarely engage in such attention to detail. It thus may be beyond the capabilities of many persons with brain injuries. Of related concern is the fact that in order for imagery to be beneficial, the individual must retain the image. Studies with amnesics have shown that they forget the associated information unless the experimenter provides them with the image at time of retrieval, yet this diminishes the practical value of the technique.

Despite these drawbacks, clinicians may attempt to use imagery as a therapy technique since some patients can benefit from it particularly when it is combined with other strategies. Crovitz has emphasized several factors which are important in the use of imagery. He stressed that it was important to give patients sufficient time to form the image. Secondly, he believed that images generated by the patient were more beneficial than those provided by the examiner. Thirdly, Crovitz argued that the plausibility of the visual image was important.

Other Cognitive Retraining Programs

Other psychological methods for memory improvement emphasize effective ways to minimize cognitive deficits. Some of these have been loosely referred to as cognitive retraining programs since they attempt to provide persons with brain injury with new cognitive strategies to circumvent those no longer available. Luria, a pioneer in retraining theory, recommended that restorative therapy be individually tailored to the assets and liabilities of the brain injured person. He placed particular importance on the cognitive mediation of behavior and believed that a disruption in covert mediation or private speech was often a consequence of brain injury. He advocated that external mediation in the form of self-instruction would mitigate cognitive deficits.

Other researchers have applied Luria's ideas in studies with amnesics. Webster and Scott believed that self-instruction facilitated the organization of incoming information and thus resulted in better retention of material. Structuring cognition in this way was thought to lessen the frequency of thought intrusions, poor inhibition, and perseverative tendencies which often interfere with memory. Barbara Wilson has combined a number of cognitive strategies in rehabilitation programs. She employs the "PQRST" method (which requires that the patient "Preview, Question, Read, State and Test") and in addition, incorporates relevant information from the patient's life in the therapy session. Thus, the patient is able to learn specific information useful in his daily activities even though he may not spontaneously utilize the PQRST method in situations outside of the therapy session.

Behavioral Techniques

Several studies have shown that amnesics are capable of classical and operant conditioning whereby environmental stimuli (e. g., attention, affection, permission to watch television, favorite foods, etc.) may be used to reinforce certain classes of behavior. The first step in designing a behavioral program involves conducting a "functional analysis" of the patient's behavior. Once meaningful reinforcers (which vary with each individual) and desired behaviors (e.g., a decrease in disruptive activities, an increase in responsible activities, or a completely new behavioral repertoire) are specified, the therapist designs a program which emphasizes the association between the reinforcers and the behavior. This type of technique has a great deal of therapeutic potential especially when it is creatively integrated with the patient's home environment and carried out in a consistent manner. Obviously, the family's active involvement in the behavioral program is of critical importance.

Computerized Rehabilitation of Amnesia

Computer technology has recently been used to meet the needs of persons with brain injuries. In some instances, computer based rehabilitation methods focus on isolated operations involved in cognition, including selective attention, vigilance, discrimination, inhibition, and the generalization of responses. In other instances, they mechanically simulate the therapy programs described above.

The advantages of computerized rehabilitation include the possibility that therapy can be conducted at home with the computer serving as an extension of the therapist, the fact that the patient receives prompt and accurate feedback, and the possibility that computer intervention might provide the patient with a sense of autonomy. The drawback of this type of program is that with few exceptions, these programs have not introduced any new mnemonic techniques which go beyond those already in practice. In addition, they may delete the very factor which the patient finds rewarding—close and consistent personal contact with the therapist.

One computer-based memory retraining technique which departs from traditional therapies was introduced by Glisky, Schacter and Tulving (1986). Their method of "vanishing cues" involves the repeated presentation of word fragments on a computer screen. If the patient is able to correctly identify a word, one letter is deleted on the next trial and the patient is repetitively exposed to successive deletions of the word until he no longer needs any letter cues. Although it still takes many trials for the patient to learn new words, these investigators have reported success in teaching several amnesic patients new vocabularies which they are able to retain across a six week interval. This therapy does not restore memory functions but assists the patient in the acquisition of a specific body of knowledge.

External Memory Aids

Other aids for memory improvement are directly linked to the environment. Harris has given the name 'external memory aids' to this category. Included in this group are shopping lists, diaries, timers, and activities such as relying on another person, and leaving something in a special place. Harris highlighted several features he believed were essential for optimal memory aid. He noted that active cues were preferable to passive ones and that specificity, temporal contiguity, and accessibility of the cues were important.

One device which meets these criteria and was described recently in the memory rehabilitation literature, is the digital alarm clock/watch. Gouvier has found this instrument efficient for brain injured clients when supplemented by a personal appointment calendar. In effect, the clock is set to beep hourly, reminding the person to consult his daily schedule book. This device is both convenient for amnesics to use and allows them to be more independent in their daily routines.

Practical Tips

Beyond considering the therapeutic techniques mentioned above, the following practical recommendations are offered to assist the clinician.

Dealing with Denial

A significant problem in rehabilitating patients with serious memory deficits is that they tend to deny or be unaware of the severity of their problem. As a result they frequently reject the need for rehabilitation of memory or feel that it is insulting to be required to write things down which they are sure they will not forget. Even patients who are aware of memory problems find the techniques to be reminders of the deficits that they now face. They therefore may attempt to avoid them.

In order to gain a patient's cooperation, a variety of approaches can be taken. Simply confronting the patients repeatedly with his failures is unlikely to gain their cooperation. This is a mistake frequently made by the rehabilitation staff and family members. While some degree of confrontation is inevitable, it must always be presented in the context of attempts to assist the patient. With some patients, an effective technique is to persuade them to write down (if only for the therapist's sake) a brief description of what they have just done in therapy, including the date, time of day, location, and therapist's name. At a later time, the patient is asked what he did during that specific therapy time. When he is unable to produce the correct response he is referred to the written entry, which, because it has been written in his own handwriting, cannot be dismissed. Repetition of this technique may eventually induce awareness of the memory problem. Since memory lapse is pointed out concurrently with a solution (i.e., to remember things they must be written down) this has often been found effective even in profoundly amnestic and agitated patients.

Keep Material Simple and Meaningful to the Patient

Presentation of a complex mnemonic strategy to be practiced with meaningless material will simply create resistance, both because of the amount of mental effort needed and the patient's expectation that he might fail. Therapists should therefore take pains to ensure that when a strategy is being taught for the first time, material which guarantees success is carefully selected.

Provide an Early Framework

Frequent mention is made of so-called anterograde amnesia following brain injury. This is a poorly defined construct which refers to the patient's inability to learn new information following the injury. The period of anterograde amnesia is considered over when the patient is oriented to person, place, and time and is aware of what is happening on a daily basis. Naturally, patients do not go to bed with anterograde amnesia one night and wake up without it the next morning. Instead, they typically progress from total disorientation to a general awareness of having sustained an injury, to an awareness of their surroundings, to a realization that they are receiving therapy, to a recognition of their therapists, and so on. It is not uncommon for patients who are supposedly past the anterograde amnesia stage to occasionally forget what they have done the day or even the hour before, depending on their level of fatigue, etc. In order to facilitate the rate of recovery, the emphasis should be on providing them with the broader outlines of their situation before presenting them with specific information (such as word lists or names of therapists). As their reference framework is developed, their ability to recall such specific information should improve.

Monitor Medications

Particularly during the acute stage of recovery, medications that have sedative properties (e.g., Dilantin) can significantly undermine recovery of memory functions. Dosages should be carefully monitored. One clue to the negative effects of the medication is a prolonged confusional state which should not be mistaken for anterograde amnesia. Alternative medications that perform the same functions without sedative properties should be considered.

Chapter 22

Depression, Antidepressants, and Traumatic Brain Injury

Survivors of traumatic brain injury (TBI) are susceptible to a variety of neurobehavioral disorders that are amenable to successful treatment with antidepressant medications. There are a number of classes of such agents, and research and clinical experience demonstrate that these agents can also be used to treat more than just depressive disorders.

This chapter will provide a brief survey of the uses, both new and old, of antidepressants in survivors of TBI and also of some of the newer theories of the physiology of depression in these patients, as they allow a somewhat rational approach to medication choices.

The principal classes of antidepressants include the tricyclic antidepressants (TCAs), newer heterocyclic antidepressants, selective serotonin reuptake inhibitors (SSRIs), and monoamine oxidase inhibitors (MAOIs). Less frequently used but effective agents include the stimulant and dopaminergic drugs. Table 22.1 lists some other "unconventional" agents that may be helpful in certain subtypes of depression.

Use of Antidepressant Agents

Antidepressants are principally used to treat the depressive disorders and depressive spectrum disorders. However, antidepressants

Journal of Head Trauma Rehabilitation 1995;10(2):90-95. Copyright Aspen Publishers, Inc.; reprinted with permission.

have also had demonstrable effectiveness in treating attention deficit disorders, arousal disorders, impulse control disorders, sleep disorders, some psychotic disorders, and disorders of violent behavior (see list, "Premorbid or Posttraumatic Neurobehavioral Syndromes That Can Be Treated with Antidepressant Agents in Survivors of Traumatic Brain Injury").[1,2]

Table 22.1. Some antidepressant agents

Agents	Representative examples
Conventional agents	
Tricyclic antidepressants	Desipramine, protriptyline
Heterocyclic antidepressants	Trazodone, maprotiline
Selective serotonin reuptake inhibitors	Fluoxetine, sertraline, paroxetine
Monoamine oxidase inhibitors	Phenelzine, tranylcypromine
Newer agents	Bupropion, venlafaxine
Stimulants	
Classic stimulants	Amphetamine, methylphenidate, pemoline
Dopaminergics	Levodopa, amantadine, bromocriptine
Dopaminergic/MAOI	Selegiline
Other	Protriptyline, SSRIs (fluoxetine)
Anticonvulsants	
Conventional anticonvulsants	Carbamazepine, valproic acid
Unconventional anticonvulsants	Clonazepam
Unconventional agents	
Benzodiazepines	Alprazolam
Antipsychotics	Haloperidol, thorazine
Hormones	Dexamethasone, levothyroxine
Others	Lithium, buspirone, electroconvulsive therapy

The main trends in the current uses of these medications in patients with head injury can be best expressed as a series of nine clinical principles:

1. Studies in patients with TBI have demonstrated that standard psychiatric evaluation tools are effective in assessing and following depressive disorders.[3]

2. Although literature in this population is lacking, based on our own unpublished work, TCAs appear to be the most effective treatment of severe depression. However, individually, many TCAs may have sedative and anticholinergic effects and can therefore impair memory, intellect, and attention. Desipramine and nortriptyline are recommended. Protriptyline, although highly anticholinergic, is stimulant-like and may also benefit individual patients. SSRIs are very useful in mild to moderate depression; generally have fewer "cognitive" side effects, and may help attention, concentration, and arousal. Maprotiline, trazodone, amoxapine, MAOIs, and bupropion are generally not recommended owing to a high probability of significant individual side effects and because of the extremely close scrutiny required with their use. At this time, the role of venlafaxine is unclear.

3. Stimulants and dopaminergics, while relatively weak antidepressants, can be extremely useful in treating impaired memory, language, attention, initiation, and motor performance. If these features are a prominent part of the patient's depression, these agents should be considered as primary treatment of a mild depression or adjunctive treatment of a more severe depression.

4. Carbamazepine and valproic acid may be useful for rapid cycling and dysphoric states and are often very effective in agitated affective disorders, particularly those involving components of depression and dysphoria.[2] SSRIs may also be particularly useful in rapid cycling and dysphoric states.

5. Almost all conventional and stimulant antidepressants may precipitate or increase seizure activity. TCAs are more likely to cause or increase seizures than stimulant or dopaminergic drugs.[4] This does not automatically imply that these drugs

should not be used in patients with or prone to seizure disorders. Rather, if an increase in seizure activity is noted, the physician should do a risk-benefit analysis and, if the medication is found to be very helpful for the patient, consider adding a minimally sedating anticonvulsant such as valproate, carbamazepine, or gabapentin. Another approach could be changing to a different antidepressant of the same clinical family, which might not be as epileptogenic for the patient.

6.   Almost all antidepressants, except antipsychotics and lithium, can cause manic states, and all of them can cause agitated states by a number of different mechanisms. TCAs, SSRIs, stimulants, and dopaminergics are particularly prone to this. In these cases withdrawing the antidepressant is usually helpful.

7.   Akathisia, a combination of motor and psychic restlessness that is often accompanied by agitation, anger, irritability, and dysphoria, is another less frequent but troubling antidepressant side effect and is most frequently associated with SSRIs and also occasionally seen with benzodiazepines.[5] It is, of course, a more common side effect of antipsychotic drugs, but since these are rarely used as antidepressants, this is not usually a practical concern. Treatment usually consists of withdrawing the causative agent.

8.   Surprisingly, paradoxical depression may occur with a variety of antidepressants via different mechanisms and is most commonly seen with TCAs and SSRIs. With TCAs and to some extent SSRIs (especially fluoxetine) depression may recur or worsen because of a "window" effect in which patients improve and then, as the serum concentration increases, become more depressed. Rather than push the dose higher, the treatment is to reduce the dose to within the individualized antidepressant range for each patient. In this regard, TCA serum concentrations have more clinical relevance than SSRI concentrations, and it is useful to routinely monitor them.[6] Currently, monitoring of SSRI concentrations is not particularly helpful. Often depression in conjunction with SSRIs may appear with features of akathisia, dysphoria, Parkinsonism, psychomotor retardation, or obsessive-compulsive disorder. In these cases it is usually necessary to discontinue the SSRI.

9.   Sedation with concomitant memory, attentional, and cognitive impairment is also a very important practical problem, because it is common and because it retards general and cognitive rehabilitation, which is often the main focus of treatment. Sedation most often occurs with cyclic antidepressants, anticonvulsants, and benzodiazepines and can be minimized by choosing the lowest effective dose or a less sedative alternative class of medication. Another approach is to use a lower than usual dose of a stimulant TCA, such as protriptyline, with an adjunctive stimulating agent such as a dopaminergic, methylphenidate, dextroamphetamine, or pemoline.[7]

In summary, treatment can involve a variety of medications best chosen to help the patient's main target symptoms. A consensus is emerging that TCAs, SSRIs, valproate, and carbamazepine are reliable initial medications for most patients.

Pathoetiology of Depression

With regard to understanding the pathoetiology of depression in these patients, it is noteworthy that in recent years significant progress has been made in elucidating the origin of depressive states after TBI and other neurological disease.[8] Four such developments can be briefly outlined as follows:

1.   Evidence from the clinical and basic sciences is beginning to allow the conceptualization of depression and depressive states in general and also after TBI, as related to bilateral dysfunction of the frontal and temporal lobes and the disruption of deep diencephalic structures and networks. The disruption of normal neuronal networks and neurotransmitter levels in these anatomical areas is thought to be causative, and depression can be seen as the expression of a final common pathway.[9]

2.   It is also beginning to be appreciated that post-TBI depression may often occur in individuals who already have a premorbid genetic vulnerability to or an individual history of an actual depressive spectrum disorder, such as attention deficit hyperactivity disorder, alcohol or substance abuse, depression, or one of several types of personality disorders.

3. New models are also beginning to suggest a close theoretical and clinical association among mood, movement, and thought in many patients.[9] For example, depressed TBI patients are often psychomotor retarded and have difficulty with initiation and perseveration. Manic and agitated patients, on the other hand, may be psychomotor accelerated, think too fast to concentrate or pay attention, and be impulsive.

   This relationship between mood and movement may be mediated in part by the cortico-limbic-striatal circuit of Nauta.[10] This model can be useful in understanding the relationship among mood, movement, and cognition in individual patients and in selecting the appropriate antidepressant according to the principles discussed earlier.

4. Many people with TBI also show associated difficulty with memory, processing, attention, and language. These particular functions are often targeted in cognitive rehabilitation programs. Dopaminergics, stimulants, SSRIs, and even TCAs can be especially fruitful in helping patients maximize their rehabilitation potential in these areas.

The antidepressants discussed here can also be effective in TBI patients suffering from the other disorders listed, but a discussion of these is beyond the scope of this review.

Finally, it is worth noting that iatrogenic complications of treatment with other psychoactive medications may cause or intensify depressive states and impair cognitive, attentional, and memory functioning. There are many such classes of medication. They include anticonvulsants such as phenytoin and phenobarbital, antihypertensives such as beta-blockers and alpha-methyldopa, antipsychotics, steroid withdrawal regimes, antispasticity drugs, hypnotics and sedatives, cholinergics and anticholinergics, and aspirin type nonsteroidal antiinflammatories. It is always worth trying to minimize the number and dosage of such medications in patients with TBI.

Sometimes introducing a gradual discontinuation or therapeutic substitution of the causative agent will preclude the need to start an antidepressant.

Premorbid or Posttraumatic Neurobehavioral Syndromes That Can Be Treated with Antidepressant Agents in Survivors of Traumatic Brain Injury

Depressive disorders
- Major depressive disorder
- Dysthymic disorder
- Atypical depression
- Bipolar depression
- Cyclothymic depression
- Dysphoric mania
- Bipolar mixed states
- Personality disorder-associated depression
- Medication-induced depression
- Posttraumatic depression
- Seizure disorder-associated depression
- Psychotic depression
- Seasonal affective disorders

Depressive spectrum disorders
- Anorexia
- Bulimia
- Attention deficit hyperactivity disorder
- Attention deficit states
- Obsessive compulsive disorders
- Catatonia
- Bipolar mania
- Rapid cycling affective disorders
- Cyclothymic hypomania
- Anxiety and panic disorders
- Phobias
- Chronic fatigue syndrome
- Chronic pain syndrome
- Posttraumatic stress disorder

Other disorders
- Impulse control disorders
- Explosive disorder
- Paraphilias
- Hypersexuality
- Impotence

Sleep disorders
Narcolepsy
Underarousal
Agitated states
Assaultive states
Chronic screaming
Postconcussive migraine
Postconcussive syndrome/ minimal head injury syndrome
Cognitive impairment
Startle disorders
Tic disorders
Tourette's syndrome
Post-head injury movement disorders
Akinesia
Parkinsonism
Bradyphrenia
Amnestic disorders
Thought disorders
Aphasia
Language disorders

—by Anthony B Joseph, MD
and Bruno Wroblewski, MSPharm

Anthony B Joseph, MD, is Assistant Clinical Professor of Psychiatry, McLean Hospital and Harvard Medical School, Boston, Massachusetts, Medical Director, Center for Neurobehavioral Rehabilitation at Middlesex Hospital Waltham, Massachusetts, Director, Neuropsychiatry and Neuropharmacology Physician Training Program of the Massachusetts Statewide Head Injury Program, Boston, Massachusetts

Bruno Wroblewski, MSPharm, is Clinical Pharmacist, Greenery Rehabilitation Center, Assistant Professor of Pharmacy, Massachusetts College of Pharmacy, Clinical Instructor, Department of Rehabilitation Medicine, Tufts University School of Medicine, Boston, Massachusetts

References

1. Mysiw WJ, Jackson RD. Tricyclic antidepressant therapy after traumatic brain injury. *J Head Trauma Rehabil.* 1987;2(4):34-42.

2. Cassidy JW. Neuropharmacologic management of destructive behavior after traumatic brain injury. *J Head Trauma Rehabil.* 1994;9(3):43-60.

3. Jurge RE, Robinson RG, Arndt S. Are there symptoms that are specific for depressed mood in patients with traumatic brain injury? *J Nerv Ment Dis.* 1993;181:91-99.

4. Wroblewski B. Epileptic potential of stimulants, dopaminergics, and antidepressants. *J Head Trauma Rehabil.* 1992;7(3):109-111.

5. Joseph AB, Wroblewski BA. Paradoxical akathisia caused by clonazepam, clorazepate and lorazepam in patients with traumatic encephalopathy and seizure disorders: a subtype of benzodiazepine-induced disinhibition? *Behav Neurol.* 1993; 6:221-223.

6. Preskorn S, Fast G. Therapeutic drug monitoring for antidepressants: efficacy, safety, and cost effectiveness. *J Clin Psychiatry.* 1991;52:23-33.

7. Wroblewski B, Glenn MB, Cornblatt R, Joseph AB, Suduikis S. Protriptyline as an alternative stimulant medication in patients with brain injury: a series of case reports. *Brain Injury.* 1993;7(4):353-362.

8. Silver JM, Hales RE, Yudofsky SC. Psychopharmacology of depression in neurologic disorders. *J Clin Psychiatry.* 1990;51(1,suppl):33-39.

9. Joseph AB. Disorders of mood and movement: an overview. In: Joseph AB, Young RR, eds. *Movement Disorders in Neurology and Neuropsychiatry.* Boston, Mass: Blackwell; 1992.

10. Nauta WJH. Reciprocal links of the corpus striatum with the cerebral cortex and limbic system: a common substrate for movement and thought? In: Mueller J, Yingling C, Zegans L,

eds. *Neurology and Psychiatry: A Meeting of Minds.* Basel, Switzerland: Karger; 1989.

Chapter 23

Pharmacologic Treatment of Acute Traumatic Brain Injury

During the past several years, results of clinical trials have generated considerable optimism about the prospects for effective treatment of acute central nervous system (CNS) injuries. A multicenter trial demonstrated the effectiveness of methylprednisolone, as well as naloxone hydrochloride, in improving neurologic recovery after spinal cord injury. In ischemic stroke, early treatment with tissue plasminogen activator or treatment with low-molecular-weight heparin led to improved outcome for some patients. To date, however, no effective pharmacotherapy has been developed for head injury.

One of the more promising experimental strategies for treatment of acute CNS injury has been the use of antioxidants or free-radical scavengers. This approach is based on the concept that oxygen free radicals are generated in response to the insult, thereby overwhelming endogenous antioxidant or free radical-scavenging systems such as superoxide dismutase (SOD), catalase, glutathione, ascorbic acid, and (α-tocopherol. Free radicals are believed to contribute to subsequent tissue damage through a variety of proposed mechanisms, including peroxidation of lipid membranes, microvascular damage, edema formation, and subarachnoid hemorrhage including vasospasm. There is strong experimental support for this hypothesis: superoxide, hydroxyl, and nitric oxide radicals are produced in response to CNS injuries; treatment with antioxidants or free radical scavengers, such as SOD or α-tocopherol, limits secondary damage and promotes

Editorial, *Journal of the American Medical Association*, August 21, 1996, Vol 276, No. 7, 569-70; reprinted with permission.

recovery in experimental models of spinal cord trauma, cerebral ischemia, and brain trauma. Even more convincing support for this concept has come from recent studies using transgenic mice. Animals that overexpress Cu Zn-SOD, which is a cytosolic enzyme encoded by the human transgene SOD-1, show improved recovery following brain surgery; moreover, knockout animals that lack the mouse gene for Cu Zn-SOD (SOD-1) or Mn-SOD (SOD-2) show larger infarcts following ischemic injury than control animals.

Given this experimental literature, as well as the promising results from the earlier phase 2 study with polyethylene glycol-conjugated SOD (pegorgotein), the results from the phase 3 study by Young and colleagues in the August 21, 1996 issue of the *Journal of the American Medical Association* are disappointing. These investigators studied 463 patients with severe, closed head injury in a randomized, placebo-controlled, multicenter study. Patients received a single intravenous dose of a placebo or 1 or 2 doses of pegorgotein within 8 hours of injury. The primary endpoint was the Glasgow Outcome Scale (GOS) score at 3 months after injury. Secondary endpoints included the Disability Rating Scale (DRS) and mortality rate. Although pegorgotein was well tolerated at the doses used, and there was a higher percentage of favorable outcomes in patients treated with the drug, particularly at the lower dose, there were no statistically significant beneficial effects for treatment with regard to the GOS score, DRS score, or mortality at 3 or 6 months.

There are several possible explanations for this negative result. Although the sample size, based on the earlier phase 2 study, was chosen to provide 90% power to detect a treatment difference of 14% or more, it may have been insufficient to detect a smaller but clinically important difference. Another issue is whether "severe" head injury represents the optimal trauma group in which to examine a potential treatment effect. For example, in studies with transgenic animals, mice overexpressing SOD-1 showed reduced infarct size after a moderate ischemic insult but not after a severe one. Time at which treatment is begun and duration of treatment also may be important variables. On average, patients in the study by Young et al. were treated approximately 6 hours after head injury. In animal models, free radicals are released relatively early after trauma, and most effective clinical treatment requires early intervention. In the present study it would be helpful to know whether patients treated within the first 3 to 4 hours of injury fared better than those treated at later time points. The optimal duration of the treatment with antioxidants or free-radical scavengers is presently unknown, even in experimental models. However, the secondary injury process in animal models of brain trauma continues for at least several days.

Although an important pathophysiological role for oxygen free radicals in clinical brain trauma on the basis of the pegorgotein trial cannot be excluded, 2 recently concluded phase 3 studies with the antioxidant tirilazad mesylate in head injury also did not show unequivocal evidence of efficacy (oral communication, Larry Marshall, MD, July 1996). However, the tirilazad trials apparently suffered from unequal randomization of patients with associated shock, which may have skewed the results against drug treatment. Other methodological problems were also encountered in the international trial of tirilazad, which points out the substantial difficulties in undertaking multicenter trials with this class of patients.

These negative studies continue a long history of drug treatment trials in severe head injury that have failed to show significant clinical benefit. Such interventions have included administration of corticosteroids, barbiturates, a lactate buffer (tromethamine), the calcium channel antagonist nimodipine, and citicolene (cytidine diphosphate choline), among others. Why has it been so difficult to demonstrate effective drug treatments for clinical head injury, in contrast to studies of stroke or spinal cord injury?

One possible explanation is that patients with severe brain trauma reflect a heterogeneous population in terms of underlying mechanisms of secondary injury. The latter often include hypoxia, ischemia, contusion, diffuse axonal injury, edema, and the presence of an associated hematoma. In assessing therapeutic strategies, investigators may need to better define the subpopulation of head-injured patients being studied. For instance, despite 2 earlier negative trials with nimodipine in head injury, subgroup analysis indicated a potential beneficial effect for patients with traumatic subarachnoid hemorrhage. This suggested benefit has now been confirmed in a relatively small study that included patients with mild or severe head injuries. Data from the international tirilazad trial also apparently indicate a beneficial effect for men with traumatic subarachnoid hemorrhage (oral communication, Larry Marshall, MD, July 1996).

A more fundamental question is whether a treatment strategy directed at a single pathophysiological factor can substantially improve outcome in a disease that is so clearly multifactorial. For example, experimental studies have implicated a large number of interactive biochemical processes in secondary tissue damage; these include phospholipid hydrolysis, release of excitatory amino acids, and inflammatory/immune responses, among others. Therefore, what may be required for optimal treatment are either drugs that affect multiple sites of the secondary injury cascade or use of combination drug strategies. For example, thyrotropin-releasing hormone (TRH) or TRH analogs have shown effectiveness in animal models of neurotrauma, including spinal cord injury and traumatic brain injury. A small pilot clinical study of TRH in spinal cord injury was also promising. Proposed mechanisms of action for TRH are multifactorial, including modulating effects of endogenous opioids, peptidoleukotrienes, platelet-activating factor, and excitatory amino acids, as well as improving cerebral blood flow and bioenergetic state. Another possible example may be dexanabinol (HU-211), a cannabinoid that appears to function as an N-methyl-D-aspartate antagonist, an antioxidant, and an inhibitor of tumor necrosis factor-α release.

Relatively few studies in experimental animal models of neurotrauma have investigated combination treatment strategies, and the technical and logistical issues for developing multidrug clinical trials are substantial. However, this approach has been effectively accomplished with considerable success in the treatment of cancer and infectious diseases. During the last several years the National Institutes of Health has funded a multicenter preclinical consortium of spinal cord research centers, 1 objective of which is to evaluate combination treatment approaches. Leaders of experimental brain injury research programs have met to attempt to develop a similar multicenter drug evaluation strategy.

Despite the absence of a demonstrated effective treatment for human traumatic brain injury to date, basic research in this area is accelerating, and a number of clinical trials are under way or in the late planning stages. Furthest along are studies using N-methyl-D-aspartate blockers, including competitive and noncompetitive receptor antagonists, as well as modulators of the polyamine and glycine sites on this receptor, data from some of these trials should be available in the near future. Improved prospective identification of patient populations likely to benefit from such multifaceted and novel approaches may lead to reductions in the substantial morbidity and mortality associated with severe head injury. Until then, our optimism must remain guarded for the prospect of pharmacologic therapy to substantially improve outcome for patients with acute traumatic brain trauma.

—by Alan I. Faden, MD

From the Institute for Cognitive and Computational Sciences, Georgetown University Medical Center, Washington, DC.

Chapter 24

Alcohol Abuse and Traumatic Brain Injury

The role of alcohol and other drug abuse in traumatic brain injury is well documented, with an incidence of intoxication at injury of approximately 50 percent. Because of cognitive, behavioral, and functional deficits, brain injury survivors pose unique challenges to the alcoholism treatment field.

Head Injury and Alcohol Abuse

Alcohol consumption is a strong predisposing factor in traumatic brain injury (Kerr et al. 1971; Field 1976; Parkinson et al. 1985). In studies addressing head injury and alcohol use specifically, elevated blood alcohol levels were present in more than 40 percent of the patients seen in emergency rooms or admitted to hospitals because of traumatic head injury (Galbraith et al. 1976; Rutherford 1977; Brismar et al. 1983; Parkinson et al. 1985). In the most recent study of head-injured patients at a North American trauma center, 67 percent of those tested for blood alcohol levels showed evidence of alcohol use and more than one-half (51 percent) were intoxicated, using a definition of 100 mg/100 ml (100 mg/dl) (Sparadeo and Gill, in press). This is consistent with a Swedish study showing a 58 percent rate of intoxication among those tested (Brismar et al. 1983).

In a study of neuropsychological deficits in alcoholics, psychometric test performance was significantly lower among head-injured alcoholics

Alcohol World: Health & Research, National Institute on Alcohol Abuse and Alcoholism, Vol. 13, No. 2, 1989.

than among those who had not experienced head injuries (Hillbom and Holm 1986). Both groups scored lower than the general population on most test items. Results of the study also suggest that the incidence of head injury in alcoholics is two to four times higher than in the general population.

Other studies have documented the role of alcohol and other drug abuse in traumatic brain injury. Alterman and Tarter (1985) found the risk for head injury in patients with familial alcoholism to be almost twice that of patients without such history. In a study of 75 severely brain-injured patients (Tobis et al. 1982), 51 had histories of alcohol abuse and 29 had histories of illicit drug use. The number of patients using both alcohol and other drugs was not specified. Sparadeo and Gill (in press) found that 25 percent of their sample had alcohol histories documented in their medical records. A recent survey of brain injury rehabilitation programs around the country reported that approximately 55 percent of patients had some alcohol or other drug abuse problems before the brain injury and 40 percent had abuse problems described as moderate to severe (NHIF 1988).

Psychosocial Consequences of Head injury

Traumatic brain injury can mean many long-term psychological and behavioral difficulties. Because every head injury is different, it is impossible to predict the exact outcome for the survivor. While generalizations can be made, it is important that treatment professionals and other concerned persons note that individuals may present few problems or a combination of several problems. Some deficits following head injury are painfully obvious; other are extremely subtle and become evident only during intensive clinical evaluation (Lezak 1978b). Alcohol and other drug abuse professionals working with head injury survivors commonly deal with clients who appear to function normally in most settings but who are unable to understand the concepts of alcohol or other drug addiction or to benefit from traditional treatment modalities.

To work effectively with survivors of traumatic brain injury, it is vital that alcohol and other drug abuse professionals acquaint themselves with the unique problems these clients present. The following discussion of the more common consequences of head injury is drawn from general knowledge in the field of brain injury rehabilitation. For more detailed information, the reader is directed to Levin and colleagues (1982), Edelstein and Couture (1984), Lezak (1978*a*, 1978*b*, 1983), and Brooks (1984).

Impairment of Memory

Post traumatic amnesia is one of the most common consequences of head injury. For many survivors, memory for events and conditions prior to their injury is generally intact while short-term memory for recent events is disrupted. In practical terms, this means that brain injury survivors might remember the events of their high school prom in great detail but forget what was served for breakfast this morning. Some survivors may try to fill in the gaps with confabulation, a usually sincere attempt to mask memory deficits that is sometimes misinterpreted as dishonesty. Impairment of recent memory makes it difficult for many survivors to retain information and generalize new learning from one setting to another.

Decreased Self-Awareness and Insight

Many survivors of traumatic brain injury experience a reduced capacity for insight, self-monitoring, and awareness. They may have difficulty seeing the relationship between their behavior and the resulting consequences and may experience confusion or frustration in their attempt to understand situations.

Impairment of Abstract Reasoning

The ability to integrate information and to reason in the abstract are vital skills in our "information age." Unfortunately, many brain injury survivors experience a reduction in these skills and a corresponding increase in concrete thought. In assessment, these problems are sometimes detected in proverb interpretation tasks, where clients may be unable to move beyond the concrete content of a simple saying to its more abstract meaning (Lezak 1983).

Deficits of Attention and Concentration

Many brain injury survivors have difficulty attending to complex tasks. They are more easily distracted by extraneous stimuli and have a reduced ability to concentrate and focus.

Inappropriate Social Behavior

Problems with impulsiveness and disinhibition are common among survivors of traumatic brain injury. They may giggle or make inappropriate comments; they may interact in a rude or aggressive manner. Excessive flirting or more overt sexual gestures are sometimes observed. Some survivors become withdrawn and isolated; others demonstrate behavior that is self-centered and perceived as immature. They may have a low tolerance for stress and be easily frustrated.

Changes in Mood and Affect

Some brain injury survivors experience changes in emotional responses. Affect may become flat or blunted with little expression of either joy or sadness. Emotions may become labile, with broad swings of mood. Anger, along with feelings of profound grief, may be accompanied by a clinical depression.

Language and Communication Deficits

Damage to the brain may result in oral-motor problems, such as slurring of speech and difficulty forming words (dysarthria). Of a more serious nature are deficits of comprehension or language disorders known as aphasia. The brain injury survivor may not understand everything heard and may not be able to find the words or formulate the sentences necessary to respond. These problems may result in increased frustration or confusion for survivors and concerned persons alike.

Sensory Deficits

There is a high incidence of visual-perceptual problems following head injury; reading and writing abilities may be impaired. Tinnitus (ringing in the ears) or other disorders may affect hearing.

Goal-Formulation and Problem Solving Difficulties

Unrealistic or undefined goals are common among brain injury survivors. When they do have clear and reasonable objectives, many survivors have a reduced ability to solve problems and to achieve their goals without sufficient structure and support.

Vocational/Educational Problems

Because of the permanence of brain damage and the long-term nature of its consequences, few head injury survivors are able to return to their premorbid (preinjury) level of vocational or educational placement. Those who have survived mild injuries often retain the cognitive skills necessary to return to work but may experience reduced tolerance for stress and increased fatigue.

Impact on the Family and Community

The functional impairments from traumatic brain injury, though serious, do not usually require that survivors be institutionalized. In their study of severely brain-injured patients, Tobis and colleagues (1982) reported that 72 percent had been discharged to return home; the rate of community discharge is even higher among survivors of moderate and mild injuries. As a result, families and communities must face the issue of the reintegrations of survivors who may have experienced profound changes in their abilities and personalities.

There is a high incidence of divorce following head injury. Reports of depression and somatic disorders among spouses or children of survivors are common. Many survivors experience social isolation and marginalization as a result of their injuries; peer relationships and support systems are often radically altered.

Alcohol and Other Drug Abuse Following Head Injury

When the complex variable of alcohol or other drug abuse is considered within the context of the social reintegration of brain injury survivors, the potential for serious problems seems clear. Given that the population as a whole has a high rate of documented alcohol abuse prior to injury (and that alcohol abuse is a key factor in the etiology of brain injury), it is reasonable to suggest that alcohol consumption following injury would also be a problem. This is especially so, considering that the great majority of brain injury survivors are discharged into the community, where alcohol and other drugs are readily accessible. Reilly and colleagues (1986) have identified four factors that increase the risk of alcohol abuse after traumatic injury: 1) increased discretionary time and boredom, 2) increased enabling from family and friends, 3) uncertainty over the ability to return to work or to function effectively at work, and 4) physical limitations and posttraumatic mood change. All of these factors can be found among most brain injury survivors.

While anecdotal reports are numerous, there are few data on the incidence of alcohol and other drug abuse after brain injury. In one of the first attempts to document postinjury use patterns, Sparadeo and Gill (1988) found that 54 percent of the survivors they surveyed had returned to alcohol use after completion of rehabilitation. This was in spite of the fact that the majority had been injured in motor vehicle accidents while under the influence of alcohol or other drugs. The two major factors influencing abstinence in the remaining 46 percent were the presence of a seizure disorder or placement in long-term, supervised living situations.

Clinical Considerations for Alcohol and Other Drug Abuse Professionals

Brain injury survivors present unique problems for counselors and other professionals because the psychosocial and functional consequences of brain injury complicate the already difficult tasks of evaluation and treatment. Given what is known about traumatic brain injury and alcohol abuse, it is likely that most professionals will occasionally encounter brain injury survivors; those practicing in urban areas or among minority populations should give special attention to the incidence and consequences of brain injury. Cognitive and neurobehavioral problems may have an impact on the following areas of practice.

Assessment and Diagnosis

Memory deficits tend to make brain injury survivors poor historians, and subjective reports of alcohol or other drug use patterns may be inaccurate. Impaired insight may keep survivors from recognizing that their use patterns are problematic. Because many mild head injuries go unreported (Hillbom and Holm 1986), it is recommended that evaluators inquire about previous accidents or injuries. A simple question such as "Have you ever been knocked unconscious?" may be helpful in a preliminary screening for possible head injury status.

Because brain injury survivors sometimes have difficulty with abstract thought and more complex concepts, long or complicated assessment tools may be ineffective. Consideration should be given to the use of a brief diagnostic tool such as the CAGE Questionnaire

(Ewing 1984). Utilization of data from neuropsychological or rehabilitation evaluations is also suggested.

Changes in functional abilities are often the most reliable and measurable symptoms of alcohol or other drug abuse by head injury survivors. Once the practitioner has determined that such changes are not the result of other medical conditions and can be associated with known incidents of consumption, decreasing skills or increasing patterns of maladaptive behavior may provide observable diagnostic criteria for alcohol abuse. For the survivor, these declines in functional ability can be devastating, limiting involvement in rehabilitation or vocational programming. Threatening to discontinue essential services may motivate the brain injury survivor to respond to intervention.

Intervention and Treatment

Insight-oriented approaches are prevalent among treatment models for alcohol and other drug abuse (Logan et al. 1987). However, the usefulness of psychodynamic approaches with brain injury survivors is questionable because of the high incidence of cognitive deficits, such as impaired abstract reasoning and decreased insight. Behavioral difficulties of survivors, such as impulsiveness and disinhibition, may cause conflict or tension in group sessions, reducing the effectiveness of the sessions. Rather than receiving support and affirmation from group members, brain injury survivors may be stigmatized or characterized as disruptive. These problems also may be experienced in meetings of self-help groups, such as Alcoholics Anonymous, where significant neurobehavioral problems attributable to head injury may be viewed as "character defects."

In the case of brain injury rehabilitation, the prevailing behavioral model of intervention relies on achieving positive long-term outcomes through a series of short-term goals (Goldstein and Ruthven 1983; Wood 1987). This approach may be more effective with inpatients than with alcohol- or other drug-abusing outpatients who live in community settings where factors influencing behavior cannot be as easily monitored.

In a manual examining methods of counseling head injury survivors in the community, Blanchard(1984) emphasizes the need for practitioners to understand the cognitive and behavioral consequences of head injury and to rely more on such basic counseling techniques as respect, authenticity, and empathy.

Case Management

Agencies and individual practitioners serving brain injury survivors who abuse alcohol or other drugs are responsible for addressing their often complex needs and either providing necessary services or making appropriate referrals. Effective case management usually requires an interdisciplinary approach involving social workers, psychologists, occupational and physical therapists, vocational counselors, and specialists in community reentry. Professionals must acquaint themselves with available programs, since referrals to economic or housing assistance programs and consultation with medical or public health professionals may be necessary. Services for spouses or families of clients also should be considered, because the dual problems of disability and alcohol or other drug abuse put intense pressure on family systems.

Future Directions

The outlook for future development in the area of alcohol or other drug abuse and brain injury is mixed but hopeful. There remains a troubling avoidance of the problem on the part of clinicians who provide acute care to brain-injured persons. In a recent and quite revealing survey of 154 trauma centers in 43 States, only 55.2 percent regularly measured blood alcohol levels upon admission (Soderstrom and Cowley 1987). In a retrospective chart review of 379 trauma patients seen in the emergency room of an urban teaching hospital, Chang and Astrachan (1987) found that although 43 patients were suspected or known to have used alcohol or other drugs, none was referred for further evaluation.

Rehabilitation providers, on the other hand, have responded to the problem of alcohol abuse and brain injury with a positive initiative. In 1987, the Professional Council of the National Head Injury Foundation convened a Substance Abuse Task Force. The work of this group, though preliminary, has helped to define the problem from both an etiological and clinical perspective and to suggest potential solutions. A positive finding of the task force is that 50 percent of acute and 83 percent of the postacute rehabilitation programs surveyed are addressing alcohol and other drug abuse within their range of services (NHIF 1988).

Better identification and intervention strategies for those with traumatic brain injury will succeed only if a corresponding initiative

220

is undertaken within the alcohol and other abuse treatment field. Recommendations for development of effective services for brain injury survivors include improvement in the following areas.

Research

The number of brain injury survivors being served within the current alcohol and other drug abuse treatment system is not documented. To determine the effectiveness of current programs and methods, it is essential that this population be profiled. While it may be reasonable to suppose that brain-injured persons who abuse alcohol or other drugs have a high incidence of discharge from treatment centers for failure to meet treatment goals and are more prone to relapse than those without brain injuries, this has not been established.

Education

Perhaps the greatest barrier to the effective identification and treatment of brain injury survivors with alcohol or other drug abuse problems is the continued lack of awareness among professionals. Medical and rehabilitation professionals would benefit from additional training in assessing alcohol and other drug abuse. Professionals treating clients who abuse alcohol and other drugs need more information about brain injury and its consequences. Alcohol and other drug abuse counselors should be encouraged to familiarize themselves with the brain injury rehabilitation programs and services in their communities.

Interdisciplinary Dialogue and Cooperation

Communication between the rehabilitation and alcohol and other drug abuse fields merits further development, especially where brain injury is concerned. Professionals in both fields have much to learn from each other.

Preliminary attempts to examine and integrate information from various fields have contributed much to the effort. With additional research, education, and improved interdisciplinary cooperation, the outlook is hopeful.

References

Alterman, A.I. and Tarter, R.E. Relationship between familial alcoholism and head injury. *Journal of Studies on Alcohol* 46(3):256-258, 1985.

Blanchard, M.K. *Counseling Head Injured Patients.* Albany, NY: New York State Head Injury Association, 1984.

Brismar, B., Engstrom, A., and Rydberg U. Head Injury and intoxication: A diagnostic and therapeutic dilemma. *Acta Chirurgica Scandinavica* 149:11-14, 1983.

Brooks, N. *Closed Head Injury: Psychological, Social and Family Consequences.* Oxford: Oxford University Press, 1984.

Chang, G. and Astrachan, B. Identification and disposition of trauma patients with substance abuse or psychiatric illness. *Connecticut Medicine* 51:4-6, 1987.

Edelstein, B.A. and Couture, E.D. *Behavioral Assessment and Rehabilitation of the Traumatically Brain-Damaged.* New York: Plenum Press, 1984.

Ewing, J.A. Detecting alcoholism: the CAGE questionnaire. *Journal of the American Medical Association* 252(14):1905-1907, 1984.

Field, J.H. *Epidemiology of Head Injury in England and Wales: With Particular Application to Rehabilitation.* Leicester: Printed for H.M. Stationary Office by Wilsons, 1976.

Galbraith, S., Murray, W.R., Patel, A.R., and Knill-Jones, R. The relationship between alcohol and head injury and its effect on the conscious level. *British Journal of Surgery* 63:128-130, 1976.

Goldstein, G. and Ruthven, L. *Rehabilitation of the Brain-Damaged Adult.* New York: Plenum Press, 1983.

Hillbom, M. and Holm, L. Contribution of traumatic head injury to neuropsychological deficits in alcoholics. *Journal of Neurology, Neurosurgery, and Psychiatry* 49:1348-1353, 1986.

Kerr, T.A., Kay, D.W.K., and Lasman, L.P. Characteristics of patients, type of accident and mortality in a consecutive series of head injuries admitted to a neurosurgical unit. *British Journal of Preventive and Social Medicine* 25:179-185, 1971.

Levin, H.S., Benton, A.L., and Grossman, R.G. *Neurobehavioral Consequences of Closed Head Injury*. New York: Oxford University Press, 1982.

Lezak, M.D. Living with the characterologically altered brain injured patient. *Journal of Clinical Psychiatry* 39:592-598, 1978*a*.

Lezak, M.D. Subtle sequelae of brain damage: perplexity, distractibility and fatigue. *American Journal of Physical Medicine* 57(1):9-15, 1978*b*.

Lezak, M.D. *Neuropsychological Assessment*. 2nd ed. New York: Oxford University Press, 1983.

Logan, S.L., McRoy, R.G., and Freeman, E.M. Current practice approaches for treating the alcoholic client. *Health and Social Work* 12(3):178-186, 1987.

National Head Injury Foundation (now Brain Injury Association, Inc.). Professional Council Substance Abuse Task Force. *White Paper*. Southborough, MA: NHIF, 1988.

Parkinson, D., Stephensen, S., and Phillips, S. Head injuries: A prospective, computerized study. *Canadian Journal of Surgery* 28(1):79-83, 1985.

Reilly, E.L., Kelley, J.T., and Faillace, L.A. Role of alcohol use and abuse in trauma. *Advances in Psychosomatic Medicine* 16:17-30, 1986.

Rutherford, W. Diagnosis of alcohol ingestion in mild head injuries. *Lancet* 1:1021, 1977.

Soderstrom, C.A. and Cowley, R.A. A national alcohol and trauma center survey. *Archives of Surgery* 122(9):1067-1071, 1987.

Sparadeo, F.R. and Gill, D. "Alcohol Use After Head Injury." Paper presented at the annual conference of the American Psychological Association, Atlanta, GA, August 1988.

Sparadeo, F.R. and Gill D. Effects of alcohol use on head injury recovery. *Journal of Head Trauma Rehabilitation* (in press).

Tobis, J.S., Puri, K.B., and Sheridan, J. Rehabilitation of the severely brain-injured patient. *Scandinavian Journal of Rehabilitation Medicine* 14(2)83-88, 1982.

Wood, R.L. *Brain Injury Rehabilitation: A Neurobehavioral Approach.* Rockville, MD: Aspen Publishers, 1987.

—by Gregory A. Jones

Gregory A. Jones is program director for chemical health at the Vinland National Center in Loretto, Minnesota. The author thanks Francis R. Sparadeo, Ph.D., for generously providing information and manuscript material necessary to the completion of the article.

Chapter 25

Disruption of Sexuality Can Have Traumatic Effect

The devastating effects of traumatic head injury on the lives of those injured and their families is well known. Only recently however, has attention been focused on the disruption of sexual behavior that occurs with head injury. Since sexuality is such an important aspect of everyone's life, disruption of sexual behavior and relationships can have profound effects on both the family system and on the overall success of rehabilitation treatment.

Sexual dysfunction is more the rule than the exception in head injury. Boller (1982) found that three out of four head injury patients had decreased frequency of sexual relations. Kostljanetz recorded sexual dysfunction in 58 percent of the patients studied. In cases of severe head injury, sexual dysfunction is observed to be nearly universal.

There are several different classes of sexual behaviors seen following head injury. Most of them are acting out behaviors with sexual content, rather than actual sexual dysfunction. It is important to distinguish between the different types of sexual behaviors that occur, because different behaviors require different treatments. Some behaviors are normal aspects of recovery. Others are impulsive behaviors with sexual content. There is also actual sexual dysfunction that occurs

This fact sheet, #CEM 87-001, was written by Dr. Bill Blackerby, Director of Psychology Service, Rebound, Inc. Gallatin, TN and distributed by the Brain Injury Association, Inc. (BIA). For information on ordering it or other items from BIA's current Catalog of Educational Materials, call BIA at (800) 444-6443.

as a result of the physical and cognitive effects of the head injury. Lastly, there is a class of sexual behavior that appears to be related to confusion regarding sexual identity.

According to statistics (Brooks, 1984) 85 percent of all head injuries occur to individuals below the age of 25. It is during these early, formative years that most of us develop our self-concept as sexual beings. If the process is interrupted by a head injury, sexual self-concept also becomes disrupted. This often results in a wide variety of sexual behaviors as the individual seeks to re-establish a sexual identity. This type of behavior is usually seen in the later re-entry stage of recovery, after most of the initial recovery has taken place.

If there are seizures following a head injury, sexuality can be affected. In instances of seizures that are not completely controlled with medication, interictal or between-seizure periods are often marked by loss of interest in sex. Further, when medications such as Phenobarbital are used to supplement anticonvulsants, sexual libido can be further suppressed. At this point, there is no effective method of treatment available for the problems of decreased libido related to seizures and seizure-related medication.

As the head injured individual moves into the re-entry phase of recovery, different types of disruptions of sexual behaviors occur. The behaviors can be classified into three categories which reflect the different causative factors.

1. Primary—related to the brain damage from the injury. These include: poor judgement, egocentricity or insensitivity to the partner, inability to tolerate delayed gratification, poor memory, distractibility, impaired motor functions and side effects of medications.

2. Secondary—social environment factors. These include: social isolation, depression or anxiety, altered body image and self-concept, and role changes on the part of the spouse or partner.

3. Tertiary—pre-injury social skills and experiences such as: general knowledge concerning sexuality, social skills in interacting with others, experiences with friendships, dating, marriage and sex.

The problem of role changes in the relationship deserves special mention. When the partner in a relationship also becomes the primary caretaker, sexual behavior frequently declines. It is very difficult, if not impossible to maintain the dual role of sexual partner and caretaker in a relationship. If the caretaker role is prolonged, it becomes extremely difficult to revert to the original role of sexual partner in the relationship.

The recovery process can be roughly divided into three overlapping stages. Each stage can be characterized in terms of the sexual behaviors which are most commonly observed.

- *Acute stage*—Genital exposure and fondling, public masturbation, sexual delusion and confabulation.

- *Post acute stage*—Confabulation, physical or verbal approaches, inappropriate joking, repeated sexual references, and drive disturbance.

- *Re-entry stage*—Insensitivity to others, distractibility, poor judgment, memory disturbance, spouse or family role change, depression, social isolation, anxiety, medication effects, altered body image and self-concept.

In the acute stage, as the patient gradually awakens and becomes more alert, the self-stimulation that occurs represents a part of the normal adaptive awakening process, rather than actual sexual dysfunction. The behavior that occurs in this stage may actually aid in the improvement in level of consciousness. Often, patients in this stage are only able to consistently respond to extreme stimuli such as pain, loud noise or sexual stimulation. Therefore, the self-stimulation behavior may be very therapeutic.

The problem, of course, is that the behavior occurs in public. Patients that can be redirected can begin learning to discriminate the appropriate context for these behaviors. For those individuals whose cognitive functioning does not permit them to respond to redirection, sufficient privacy should be provided so that public aspect of the behavior is minimized.

In the post-acute stage, the sexual behaviors that occur usually represent disinhibited responses that, again, occur in an inappropriate context. These behaviors do not constitute actual sexual dysfunction but are inappropriate to the situations in which they occur. A treatment procedure that seems to be effective at this stage is a teaching process composed of the following simple components:

1. describe the inappropriate behavior
2. explain why it is inappropriate and the effects of this behavior on others
3. describe an appropriate behavior to replace the inappropriate one
4. ask the individual to repeat the original interaction, substituting the appropriate behavior
5. praise the individual for successfully changing the interaction.

This simple procedure is easily learned by hospital staff and by families and has proven to be very effective from preliminary results of the Timber Ridge Sexuality Research Project.

A note regarding sex drive disruption is relevant at this point. Actual change in the sex drive following a head injury is fairly rare. The areas of the brain that are involved in sex drive are located deep inside the brain and are not often damaged in traumatic injuries. Sometimes, other complications, such as hypoxia (lack of oxygen) or hydrocephalus (increased pressure caused by excessive fluid), can cause primary disturbance.

However, it rarely occurs from the head trauma alone, unless there is penetrating injury (Boller, 1982). Much more common is the loss of interest in sex that often occurs in both men and women following a head injury. This apathy and loss of interest in sex is believed to be related to injury to the frontal areas of the brain, which regulate major aspects of motivation and initiation of behavior. There are several treatment approaches to this problem currently under investigation in the Timber Ridge Sexuality Research Project. One of these is to provide the external structure in the environment to overcome initiation difficulties. This is coupled with education and counseling with the relationship partner and traditional, behavioral sex therapy methods. Preliminary results suggest that this is a promising approach for treatment of these problems.

The treatment for these problems requires multiple approaches. For the primary factors, the most effective approach seems to be a combination of cognitive retraining and development of compensatory strategies and aids. This is coupled with directed practice using the traditional behavior sex therapy techniques. For the secondary factors, the approach seems to be that of individual, group and family education and counseling. Behavioral sex therapy is employed, carefully ensuring that both partners experience sufficient success reinforcement and social contact to combat the depression, anxiety and self-concept problems.

The tertiary factors in sexuality disruption are extremely important in recovery from head injury. Personality characteristics and social behavior patterns existing prior to the head injury can have profound effects on post-traumatic sexuality. Lishman suggests that premorbid factors such as the existence of instability and antisocial behavior affect the probability of sexual behavior problems following head injury. The research literature clearly shows that head injury is frequently associated with young males from lower socio-economic conditions, who were socially unstable, with histories of alcohol and drug abuse, and social support systems. These factors often seem to be associated with post-traumatic inability to satisfy the partner's need for affection and emotional intimacy.

Premorbid characteristics which affect post-traumatic sexuality problems are perhaps the most difficult to treat successfully. Often they are the products of years of previous inadequate learning and behavior and are very difficult to alter, even without the presence of a head injury. Intensive trainings in social skills, sexuality education, counseling and behavioral sex therapy seem to offer the best hope for improvement.

Chapter 26

Community Integration of Individuals with Traumatic Brain Injury

Each year, an estimated 50,000 to 70,000 Americans sustain head injuries serious enough to leave significant residual impairments. More than a million individuals in the United States are estimated to have continuing symptoms from their traumatic brain injuries (TBIs), including interference with basic activities of daily living. The highest incidence is among young people between the ages of 15 and 24, and two-thirds to three-fourths of those injured are male. Approximately one-half of these traumas are caused by motor vehicle accidents, including motorcycles.

Some good news is reported. The incidence of drunk driving (a factor frequently linked to these accidents) appears to be declining slightly, and the use of safety devices (seat belts, airbags) is on the rise. With increased effectiveness in emergency medical care and neurosurgical services, many injured individuals who would previously have died are now surviving, albeit with permanent severe disabilities.

After completion of inpatient rehabilitation, individuals begin the lengthy process of reintegration into their community lives. Estimates of the cost of health care *after* hospitalization are staggering, and costs of treatment for injured individuals are among the highest for any disability group.

REHAB: Bringing Research into Effective Focus, Vol. XVI, No. 8. (1994), a publication of the National Institute on Disability and Rehabilitation Research. Prepared by Conwal Incorporated, 510 N. Washington St., Suite 200, Falls Church VA 22046; reprinted with permission.

The National Institute on Disability and Rehabilitation Research (NIDRR) is funding research into the complexities of this process at numerous sites. Findings from three of these research programs are featured in this *BRIEF*: the Rehabilitation Research and Training Center on Community Integration of Individuals With Traumatic Brain Injury at the State University of New York at Buffalo, the Comprehensive Model of Research and Rehabilitation for the Traumatically Brain Injured at the Department of Physical Medicine and Rehabilitation at the Medical College of Virginia, and the Rehabilitation Research and Training Center on Head Trauma and Stroke at the New York University Medical Center. The reported findings are organized by topic rather than by the research programs from which they came. The settings from which they originate are briefly identified as the Community Integration, Comprehensive Model, and Head Trauma/Stroke projects so interested readers can seek further information from the contact people listed under Sources.

Assessment of Community Integration

Five rehabilitation facilities—model systems brain injury centers—are compiling data on people with traumatic brain injuries: State University of New York at Buffalo, Medical College of Virginia, Rehabilitation Institute of Michigan, Mt. Sinai Medical Center in New York, and Santa Clara Valley Medical Center in San Jose, California. One of their purposes is to assess how well individuals have become reintegrated into their communities. As reported by Willer et al., (1991) the Community Integration Questionnaire (CIQ) was developed as a tool to provide this measurement. As a starting point, its developers used the World Health Organization (WHO) definition of *handicap*: a disadvantage resulting from an impairment or a disability, that limits fulfillment of a role that is normal (depending on age, sex, and social and cultural factors) for an individual. WHO describes six areas of role performance with which an impairment or disability can interfere: orientation (correct understanding of time, place, and person), physical independence, mobility, occupation, social integration, and economic self-sufficiency.

The Community Integration Questionnaire measures the degree to which a disadvantage is present by assessing a person's integration into the life realms of home, social networking, and productive activities. The 15 questions on the questionnaire include "Who usually prepares meals in your household?" "Who usually looks after your personal finances, such as banking or paying bills?" "How often do you travel outside the home?" The CIQ was found to be a reliable instrument and capable of discriminating between individuals with TBI and those with no apparent disabilities. Its developers note that the CIQ measures integration outcomes but not skills or skills deficits; nor does it assess an individual's feelings, such as sense of control or degree of satisfaction. They see it as a tool to be used in concert with other assessments of individual functioning.

A neuropsychological testing protocol has been developed and used by the five model systems programs to evaluate levels of function among individuals with traumatic brain injuries. Described by Kreutzer et al. (1993), this battery of tests includes portions of the Halstead-Reitan Neuropsychological Test Battery, the Wechsler Memory Scale–Revised, and the Wechsler Adult Intelligence Scale–Revised. Typically administered within 10 days of hospital discharge, results from 243 individuals tested showed diverse impairment, with greatest losses in attention, motor speed, and verbal learning. Retesting of 49 individuals one year postinjury showed significant improvement in a number of areas, including attention, verbal learning, verbal memory, and visuoperception. Researchers are optimistic that longitudinal data from this project will provide much-needed information about potential for improvement in cognitive function beyond the acute rehabilitation phase.

Behavioral Changes

Return to the family setting may be negatively affected by changes in the personality and behavior of the head-injured person. Few families understand or know how to cope with the changes they will face.

A series of studies was conducted by the Community Integration project with volunteer participants in *retreat weekends*, which focused on family and psychological issues. Interviews were conducted with married couples in which one spouse had sustained a brain injury and with families in which a child had been injured. Spouses and parents were asked to assess the injured individuals on a 40-item behavior rating scale that contained such items as "Sometimes lets frustration lead to anger," "Is moody," "Often finds it difficult to make decisions," "Is occasionally socially isolated." The most *frequent* problem mentioned was fatigue, but changes in personality, emotionality, and social behavior caused more concern. Deficits in cognitive functioning were sometimes perceived as personality changes (e.g., apparent laziness that reflected a memory deficit). Following a traumatic brain injury, depression and anxiety are common, but socially inappropriate behaviors appear to cause the most family disruption.

A study of the effects of parental injury on the behavior of children and uninjured spouses found children described as displaying increased acting-out behaviors, emotional problems, or relationship difficulties. Sample reports included "Had problems in school," "Received poor grades," "Had temper tantrums." Negative parenting performance (e.g., "Yelled at children," "Did not show interest in children," "Impatient with children") by *both* injured and uninjured parents was reported in most families. Most of the families reporting substantial breakdowns in relationships between children and their injured parent involved injured fathers. Most (17 out of 24) noninjured parents reported substantial depression, which correlated significantly with negative parenting performance and negative behavior by children.

Both men and women with traumatic brain injuries reported that the loss of autonomy and independence was their highest-rated problem, and both mentioned personality changes and memory deficits as significant. Among married couples, nondisabled wives identified their brain-injured husbands' personality changes and cognitive deficits as primary problems. Nondisabled husbands, by contrast, placed their spouses' loss of autonomy and mood swings at the top of their lists. Families in which husbands sustained brain injuries placed higher importance on job loss and income change as problem areas than did families in which wives were injured. Women with brain injuries and nondisabled wives valued support groups and other emotional support methods as coping strategies, whereas the men stressed problem-focused and goal-oriented strategies.

A retreat for 12 families with injured sons living at home found that problems of daily living were of primary concern to the sons. This included their relationships with peers; and they were aware of their behavioral problems and their impact on their families and school performance. Taking responsibility for their own rehabilitation was their main coping strategy. Mothers listed difficulty in obtaining needed services as their primary problem, followed by their sons' behavior and personality changes and their impact on the rest of the family. Their coping strategies were development of a positive outlook and acceptance of the sons' postinjury limitations.

Married couples, in which one partner had a brain injury, were questioned about levels of disability and psychological distress. Two-thirds of those with brain injuries were male. All participants rated injured individuals' cognitive disability (fatigue, memory problems, difficulty with decision making, problems with written or oral directions) and social aggression (anger, verbal and physical outbursts, aggressive behavior, and the tendency to make obscene gestures). All participants also evaluated their own levels of psychological distress.

Brain-injured individuals with higher ratings of cognitive and social dysfunction were more likely to be depressed and anxious. Noninjured spouses also showed increased anxiety and depression, with wives more affected than husbands. Severity indicators such as posttraumatic amnesia or length of coma were not correlated with the presence of affective symptoms. The researchers at the Community Integration project noted that social aggression and inappropriate behaviors by brain-injured individuals and duration of marriage might be useful predictors of psychological distress in noninjured spouses.

Family Burden

The concept of burden has been given special attention by researchers studying the relationships between individuals with disabilities and their caregivers or family. The Community Integration project conceptualized burden as "resulting from the stress associated with caring for a person with a disability." In a review of research on the effects of traumatic brain injuries on marital relationships, they found that there has been little attention to self-evaluation of degree of impairment by individuals with traumatic brain injury or of the relationship of this self-evaluation to marital satisfaction and spousal perception of burden.

A study by the Community Integration project of pairs of individuals—one with a brain injury and the other a spouse or parent—showed that, overall, high levels of burden were felt both by parents and spouses. Parents expressed higher concern regarding life-long care of the brain-injured person; spouses reported less personal reward in providing care than did parents. Spouses described burden as emotional, whereas parents described stresses involved in accomplishing goals. Inappropriate social behavior and, to a lesser extent, cognitive disability were described as major aspects of burden with both groups of caregivers. Severity of injury and physical disabilities showed less impact on perception of burden.

The Head Trauma/Stroke project looked at 31 pairs of individuals with traumatic brain injuries and their mothers, spouses, or significant others. Depending on their responses to a problem checklist, pairs were classified as high- or low-agreement families. High agreement families were divided by whether the significant other or the individual with traumatic brain injury listed at least twice as many problems as their partner.

Participants noted physical, cognitive, and behavioral problems, but those described by significant others as causing the greatest burden were behavioral: irritability, mood swings, and changed personality. The greatest burden was felt by the high-agreement families. This might be because the problems are more severe and obvious, or the pairs may be more focused on their struggles with existent problems.

Interestingly, of the pairs in which the partner with a traumatic brain injury mentioned more problems than the significant other, the return-to-work/school rate was highest. This could be due to the ability of the injured individual to recognize problems and compensate for them, or returning to work could result in daily confrontation with these problems. Other explanations offered were that significant others perceived brain-injured individuals as functioning well because of their return to work or that their particular deficits did not interfere with family life.

Family Intervention

The Community Integration project has identified a number of areas in which managing behavior problems in the home could be facilitated by professional followup and support:

- understanding the unique nature of each individual circumstance;
- clarifying the source of the behavior change;
- applying behavior modification techniques with consistency; and
- assisting the injured individual to achieve awareness to the degree of impairment.

The need for enhancing family intervention strategies is addressed by the Comprehensive Model project, which recommends seven different but overlapping approaches: family education; support groups; family networking; advocacy; family therapy; marital therapy; and sexual counseling. An individual with a traumatic brain injury is surrounded by multiple systems which typically include the family, rehabilitation team, third-party payers, and community support groups, making effective family coordination of these resources crucial to maximize their complementary functioning.

Return to Work After TBI

The ability to hold a job is one of the most potent measures of community integration. Staff at the Head Trauma/Stroke project identified factors that might predict which individuals with traumatic brain injuries would benefit vocationally from a neuropsychological rehabilitation program. Fifty-nine people with moderate to severe brain injuries participated in the study. It was found that measurements obtained *after* completion of a 20-week intensive neuropsychological remediation program were more accurate than those obtained before the program in predicting employability and actual work status six months postprogram. The single most important factor in predicting return to work was a capacity for acceptance, as reflected by staff ratings in:

- complying with program routines and objectives,
- actively participating in the therapeutic community,
- publicly acknowledging problems, and
- endorsing staff recommendations for the vocational aspects of the program.

The second best predictor was the injured individual's self-awareness. The ability to regulate affect was rated as a significant factor in employability, as were length of coma and verbal aptitude. Perhaps surprisingly, cognitive deficits in attention, memory, and concentration did not appear to contribute significantly to predicting return to work.

Supported employment has been successful in helping individuals with traumatic brain injuries return to work. Forty-one individuals who had sustained severe brain injuries were placed in competitive employment by the Comprehensive Model project using an onsite employment specialist who provided ongoing case management. Before this intervention, the injured individuals had worked only 15 percent of the total months in which they had been available for work postinjury; subsequent to the services, they worked 75 percent of total available months. All placements were in competitive positions paying at least minimum wages. Most work terminations were related to impaired work habits and inappropriate behavior on the job. The researchers reported a job retention rate of 71 percent and offer cautious optimism that the supported employment model provides one means of enhancing the employability of individuals with traumatic brain injuries.

Substance abuse has a dramatic impact on obtaining and maintaining employment. The Comprehensive Model project found the incidence of intoxication among individuals admitted for inpatient treatment of traumatic brain injury to be at least 50 percent. Preinjury substance abuse is said to be relatively common with this group, and postinjury substance abuse is believed to be equally common. The use of alcohol and nonprescription drugs can be particularly dangerous for a head-injured person who is likely to be more susceptible to their effects and might have seizures. With adjustment to employment already compromised by cognitive and behavioral problems, abstinence from alcohol, rather than controlled consumption, is recommended.

Circles of Support

In an effort to reconstruct support networks for individuals with traumatic brain injuries, the staff at the Community Integration project propose creating *circles of support*. These unique networks contain individuals selected by the *focus person*—the individual with the injury. A facilitator functions as group coordinator and resource specialist, helping the group to keep on track and maintain momentum and reminding members to work toward empowering the focus person. The composition of the circle changes over time. Some members leave because of lack of commitment or conflicts of interest; others may lack continued purpose, as when a professional joins on a short-term basis to assist in accomplishing a specific goal. The purposes of the circle are to enable the focus person to express his/her positive self-image, and to identify personal strengths which can transform the dreams into attainable goals. The facilitator has the crucial assignment of helping members accept their tasks and work toward solutions. This semistructured approach uses natural processes found in friendships to establish an individualized, sensitive support group. The group, in turn, offers a potentially effective way to help people with traumatic brain injuries to enhance their community integration.

Implications

Desire for community integration reflects a universal human need to be accepted and productive. People who have had traumatic brain injuries face major challenges to fulfillment of this wish because their needs span the full range of physical, cognitive, and emotional functioning. However, efforts to contain health-care costs and reduce tax-dollar expenditures for individuals with special needs have brought political scrutiny to funding the needed safety net. This public funding crisis gives added urgency to the community integration problems faced by individuals with traumatic brain injuries. Research findings described suggest that resources already exist that could enhance their integration; what is frequently needed is imagination and assertive networking with community service providers who are accustomed to serving people with different, but similar, disabilities. A focus on consumer empowerment may be an important first step. It sets the stage for greater involvement of consumers, their families, and ever-widening circles of voluntary helpers to take over some of the rehabilitative work previously borne by paid professionals. The payoff may be double. Public dollars are saved, and the work is more effective because it is done by people who are natural, long-term members of a person's social network.

Sources

The Rehabilitation Research and Training Center on Community Integration of Individuals With Traumatic Brain Injury at the State University of New York at Buffalo, 197 Farber Hall, 3435 Main Street, Buffalo, NY 14214. For more information contact Barry Willer, Ph.D., Director, (716) 829-2300.

The Comprehensive Model of Research and Rehabilitation for the Traumatically Brain Injured at the Department of Physical Medicine and Rehabilitation at the Medical College of Virginia, West Hospital 3rd Floor Room 3-102, 1200 E. Broad St., Richmond, VA 23298. Jeffrey Kreutzer, PhD., Director. For more information contact Jennifer Marwitz, (804) 371-2374.

The Rehabilitation Research and Training Center on Head Trauma and Stroke at the New York University Medical Center, Department of Physical Medicine, 400 E. 34th St., New York City,

NY 10016. Leonard Diller, PhD., Director. For more information contact Marie Cavallo, (212) 263-6161.

Willer, B., Rosenthal, M., Kreutzer, J., Gordon, W., & Rempel, R. (1991). Assessment of community integration following rehabilitation for traumatic brain injury. *Journal of Head Trauma Rehabilitation*, 8(2) pp. 75-87.

Kreutzer, J., Gordon, W., Rosenthal, M., & Marwitz, J. (1993). Neuropsychological characteristics of patients with brain injury: Preliminary findings from a multicenter investigation. *Journal of Head Trauma Rehabilitation*, 8(2) pp. 47-59.

Whatever It Takes

The Community Integration project has developed a service model titled Whatever It Takes (WIT). Ten principles emphasize practical approaches to accomplish the goal of community integration.

- No two individuals are alike.
- Skills are more likely to be acquired when taught in the environment where they are to be used.
- Environments are easier to change than people.
- Individual program plans must include assessment of environmental barriers.
- Natural supports extend assistance throughout the lifetime.
- Interventions must not do harm.
- The reimbursement system often presents its own barriers to integration.
- Respect for the individual is paramount.
- Service needs of individuals may be met through the existing community service network.

The WIT model proposed is an extension of the medical/rehabilitation model that includes aspects found in the independent living and normalization movements; it provides for practical solutions to deal with day-to-day issues facing individuals with traumatic brain injuries.

Chapter 27

The Injured and Healing Brain: Research Update

Brain disorders steal away the brightest and wisest, young and old. Brain research has made impressive strides in the first half of the 1990s, and the second half promises even more.

Neurology is no longer considered a discipline focusing on diseases for which little or no therapy can be promised. Today this dynamic specialty is the fastest growing of the life sciences. Researchers have garnered most of our information about the brain—90%—in the past 10 years. Despite an explosion of clinically relevant information, 50 million Americans are affected each year, directly or indirectly, by brain and CNS disorders. The annual impact on the national economy is $401 billion.

The Injured and Healing Brain

How can the injured brain be protected and restored? When injury occurs, whether it takes the form of trauma, stroke, or noxious episode, the brain suffers a biphasic hit. A secondary insult follows the release of the neurotransmitter glutamate, which, in high concentrations, is toxic to nerve cells. Compounds that block the secondary effect and the use of hypothermia promise an entirely new approach to therapy.

Taken from "Decade of the Brain: A Midpoint Status Report," *Patient Care*, July 15, 1995. Reprinted with permission of *Patient Care*. Copyright Medical Economics.

A goal of researchers is to create the technology to grow brain cells that could replace those damaged by trauma or disease. Up until 10 years ago, medical schools taught that the mammalian CNS had become so specialized it had lost the ability to repair itself—it was hardwired. Neuroscientists now know not only that mechanisms of recovery spring into action after insult, even in the elderly, but also that the adult human brain can grow new brain cells. The brain harbors precursor nerve cells throughout life, and these can give rise to new neurons the same way nerve cells come into being during early embryonic development. In this Decade of the Brain, researchers hope to map the entire human brain to determine the precise location of precursor cells and to learn how "rewiring" can be accomplished.

Important questions are being broached: How does a growing nerve find its target? Can functional synapses be reestablished? What are the molecular mechanisms of glial scar formation?

Traumatic Brain and Spinal Cord Injury

The cascade of events immediately following the moment of trauma results in excessive chemical activity and progressive and cumulative injury to brain cells. Secondary effects alter the way neurons function and can lead to paralysis, sensory loss, and problems with behavior and cognition. The corticosteroid methylprednisolone sodium succinate (unlabeled use) helps to minimize damage from spinal cord injury when a high dose—15-30 mg/kg IV—is administered within eight hours of injury.

The mechanism by which methylprednisolone works has yet to be fully understood, but its effectiveness has fostered hopes of developing other drugs to reduce secondary injury. A clinical trial provided evidence that the ganglioside GM_1 enhances the functional recovery of damaged neurons after one year and can act adjuvantly with methylprednisolone.

Locating damage sites is critical before treatment, and up-to-date imaging techniques are essential to neurotrauma research. MRI, positron emission tomography (PET), and single-photon emission computed tomography (SPECT) can show fiber tract damage previously unrevealed by CT. The new imaging technologies expose shearing injury and resultant reduced cerebral blood flow and metabolic dysfunction, even in areas with no apparent structural damage. Developing a protocol for combining imaging with performance tests following traumatic brain injury is a priority for the second half of this decade.

Our understanding of the inherent ability of the CNS to rescue and repair damaged nerve cells has expanded in the early 1990s. Neurotrophic factors produced by molecular engineering are being implanted into damaged CNS tissue. Further research is needed: What factors help implants form beneficial connections with nearby cells? Why doesn't the damaged spinal cord repair itself without assistance? Are chemicals present that inhibit repair? Is the immune system involved?

Federal Neuroscience Budget

Despite evidence that brain disorders are the most costly of all diseases, the federal neuroscience research budget has been erratic. It received a modest shot in the arm at the beginning of the decade, then declined between 1990 and 1994, and finally made a slight upswing in 1995 (see Figure 27.1).

Where NIH funding goes	
Diseases	**1995 funding**
NEUROLOGIC	
Alzheimer's disease	$305 million
Stroke	$116 million
Multiple sclerosis	$80 million
Parkinson's disease	$72 million
Epilepsy	$55 million
Head injury	$51 million
NONNEUROLOGIC	
Breast cancer	$377 million
Diabetes	$304 million
Kidney disease	$201 million
Arthritis	$199 million
Hypertension	$179 million
Smoking and health	$122 million
Osteoporosis	$96 million
Sickle-cell disease	$56 million
Lyme disease	$16 million
Key: NIH, National Institutes of Health.	

Figure 27.1. Where NIH funding goes.

243

The 1995 National Institutes of Health (NIH) budget (non-AIDS) is $10 billion. Within the NIH, the National Institute of Neurological Disorders and Stroke (NINDS) has been allocated $629 million. "A 4% increase in the NINDS budget was appropriated at the beginning of this decade," says Andrew Baldus, budget officer of NINDS. "But funding has evened out over the past couple of years—an indicator that federal dollars are very tight. The 1996 budget will be even more scrupulously detailed."

"Neuroscience research finds itself in competition with the multiple priorities of Congress, the administration, and the American people," says Michael D. Walker, MD, Director of the Division of Stroke and Trauma at NINDS and a consultant for this article. "All are saying we've got to bring the federal budget deficit under control while improving medical care. Just at the point when major advances in neuroscience are ready to be applied in the clinic, money is drying up. To take a compound from bench to bedside is a very expensive process—somewhere between $100 million and $700 million."

In response to the urgent need for money for brain research during this Decade of the Brain, the Dana Alliance for Brain Initiatives was founded in 1993. Fueled by $25 million from the Dana Foundation and co-chaired by James Watson, PhD, the alliance is an independent, nonprofit organization of upward of 135 neuroscientists, including Watson and four other Nobel laureates, dedicated to advancing education about the personal and public benefits of brain research.

For More Information on Brain Disorders and Brain Research

National Institutes of Health
9000 Rockville Pike
Bldg. 31, Room 8A06
Bethesda, MD 20892
(301) 496-5751

National Institute of Mental Health
5600 Fishers Lane, Room 7C-02
Rockville, MD 20857
(301) 443-4513

National Institute of Neurological Disorders and Stroke
9000 Rockville Pike
Bldg. 31, Room 8A16
Bethesda, MD 20892
(800) 352-9424

The ALS Association
21021 Ventura Blvd., Suite 321
Woodland Hills, CA 91364-2206
(800) 782-4747

Alzheimer's Association
919 N. Michigan Ave.
Chicago, IL 60611-1676
(800) 272-3900

American Brain Tumor Association
2720 River Rd., Suite 146
Des Plaines, IL 60018
(800) 886-2282

Brain Injury Association, Inc.
1776 Massachusetts Ave., NW
Suite 100
Washington, DC 20036
(800) 444-6443

Dana Alliance for Brain Initiatives
745 Fifth Ave., Suite 700
New York, NY 10151
(212) 223-4040
or
1001 G St. NW, Suite 1025
Washington, DC 20001
(202) 737-9200

National Foundation for Brain Research
1250 24th St. NW, Suite 300
Washington, DC 20037
(202) 293-5453

National Mental Health Association
1021 Prince St.
Alexandria, VA 22314-2971
(800) 969-NMHA (969-6642)

National Multiple Sclerosis Society
733 3rd Ave., 6th Floor
New York, NY 10017
(800) LEARN-MS (344-4867)

National Stroke Association
8480 E. Orchard Rd.
Suite 1000
Englewood, CO 80111
(800) STROKES (787-6537)

Parkinson's Disease Foundation
710 W. 168th St.
New York, NY 10032
(800) 457-6676

United Cerebral Palsy Research Foundation
1660 L St., NW, Suite 700
Washington, DC 20036
(800) USA-5UCP (872-5827)

—by P. Noel Connaughton, MD;
Guy McKhann, MD;
Michael D. Walker, MD

P. Noel Connaughton, MD, is Chairman, Department of Radiology, and Chief of Neuroradiology, Lancaster General Hospital, Lancaster, PA.

Guy McKhann, MD, is Director, Zanvyl Krieger Mind/Brain Institute, and Professor of Neurology and Neuroscience, the Johns Hopkins University School of Medicine, Baltimore, MD.

Michael D. Walker, MD, is Director, Division of Stroke and Trauma, National Institute of Neurological Disorders and Stroke, National Institutes of Health, Bethesda, MD.

Part Four

Special Concerns Faced by Family Members and Other Survivors

Chapter 28

Brain Injury: A Guide for Families

Family Behaviors

Up until a few years ago the primary focus of brain injury rehabilitation, from a professional standpoint, was on the patient. With the founding of the National Head Injury Foundation, (now the Brain Injury Association), there has been a realization that the family suffers as much or more than the injured party. One of our family members recently said, "When something like this happens, the whole family has a brain injury." He was, of course, referring to the extreme feeling of disorientation and confusion that results after the initial shock and medical crisis have passed. The feelings of anger, grief, guilt, denial and apprehension are quite similar to the experiences felt by persons who mourn the death of a loved one. Because of the extended rehabilitation process, the family members or significant others experience these feelings in recurring cycles.

The acquisition of new or unaccustomed behaviors is required because the old methods of dealing with the patient may no longer be effective. Moreover, subtle interrelationships of family members may be thrown off without an awareness of how to get moving in a positive direction. You may be experiencing or will soon be aware of feelings and actions in yourself that you never dreamed were possible. It

Excerpted from *Brain Injury: A Guide for Families*, copyright 1996 HDI Publishers, P.O. Box 131401, Houston, TX. 77219; reprinted with permission. To order the complete booklet or to obtain a free catalogue of available materials call (800) 321-7037.

is hoped that by knowing these possibilities you will experience less guilt, confusion, or frustration. We have described thirteen behaviors; again, you may have to deal with only some of them.

Panic

Probably the first reaction that you experienced after the accident was panic. Subsequently, this response subsides and is replaced by disorientation, inability to concentrate or focus, and an extreme feeling of loss of control. All of these feelings are valid responses to trauma associated with a life-threatening experience. The panic usually remains in some degree of intensity until your loved one is declared medically stable. At times you may think you have things under control and then "lose it" the next day. These cycles of panic are normal so do not feel that you are coping abnormally.

Resolutions to Panic

1. Acknowledge that the situation is out of your hands at this point.

2. Recognize the initial signs of panic and learn techniques for calming yourself down.

3. Do not try to take control—this will only lead to more frustration and increased episodes of panic.

4. Redirect your focus to those areas where you can have an impact, (e.g., support of other family members, care of dependent children, etc.).

5. Do not set arbitrary goals or expectations during the stage of medical stabilization.

Anxiety

Relinquishing control leads to decreased panic but increased anxiety. Initially, your anxiety was almost exclusively limited to whether your loved one would survive. You may have said things like, "If only he will live—that's all that matters." However, the closer the patient gets to safety, the greater your requirements. Once you see that the patient will live, you focus on his ability to eat, then to walk, then to talk, then for self-care, and then the question of returning to school or earning a living. There is anxiety of varying levels associated with all these rehabilitation stages.

Resolutions for Anxiety

1. Learn relaxation techniques.

2. See your psychologist, social worker, or counselor for individual or group therapy.

3. Take time for yourself. Give yourself permission to divert your attention by either relaxing or engaging in pleasurable activities.

4. Don't try to be everything to everybody—delegate responsibilities to others. People often want to help but do not know how to assist you.

5. Stay clear of people who provoke anxiety.

Denial/Overoptimism

Denial is a defense mechanism that we all use at times to keep us from dealing with the facts. It is often adaptive at first because it helps alleviate the intensity of the emotional pain and suffering we are experiencing. There is nothing wrong with optimism and hope, but there does come a point when denial can be a negative influence in the effective rehabilitation of your loved one.

One of the symptoms of denial is that of setting arbitrary dates to gauge the patient's progress. We have seen families say such things as, "Mom will be out of the wheelchair by Thanksgiving, off the walker by Christmas, and she will throw away her cane by Easter." Such predictions are usually unrealistic and can result in increased anxiety and/or anger as the date approaches. The patient who fails to meet these goals will often become depressed and feel guilty. The inadvertent message here is that the patient is not acceptable in his current condition and he may fear that you will withdraw your support if he cannot comply. Instead, goals should relate to the patient's documented progress and projected potential as determined by the therapists involved.

Resolutions for Denial

1. Take it day by day—deal with today's problems without letting your expectations for the future affect immediate needs.

2. Deal with the patient as he is today. This does not mean that you are satisfied with the progress and are giving up on the future.

3. Seek emotional support to handle the increased anxiety or anger that occurs as a result of decreasing denial.

Anger

Letting go of denial very often leads to freely expressed anger. This is directed at a variety of individuals, including the person responsible for the accident, witnesses at the scene of the accident, staff in the hospital, other family members, and the patient himself. There may be a generalized anger toward more abstract groups such as motorcycle manufacturers, legislators, God, and the medical profession as a whole.

This is a stage that you are going through, just as the patient has various stages he will experience. Recognize it as such and attempt to re-channel your emotions in a positive direction.

Resolutions for Anger

1. Recognize that you are angry about what happened.

2. Identify the stimulus for anger and avoid it if possible (e.g., specific nurse, particular friend of patient, etc.).

3. Substitute a vigorous and/or productive activity for anger (e.g., exercise, house-cleaning, yard work).

4. Do not allow the anger to eat away at you and affect your own health.

5. Seek counseling to deal effectively with anger.

Frustration

Frustration is usually the result of unachieved expectations and often goes hand in hand with anxiety and anger. If you are a person who is used to being in control, the occurrence of a brain injury in your family will be one of the most frustrating times of your life. Recovery does not follow a "normal" pattern and thus, tends to be very individualized. Consequently, definitive answers are at a premium, and frustration often follows.

Resolutions to Frustration

1. Set small, realistic goals for the patient.

2. Try to determine the doctor's rationale for a decision and discuss your ideas with him in a nonconfrontational manner.

3. Find out if there are alternate or back-up support systems.

4. Recognize those things that are essentially outside your control; there are some things you just cannot change.

Fatigue

There is probably no other time when you have been this fatigued for any extended period. You have just been through the trauma of life versus death, which brings with it many sleepless nights. In addition, the demands on you during waking hours increases. The responsibility for the care of an individual who is brain injured is often a 24-hour job and is similar to the care of a new baby. Moreover, all the tension resulting from anxiety and anger are very tiring and add to the overall debilitating effect of fatigue.

Resolutions for Fatigue

1. Utilize relaxation techniques for insomnia. If you are unfamiliar with these, consult a psychologist.

2. Put off until tomorrow what is not absolutely necessary.

3. Delegate responsibilities. Others will usually be glad to help.

4.   Do not feel that you have to constantly be by the patient's side. Ignore accusations that you do not visit enough.

Irritability/Impatience

Patients with brain injury are not the only ones who become irritable or impatient—family members behave this way also. Irritability is a manifestation of the previously described reactions including anxiety, anger, and fatigue. Issues of little importance become very significant. Families will at times lose sight of the overall picture and focus great amounts of energy on problems that are not particularly important or productive. Try to step back and take a new look at your goals for the patient. You may be using impatience as a means of feeling involved, since you have a reduced ability to impact upon larger issues. Your tolerance for human error or what appears to be human error is nil.

On the other hand, you may find yourself at odds with others who complain about problems that appear minute in comparison to the magnitude of the issues you must address. Be aware of this possible side-effect and recognize that you may find it difficult to be sympathetic to others at this time.

As time passes and your loved one has been at home for a while, this impatience can easily be directed toward the patient himself. Memory problems, slowed responses, and inappropriate behavior are often reasons for becoming short-tempered. There will be times when you will feel that the injured individual does not comprehend or appreciate all the trauma you experienced and the time and effort you have put into the rehabilitation program. Unappreciative behavior on his part can easily add to irritability and impatience in family members.

Resolutions for Irritability/Impatience

1.   Look at the "big picture." Focus on long term goals.

2.   Recognize your impatience and apologize ahead of time.

3.   Do not set preconceived time frames for the patient accomplishing a task. Patients who are brain injured cannot be rushed.

4.   Be open and honest about your feelings.

Criticism of Primary Caretaker

Taking care of a patient who is brain injured is like running a restaurant—everybody thinks they can do a better job! This category adds a new dimension to the previously described behavior of family abuse. You may receive grief not only from the patient, but also from other family members. This criticism tends to surface particularly when things are not going well at home. Additionally, the primary offenders are those who only have periodic contact with the patient.

A specific example, involving a family whose 50 year-old father was injured in a tractor accident, may serve to illustrate this problem. Prior to the accident, this father of seven children had been a mild-spoken man who was the sole bread winner in the family. Four of the seven children were out on their own and three lived at home, spending varying amounts of time in the house. At six months post-injury the patient continued to need round-the-clock nursing care, primarily because of combative and verbally abusive behavior. All but one of the children blamed the mother for their father's personality change, intimating that she was not treating him fairly. Over an additional three-month period, with our professional assistance, they began to see that it took little to no provocation to set him off. However, the excessive criticism of the mother definitely took its toll on her ability to both accept her husband's changes and learn to ignore abuse from both family and patient.

Before the patient leaves the hospital it is best to designate one individual as the primary caretaker. If you are not that person, you can most effectively assist in the patient's care by being supportive of that individual rather than working at cross purposes with them.

Resolutions for Criticism

1. Invite the critical individual to take your place for a day.

2. Use these criticisms as an opportunity to obtain assistance.

Feeling of Hopelessness

There may come a point during the rehabilitation process when you will be overcome by a feeling of despair. The first symptom usually revolves around the realization that your life may never return to its original pattern. This thinking may be set off when the patient reaches his first prolonged plateau, or it may be associated with a noticeable slowing of recovery. As you begin to readjust your thinking and realize that your life plans have to be changed, an extreme feeling of hopelessness is a common response. Do not think that you are reacting abnormally. This is a stage that must be worked through.

Resolutions for Hopelessness

1. Do not set arbitrary time limits on recovery—you are setting yourself up for disappointment.

2. Modify your goals and expectations. Very few patients who are seriously brain injured return to their former level of functioning, but this does not mean they cannot be happy at another level.

3. Make the most of the things the patient can do and try to forget the things he can no longer do.

4. If you feel that you are not moving out of the depressed state effectively, contact a social worker, counselor, or psychologist to assist.

Guilt

It is common for family members to experience feelings of guilt when caring for a patient who is brain injured. The circumstances surrounding a brain injury provide many possibilities for thinking that you have not done your best in a given situation. Guilt will arise from at least four main sources: (1) you; (2) the patient; (3) other family members; and (4) concerned others. Once you have your own guilt under control, you will have to learn to defuse the guilt-laden arrows shot at you by others.

Resolutions for Guilt

1. Accept guilt as a normal human feeling over which you have minimal control.

2. Substitute some engrossing activity to get your mind off the guilt—gardening, exercising, biking, etc.

3. Schedule your guilt sessions. For example, agree to worry only between eight and nine o'clock in the morning and then forget it the rest of the day.

Decreased Social Contacts/Lack of Leisure Time

As is often the case when a "sick" loved one returns home, the family reduces its contact with the outside world to allow the patient to have a quiet environment and to provide emotional support. The danger here is that this pattern will become a habit that will be hard to break. Studies have shown that the support of family and friends is more important than the assistance of hospital personnel, doctors, or the clergy. Thus, it is a mistake to isolate yourself from your old contacts.

Even though you may make every effort to foster old friendships, you may find that many will gradually drift away due to a variety of reasons: (1) they are not able to understand the behavioral changes of the patient; (2) they are not able to accept the patient in his post-injury condition; (3) they find that they are uncomfortable in the patient's presence because they no longer share common interests and goals. If you find this occurring with a large portion of your former friends, make every effort to form new acquaintances.

Resolutions for Decreased Social Contacts /Lack of Leisure Time

1. Do not set up an early pattern of decreased social contacts.

2. Do not quit your job unless absolutely necessary.

3. When friends call, talk about things other than the patient.

4. Schedule outings for social activities and then follow through.

5. Do not convince yourself that you are the only one who can care for the patient.

Loss of Love

One of the most all-encompassing upheavals you may face is that of losing the one you love—not physically, but emotionally. It is possible that the patient will never completely return to his original personality. The changes may be minute or they may be quite significant and long-lasting. We often hear people say such things as, "I'm married to a stranger." The whole family dynamics can be reversed. Instead of a man and woman relating on an adult-adult level, you may now be relating on a parent-child level. These changes can be equally frustrating to both the family and the patient.

Resolutions for Loss of Love

1. Talk to them the way you used to.
2. Let them make as many decisions as possible.
3. Ask their opinion (even if it is not necessarily needed).
4. Approach the situation as you would a new relationship.

Conclusion

You have taken on a big responsibility, caring for a patient who is brain injured. It won't be easy, but it can be very rewarding when you see him make some little improvement in behavior or insight, and you know it is all because you guided and helped him. Don't sell yourself short—any progress the patient makes is probably directly attributable to the assistance of the person taking care of him, and you should take credit and satisfaction from it. However, the going may get rough. Experiencing all the emotions we have described, and probably some we have not, will be taxing and tiring. You should get help when you need it.

While it would be ideal for every head injured patient's family to have an organization of other similar families to belong to; in fact, such groups are probably going to be limited to larger cities and those with rehabilitation centers. It is important for you to develop and maintain group support systems for yourself, something that will get you away from the patient for a few hours a week and give you some relief. If you are active in a church, civic club, social club, recreational or athletic group, by all means stay active in them. Do not make the mistake of giving up these valuable associations in order to devote more time to the patient. If you haven't been active in some such group activities before, find some and join them. Most communities have recreation or community centers that offer classes and clubs. Sign up for one that will get you together with other people with some of your same interests: cards, bowling, arts and crafts, book reviews, cooking classes, etc. The focus of these groups is not head injuries, and it will give you something else to focus your attention on. If there is a mental health center or Family Service Society in your community, inquire about support groups for families of mentally disturbed patients. Some of them will be going through some of the same things you are. Adult day care programs, often sponsored by county programs for the aging, may be available for the patient to go to for a few hours a week, or even daily if necessary. Some counties or states offer "respite care" or homemaker services, where someone comes to the house to relieve you while you go out for awhile. If there is a rehabilitation center nearby, see if there is a day treatment center. They offer skilled services (physical, occupational, speech and cognitive therapies) and your insurance may cover the costs. Another resource which insurance may cover is a long-term head injury residential treatment center or transitional living facility. These facilities are for patients who have completed a hospital-based rehabilitation program, but who need training in independent living and social skills and usually spend several months at these facilities.

If the patient is interested in employment and his physician does not object, he may require the services of the Vocational Rehabilitation Office in your state. These programs are set up exclusively for people with handicaps and give counseling, retraining, educational, job placement and sheltered employment services, and you can refer yourself. Just be sure the patient's doctor agrees.

Take advantage of whatever you can to get relief and do it without guilt. Good luck!

References

When your child is seriously injured: The emotional impact on families by Marilyn Lash, M.S.W. 1991. Published by EXCEPTIONAL PARENT, Department ML, P.O. Box 8045, Brick, NJ 08723.

When your child goes to school after an injury by Marilyn Lash, M.S.W. 1992. Published by EXCEPTIONAL PARENT, Department ML, P.O. Box 8045, Brick, NJ 08723.

When young children are injured: Families as caregivers in hospitals and at home by Jane Haltiwanger, M.A., and Marilyn Lash, M.S.W. 1994. Published by EXCEPTIONAL PARENT, Department ML, P.O. Box 8045, Brick, NJ 08723.

Educational Dimensions of Acquired Brain Injury edited by Ronald C. Savage, Ed.D. and Gary F. Wolcott, M.Ed. 1994. PRO-Ed, 8700 Shoal Creek Blvd., Austin, TX 78757-6897.

Head Injury: A Family Matter by Janet M. Williams and Thomas Kay 1991. Paul Brooks Publishing Company, P.O. Box 10624, Baltimore, MD 21285-0624.

Head Injury in Children and Adolescents: A Resource for School and Allied Professionals by Vivian Begali, M.Ed., Ed.S. Second edition, 1993. Clinical Psychology Publishing Co., Inc., 4 Conant Square, Brandon, Vermont 05733.

Pediatric Traumatic Brain Injury: Proactive Intervention Jean Blosser, Ed.D. and Roberta DePompei, Ph.D. 1994. Published by Singular Publishing Group, Inc., 4284 41st St., San Diego, CA 92105-1197.

Psychological Management of Traumatic Brain Injuries in Children & Adolescents by Ellen Lehr, Ph.D. 1990. Aspen Publishers, Inc., P.O. Box 990, Frederick, MD 21701.

Traumatic Head Injury in Children and Adolescents: A Sourcebook for Teachers and Other School Personnel by Mary P. Mira, Bonnie Tucker and Janet S. Tyler 1992. PRO-Ed, 8700 Shoal Creek Blvd., Austin, TX 78757-6897.

An Educator's Manual: A Teacher's Guide to Students with Brain Injuries edited by Ron Savage, Ed.D. and Gary Wolcott, M.Ed. 1995. National Head Injury Foundation, 1770 Massachusetts Avenue, Suite 100, Washington, DC 20036-1914.

Signs and Strategies for Educating Students with Brain Injuries: A Practical Guide for Teacher and Schools by Marilyn Lash, M.S.W., Sue Pearson M.A. and Gary Wolcott, M.Ed. 1995. HDI Publishers, P.O. Box 131401, Houston, TX 77219.

Resources

Brain Injury Association (BIA)
1776 Massachusetts Avenue
Washington, DC 20036
Telephone: Voice (202) 296-6443
Ask for the address and telephone number of your State chapter of BIA.

National Information Center for Children and Youth with Disabilities (NICHCY)
P.O. Box 1492
Washington, DC 20013
Telephone Voice: (800) 999-5599; TT: (703) 893-8614

Research and Training Center in Rehabilitation and Childhood Trauma
Department of Physical Medicine and Rehabilitation
New England Medical Center and
Tufts University School of Medicine
750 Washington St., #75 K-R, Boston, MA 02111-1901
Telephone Voice and TT (617) 636-5031

Chapter 29

A Family Guide to Evaluating Transitional Living Programs for Head Injured Adults

As treatment for head injuries becomes more sophisticated, new treatment approaches are developed. At one time, little rehabilitation was offered to patients after acute medical problems were resolved. Now there are extensive programs available in acute rehabilitation treatment, outpatient treatment, transitional living, and long-term care.

New treatment approaches are a reason for optimism among head injured individuals and their families. The proliferation of such programs, however, increases the problems of judging program quality. The need for careful evaluation of program quality is critical for several reasons. The tremendous cost of head injury rehabilitation necessitates every attempt to make treatment cost effective while maintaining quality. Moreover, families of head injured individuals are often the ones who must look for new facilities. As competition increases, it becomes difficult for families to know who to trust in such matters. Yet it is essential that families be actively involved in the decision making progress. In this way, they can be effective participants in the head injury treatment plan.

The present paper is designed to focus on one category of head injury treatment that appears to be most vaguely defined and most problematic to evaluate: transitional living. The paper will provide an outline for families to follow in evaluating transitional programs, and raise issues of concern for individuals managing such programs.

by Paul R. Sachs, Ph. D., CEM:88-012, Brain Injury Association, Inc.; Reprinted with permission.

In the course of describing these issues, it is hoped that the category of transitional living will be more clearly differentiated from other types of head injury treatment.

Definition of Transitional Living

Transitional living programs provide an important aspect of treatment for the recovering head injured individual. They are an essential step between inpatient treatment and independent living, or between inpatient treatment and some long-term care program. The National Head Injury Foundation's service directory describes transitional living programs as follows:

> The goal of a transitional program is to prepare individuals for maximum independence, to teach the skills necessary for community interaction, and to work on pre-vocational and vocational training. Specialized programs stressing cognitive memory, speech and behavioral therapies are usually structured to the needs of the individual. Programs of this type are being established in a variety of settings—small group homes, special educational institutions, and as part of a continuum of care in rehabilitation centers (NHIF, 1983, p. viii).

Although useful as a start and as a category in the service directory, this description is too broad. It does not differentiate transitional living programs in terms of length of stay from a long-term program that may have similar goals. The description also combines programs in group homes, special education institutions and rehabilitation facilities under one heading. There may be marked differences, however, in programs within these settings. This broad use of the term, transitional living, may reflect the current state of programming but it is ultimately confusing to the general public and weakens the impression that such programs will have on families.

To work toward a clear concept of transitional living, the following definition is offered.

> A transitional living program for head injured adults provides a short-term set of treatments that promote evaluation and development of the clients' practical independence and psychological independence within a supervised residence that challenges the clients with daily living activities and adult responsibilities,

and leads to reentry into the community or to a long-term supervised program.

Several parts of this definition should be highlighted to elaborate on the ideas contained within it.

Transitional living for head injured adults. The concept of transitional living is not unique to head injury. It has been used widely with retarded and psychiatric adults. A program for head injured adults should be specifically designed for their needs and not other diagnostic groups.

Short-term. Transitional living is not a lifetime care program. It is a time limited approach that may last anywhere from three to eighteen months, depending on the client. If within this time the client is not expected to have gained from the program, then that individual may be more suitable for another treatment modality.

A set of treatments. Transitional living is not one treatment, but rather a group of different therapeutic activities that are integrated within the transitional environment so that the activities as a whole are more helpful to the client than any of them would be if done separately.

To promote evaluation. The transitional living program should be unique enough to challenge the client in ways that they have not and could not be challenged at home or in an inpatient environment. In this way, the professional in the program can more fully evaluate the client's potential for independent living.

Development. No rehabilitation program can fairly claim that it will solve an individual's problems. A program can, however, further develop and individual's capabilities to that individual's highest level of achievement. Thus, the goal of the program should be to set in motion or accelerate a process of development that the individual will continue after completing the program. This may include a further increase in independence and simultaneously an adaptation to the long-term limitations that the client retains.

Practical independence. Independence is a complex subject. One aspect of it is the ability to be independent in practice of basic daily living skills.

Psychological independence. Independence also means thinking and acting as an independent adult. This includes taking responsibility for one's actions, making decisions, and setting personal goals.

Supervised residence. Transitional living is different from independent living and from inpatient care. The transitional living residence should be supervised in a way that enables clients to meet their goals securely yet without excessive restrictions.

Daily living activities. To achieve practical independence, the client must be presented with these activities and encouraged to try to master them.

Adult responsibilities. To achieve psychological independence, the client must have the opportunity to master responsible behavioral control that is expected of mature adults.

Reentry into the community or long-term supervised program. Transitional living is not an end in itself. It should lead to a long-term living situation that is appropriate to the level of independence that the client has achieved. For clients who are successfully able to improve their independence capabilities and to adapt to their overall strengths and weaknesses, this situation might be independent living in the community. For clients who are not able to manage independently, this situation might be long-term supervision.

Evaluating Transitional Living Programs

With this definition as a background, the specific aspects of a transitional living program can be discussed. Ten areas have been identified that appear to be important in evaluation and managing a program. All of the areas are felt to be important in evaluating the program, although the relative importance of each area will vary as a function of individual preference. These areas were selected based on their importance from this writer's experience as a director of a transitional living program. No effort was made in integrate these areas with specific certification requirements suggested by organizations such as JCAH, CARF, or State Departments of Health.

1. Location. As with any service establishment, location is an important factor in program operation. The transitional living program should be integrated into the general community in order to encourage the client's involvement in the community. This means that the clients in the residence should be able to reach, independently, the community commercial and recreational resources. In this way, it is hoped that the client will learn skills that will enable him or her to use community resources in that community or another community.

2. Physical Plant. The transitional living program should be designed to foster a feeling of independence and wellness. Therefore, a home-like rather than an institutional environment is preferred. The furnishings, bedrooms, bathrooms, and kitchen areas should all reflect this atmosphere. Clients should be encouraged and entitled to add individualized touches to the residence to increase their sense of creativity and identity.

3. Supervision and behavior guidelines. Supervision is needed to help clients structure their activities but should not be so restrictive as to inhibit the clients' ability to take individual responsibility. The transitional living program is designed to approximate independent living. Therefor supervisory staff should be prepared to handle a wide range of behaviors that might occur. Supervision should have clear behavior guidelines that reward individual responsibility and encourage support among clients. Details for managing the following areas should be in writing and available to all staff and clients: chores and responsibilities on the unit, money management, off campus privileges, sexual relationships, drug and alcohol use, automobile use, pets, vacation time, curfew, and disciplinary action. Modifications of these guidelines should be a joint effort of the staff and the clients. Families evaluating a facility should ask to see sample behavior plans and guidelines that are in writing.

4. Program. The transitional living program must incorporate and balance the varied needs of the clients. Several issues are important to consider within this area.

a. organized activity vs. free time: Head injured individuals require structure but it is also important to evaluate and develop their ability to use free time. Organized activities should have a purpose that is pertinent to the client's needs rather than added just to fill time. Such activities would include educational groups that provide essential independent living information about community resources, safety, nutrition and sexuality; recreational activities that expose clients to new skills or leisure options; or daily living responsibilities of meal preparation and hygiene. These activities should be balanced with free time in which staff are available to clients but are not providing organized activities to them.

b. rehabilitation therapy vs. independent living: Clients at the transitional living stage have a greater need for activities that train them to live away from a rehabilitation center than for continued rehabilitation therapy. The transitional living program should reflect this emphasis. The need for continued rehabilitation therapy must be carefully scrutinized to see if it will truly help the client in a way that will make a difference in a living or working situation. This issue is also discussed under vocational programming.

c. psychological therapy: Psychological stress plays an increasingly large part in a client's adjustment to the head injury with time. It is crucial that psychological therapy be a major component of the treatment program. Both individual and group therapy may be beneficial. In addition, the group atmosphere of the residence should be designed to encourage social support and sharing that will facilitate the progress of psychotherapy.

5. Medical Care. The medical needs of the clients at the transitional stage of rehabilitation differ from their needs at other stages of care. Often, clients have become dependent on medical care to a greater extent than the individual in mainstream society. Therefore, the goal of medical care in the transitional living program should be to prepare the individual for using community resources such as a family doctor or a neighborhood pharmacy, rather than relying on the transitional living program care. The program should also include the opportunity for clients to learn to evaluate and manage minor medical emergencies. Self-medication should be an option for appropriate clients. The facility should have contact with area physicians, dentists, pharmacies and medical equipment suppliers that clients may contact on their own.

6. Vocational. The extent to which a head injured individual is able to do some type of productive work has a large impact on that individual's ability to live independently and to attain psychological independence. Vocational services should be a key part of a transitional program and should include evaluation, counseling, training and placement. In keeping with the philosophy of transitional living, such vocational services should be integrated into the community at large rather than facility based. There must, however, be close communication between the transitional program and the vocational service center. Several other areas are important to consider.

a. prevocational activity: Not all clients are ready for vocational activity. Yet, these clients may benefit from some work-related activity to ease their entry into formal vocational programs. The transitional living program should offer prevocational programs for these clients. This may be in the transitional residence or in the community.

b. sheltered employment: Sheltered employment workshops have acquired an association with the retarded and psychiatric population that make people wary of them for head injured individuals. Yet, these environments offer the supervision and organized work activities that are needed for head injured adults seeking to return to work. Therefore, it is important that families carefully examine the sheltered workshops that are included in a transitional program to find out if these programs are specifically designed for the head injured adult. It may be helpful to ask how many head injured people the workshop has handled and what were the vocational outcomes of these people.

c. cognitive retraining: Cognitive retraining at the transitional living stage should be specifically directed to the individual's vocational needs rather than to simply train general cognitive skills. The cognitive retraining therapist needs to be in contact with the vocational counselor and vocational training site to truly integrate cognitive and vocational work.

7. Meals and Personal Care. These are important activities of independent living that a client must learn to handle each day. The transitional program should provide the client with the opportunity to learn and master these skills. Personal care should be the responsibility of the client. Shopping, meal preparation, and clean-up should be the responsibility of clients with instruction and supervision from staff.

8. Family involvement and Communication. Families and other interested friends should be actively involved in the client's program. It is essential that family support for the program be gained if it is to succeed. The nature of the involvement should be formal, through conferences and phone calls, and informal, through visits and family participation in the program's leisure events. A system of regular communication between staff and family should exist and be explained to families before the client is admitted. Moreover, it will be beneficial to designate one person as responsible for communicating with the family, although all individuals at the transitional living program should be available within their means to the family.

9. Goals and Discharge Planning. The goals and programming of the transitional living program differ markedly from inpatient care. The program should have a means of defining short-term and long-term goals and a mechanism for judging progress toward these goals in order to reach discharge. An estimated length of stay and projected discharge date for a client should be provided at any point in time in the program. Perhaps most important in this area is that the client should be actively involved in the process of setting goals and evaluating progress. Whereas at inpatient care stages, goals are set by the team without the patient present, at the transitional stage, the treatment planning should be a joint staff-client effort. In this way, the client's individual responsibility is further developed.

10. Costs. The cost of the program should reflect that the transitional living program, as defined here, is significantly different from inpatient care. The living arrangements are more residential and the program emphasizes paraprofessional care with vocational training, rather than intensive medical rehabilitation. In evaluating cost, it is important to look at the total figure and to consider what that fee includes and what charges are extra.

Summary and Conclusions

The transitional living program provides a unique service within the continuum of rehabilitation services. The goal of the present paper has been to clarify the purpose and program content of transitional living programs. The ten areas discussed provide a framework for families to evaluate programs, and for professionals who manage programs to consider.

For families and head injured individuals who are considering a transitional program the following recommendations are offered. Visit the facility and review the program with these ten areas in mind, as well as any others that seem important to you. Speak to staff and clients, and if possible observe the program in action. Sometimes a potential client may be able to join the program for a meal. This can be an effective, yet informal, way of learning about the program. Ask to see written information about the program guidelines, schedules and fees. Take notes and try to get a sense about how the program handles visitors. This may be a clue to how they will handle their clients.

The successful graduate of a transitional living program should be ready for some type of independent living in the community. This may be totally independent living or a more independent setting such as a supervised group home or apartment. Those clients who have learned that they are not able to manage independently may leave the transitional living program for a more highly supervised long-term living situation. Regardless of the client's outcome, transitional living should not lead to discharge to another rehabilitation program. An effective transitional living program should be a decision point for the client, the family and the staff about the client's independent living potential. This is precisely why transitional living should play such and important part in the rehabilitation of the head injured.

The concept of transitional living that has been presented here may exclude programs that consider themselves to be transitional in nature, and may include others that do not consider themselves to be transitional. It is for this reason that the area has been discussed in such detail in this paper. Programs that do not fall into this concept of transitional living may be better considered independent living programs, long-term living programs or high-level inpatient rehabilitation programs. Each of these categories also needs the clarification that has been given to the area of transitional living in this paper. It is hoped that the issues raised here will stimulate a closer examination of all head injury programs. Only in this way can a more comprehensive catalog of services to the head injured be compiled, one that avoids ambiguity and overlap and is helpful to families and head injured adults.

Chapter 30

Hiring the Head Injured: What to Expect

The brain controls far more human capabilities than the average person recognizes. An insult to the brain can be responsible for a wide range of cognitive and physical deficits. However, an employer can understand the physical limitations much more easily than the cognitive deficits because physical deficits are more obvious. The cognitive problems are not as easily recognized.

When an individual receives a head injury that does not break the skull, the brain vibrates back and forth within the skull and often suffers bruising and shearing. Frequently, there is generalized damage to both hemispheres of the brain and sometimes one side is more affected than the other. If the insult is an open head injury, the effects are usually much more localized to the side that was hit. If the damage was due to lack of oxygen to the brain (hypoxia or anoxia) or some type of infectious process such as meningitis or encephalitis, one can also expect generalized damage to both hemispheres.

From this simplistic description, one can conclude that damage to the brain can lead to cognitive problems that might affect job efficiency. The following deficits are described in detail in order to prepare you for possible problems and to provide you with techniques to avoid or at least minimize the impact. It is possible that an employee may display all of these deficits, but on the other hand only one or two may be evident.

Excerpted from *Hiring the Head Injured: What to Expect*, copyright 1989 HDI Publishers, P.O. Box 131401, Houston, TX, 77219; reprinted with permission. To order the complete booklet or to obtain a free catalogue of available materials call (800) 321-7037.

Memory Deficits

Nearly 40% of the head injured experience some degree of memory loss. A memory deficit may take many different forms and is a component of other cognitive deficits. This problem may occur when the employee attempts to immediately recall specific information (short term memory). A long term memory deficit is evident when the employee attempts to retrieve information presented to him at an earlier time (hours or days).

Memory deficits are affected by and affect auditory comprehension, new learning, sequencing and problem-solving skills which will be discussed later.

Resolutions for Memory Deficits:

1. Be aware of the employee's compensating techniques and encourage him to use them (e.g., notebook, calendar, tape recorder).

2. When giving or requesting information from the employee, do so in writing as well as verbally.

3. Provide as many environmental aids as possible to assist in memory for location of items, appointments and schedules (e.g., labeling items, bulletin boards, calendars).

Problem Solving Deficits

Problem-solving difficulties can range from minor to severe. Minor problem-solving difficulties can include not being as timely in the decision making process and experiencing mild difficulty with complex business related decisions. Severe deficits in problem-solving tasks can result in not being able to complete even simple tasks requiring problem-solving and, consequently, not being able to continue with that job. It is feasible that a person with severe problem-solving difficulties may be a "danger" in some work situations.

Resolutions for Problem-Solving Deficits:

1. For safety reasons, be aware of the possibility of problem-solving difficulties in your employee.

2. If it suits both of your needs, remove the time restraints from certain job-related tasks.

3. Respect the employee's awareness of limitations and accommodate change of responsibilities if at all possible.

Lack of Initiation

The employee may experience difficulty in the initiation of work or work-related tasks. This lack of initiation may take different forms. The problem may surface as a lack of motivation for return to work or for consideration of other work alternatives.

If an employee proceeds past this point and returns to the work situation, this lack of initiation may surface in other ways. Your employee may experience considerable difficulty beginning a work task. He may assemble all the items he needs, talk about the task, ask you questions about the job, but not get started. If he is able to start, he may not be able to move from one step to the next without confusion and delay or the need to ask more questions.

Employees who demonstrate a lack of initiation often will become "talkers" even though they were not excessive "talkers" before. They may talk their way through situations to avoid the decisions involved in initiating the tasks.

Resolutions for Lack of Initiation:

1. Establish a set of time lines for completion of work tasks.

2. Attempt to assign a series of small tasks, one at a time, in lieu of one big project.

3. If the employee is bogged down in the task, help him establish where he is in the job sequence.

4. Make job expectations explicit at the beginning of the task and reiterate expectations as needed.

Cognitive Inflexibility

Cognitive inflexibility may lead to more difficulty in the work situation than any other cognitive deficit. Cognitive inflexibility refers to the employee's inability to use divergent thinking skills. It is quite possible that your employee will make up his mind in regard to a work-related situation and not be able to consider the alternatives because he will be unable to analyze a situation from more than one perspective. In working with others, this can lead to this employee being short-tempered, argumentative and shortsighted in the decision-making and work-related process.

Resolutions for Cognitive Inflexibility:

1.   Define job role and expectations upon hiring. Explain the organization structure and chain of command for grievances. Make it clear to employee how he fits into the organizational structure.

2.   If at all possible, structure the job so that it does not include numerous small divergent tasks, but rather a series of well defined related tasks.

3.   Attempt to steer this employee clear of potential high pressure controversial situations.

Lack of Concentration (Distractibility)

The employee may experience difficulty sorting out relevant from irrelevant information. He may be unable to always screen out surrounding distractions and concentrate on the task at hand. This applies to both visual and auditory information.

An employee may appear to be disinterested in his work or your conversation, or to be a "busy body," eavesdropping on other's conversations.

Resolutions for Distractibility:

1.   Help the employee to unclutter his work environment to lessen distractions.

2.   Isolate the employee from as much visual and auditory distraction as possible.

3. With the employee's agreement, perhaps an understanding supervisor or co-worker could give a "sign" to the employee when he seems to have wandered off task.

Auditory Comprehension Deficit

An employee may have no difficulty with his hearing, but the understanding of what is being heard may be impaired.

The employee may have difficulty with long, complex sentences, or he may focus on the less important aspects of a conversation and not remember the important details.

As a result of this auditory comprehension difficulty, an employee may misinterpret information or instructions, resulting in errors and confusion.

Resolutions for Auditory Comprehension Deficit:

1. Keep oral instructions very clear and concise.

2. Accompany oral instructions with written instructions for reference, if possible.

3. Telephone messages should be written and repeated for verification while the caller is still on the telephone.

Sequencing Deficits

The term *sequencing* refers to the ordering of information into a series of steps. This information could be, for instance, directions for a task or numbers/letters in a series.

A sequencing deficit can be observed from the employee who has problems organizing and ordering his activities for the day to the employee who has trouble recalling a telephone number in the proper sequence.

Resolutions for Sequencing Deficits:

1. Frustration and error can be lessened by having step-by-step directions written in concise terms for use as a checklist.

277

2. Maps and diagrams may also be useful in certain positions. Many times visual aids prove very helpful, especially when combined with auditory instructions or physical movements.

Lag in Response Time

Although the employee may be able to resume his previous work activities, it may take him longer to perform them. It may take longer for this person to perform individual activities, even though they were once automatic responses. Difficulty may also be observed as the person is required to shift from one activity to another during the work day, causing a delay in the daily schedule.

Delays in response time may also create potential safety hazards. The employee may not respond as quickly as necessary in a dangerous situation. Safety considerations will be more relevant, of course, in some fields than others (e.g., heavy construction, driving, etc.).

Resolutions for Lag in Response Time:

1. Consider if the job is appropriate; does it represent a potential safety hazard to the employee or others?

2. Consider decreasing production demands in the beginning of reentry into the work environment, increasing demand as the employee becomes familiar with routine and responses become more automatic.

3. Help employee set up "time checks" during the day to see if production is following schedule. He may be able to monitor these himself or he may need assistance in the beginning.

Disorganization

Prior to the head injury, your employee may have been punctual, organized, and complete in his work. You may observe a difference in this behavior. Your once neat employee may have a scattered and disorganized office. His office may be representative of his entire organizational system. In order to be organized, a person must be able to integrate a number of functions and assimilate information in an orderly manner. A person with a head injury may experience difficulty with this high level cognitive skill. The result is often difficulty with finding papers, relaying information, and meeting deadlines, thus decreasing the effectiveness at work.

Resolutions for Disorganization:

1. Recognize the compensating behaviors of lists, calendars and stick-up reminders and encourage employee to use them.

2. Maintain sense of organization and order around the work environment.

3. Recognize the fact that organization is a higher level cognitive function, and that a breakdown in any of those skills (i.e., memory, sequencing, problem-solving) may lead to organizational difficulties.

New Learning Problems

New learning difficulties may occur as a result of memory, sequencing, lack of initiation or organizational difficulties. As an employee returns to work, he may soon be able to work back into his old job routine because he is using old learning of automatic tasks. Where he may experience the most difficulty is in learning a new job related skill. The memory deficit may prevent him from recalling the new procedure, the sequencing deficit may hinder him from accomplishing the task in the correct order, and his inability to initiate and organize the task may prevent him from using this newly acquired job skill in the work setting. His overall difficulty with initiation may hinder him from taking on new responsibilities at work.

Resolutions for New Learning Problems:

1. Before introducing the employee to a new job task, make sure he is comfortable in the old job.

2. Introduce new job tasks in small steps if at all possible and give the employee a new task only when the old has been mastered.

Language Deficits

Language deficits may be of either a written or verbal nature. On a verbal level, you may note that it takes the employee longer to respond, his sentences may be shorter, or he may use many words to express a very simple thought. On some occasions, you may note that he is not able to come up with exactly the right word.

Written language problems parallel spoken language problems and may be complicated by fine motor difficulties. At times, even writing a simple memo may prove difficult for the employee. Writing is a complicated task which integrates the cognitive skills of organization, sequencing and memory into a graphically presentable communication. The complexity of this and other language tasks should not be overlooked.

Resolutions for Language Deficits:

1. Be aware that certain language deficits will not improve, thus the employee is using compensating techniques in order to perform his work-related tasks. If you can, identify them. Encourage them.

2. If at all possible, allow the employee to establish and work within his own time lines.

3. If at all possible, allow the employee to establish his own system of interoffice communication, either written or oral.

Perceptual Problems

Visual perception relates to the use of visual information, but does not relate to how well a person sees. An employee with perfect eyesight may have problems with eye/hand coordination, confuse similar sizes or shapes of objects, or misjudge distances.

Visual perception may also interfere with a person's driving skills.

Resolutions for Perceptual Problems:

1. Consider whether visual perception problems present a possible hindrance to production or are a more serious threat, as in unsafe driving.

2. Encourage the employee to use compensating techniques, such as labeling for size on tools and parts. This helps eliminate visual "guessing."

3. Pressure and overstimulation from visual information may increase problems. If possible, lessen demands and hurried schedules while encouraging the employee to simplify his work area by getting rid of unnecessary equipment and belongings.

Conclusion

The vast majority of workers in our society develop an occupational identity which becomes a paramount part of their self-concept and sense of identity. Job identification is not restricted to the white collar professions, or related to status in the community, as more often than not the stone mason or construction worker takes as much pride in his work as does the attorney or surgeon. When a head injury occurs, the person experiencing the trauma may experience social as well as vocational upheaval. Deficits in both social and work skills generally become evident and job performance declines. Fatigue, diminished self-control, inflexible attitudes, distractibility, inability to accept authority are all behaviors which can make employment difficult.

Statistics compiled by the U.S. Commission on Civil Rights, 1983, indicate that the unemployment rate for adults with disabilities is 50 percent for males and 76 percent for females. Moreover, the majority of those handicapped who do have jobs are underemployed, with 30 percent living at or below the poverty level. The brain injured worker, of course, is included in these statistics. Employment or reemployment of the brain injured is a serious problem and there are no easy solutions. Unsuccessful attempts to include head injured workers in their personnel ranks have brought frustration and disappointment to the employer and psychological damage to the employee, as feelings of failure, emptiness and inferiority often develop with job rejection. Most job placement specialists who have worked with the brain injured can easily cite examples of failure. In one case, a brain injured client who was interviewing for a position on a dairy farm lay down and fell asleep on the farm manager's front lawn while job responsibilities were being discussed. Or, there was the client who continually took the newspaper off the cafeteria tray of the company president. These types of behaviors should have been corrected prior to attempted placement. A most notable example was the client who, during the first fifteen minutes of employment, charged into the corporation president's office with a cardboard box he had just completed stapling and slammed it on the desk demanding that the president inspect his work. Needless to say, these were not successful placements, but may have been if the proper steps had been taken prior to placement.

In order to resolve these perplexing problems, the following could assist the potential worker in making the transition back to employment:

1. *Cognitive Therapy*: This type of therapy can assist the client in becoming aware of and accepting the need for vocational change and in developing a rational plan to achieve vocational independence.

2. *Work Evaluation*: This is especially important as the evaluation will not only help determine appropriate vocational areas, but will also identify behaviors which could be detrimental to maintaining employment. Situational assessment is an evaluation tool which can be invaluable in identifying problem areas. In order to insure success, the client must be encouraged to assume a major role in planning his or her vocational future.

3. *Work Adjustment Training*: This should be a consideration if behavioral problems are not initially correctable and a longer period is required to prepare the individual for work. Coping skills can be developed, work competencies upgraded, endurance levels increased and the client generally reoriented to the world of work.

4. *Job placement*: This should occur only when the client is psychologically and physically ready for work and is strongly motivated toward this undertaking. Placement should be in a job that the client is capable of performing. Both management and the immediate supervisor or foreman should be made aware of potential problems, including inappropriate behaviors, that may occur. In some instances, co-workers can also be informed with the hope that they will be supportive and the employee will be made to feel part of the team. It is general

knowledge that those individuals that lose jobs do not do so because they cannot perform the required work. Jobs are generally lost because of extenuating circumstances such as no transportation, family problems, failure to accept authority on the job, dissatisfaction with job assignment, etc. Potential problems should be identified, dealt with and resolved prior to attempting job placement.

5. *Family Involvement*: It is important that family members and friends provide support and take an active part in the decision making process. Many head injured clients feel out of place even among familiar employment surroundings and may resist leaving the comfortable familiarity of home and family. He may resist the vocational reentry plan, especially if family members and friends place little value upon the established goals. Loss of support from family can cause him to suffer anxiety, depression, and a loss of motivation; thus, no vocational adjustment will be made.

6. *Counseling Services*: Ongoing counseling is essential for the purpose of assisting the client to maintain work effectiveness, reduce job-related stress and help resolve personal problems that could have a detrimental effect on job performance. "Whole Person" rehabilitation should be emphasized.

Education programs should also be initiated or expanded upon as there is a need for greater awareness and sensitivity by the public and industry toward this disability group. Course work offered both on a college or even high school level and in adult basic education programs should be considered.

The education of labor union leaders, industry leaders and, in some cases, even job placement specialists can also enhance the employability of this group. Man validates himself through work and the brain injured worker is no exception. Employment enhances both independence and self-esteem and these are essential ingredients in the rehabilitation of our brain injured population.

Let's give these individuals a second chance.

References

Bond, M.R. "Assessment of the Psychological Outcome of Severe Head Injury." *Acta Neurologica* 34, 1976, 57-70.

Corthell, D. & Tooman, M. *Rehabilitation of TBI* (Traumatic Brain Injury). Menomonie, Wisconsin: Research and Training Center, Stout Vocational Rehabilitation Institute, 1985.

DeBoskey, D. & Morin, K. A. *"How to Handle" Manual for Families of the Brain Injured*. Tampa General Rehabilitation Center, 1986.

Dunse, C., Lindeman, J. & Lowe, L. *Behavior Management: A Facility-Wide Approach*. Tampa General Rehabilitation Center, 1985.

Howard, M. & Bleiberg, J. *A Manual of Behavior Management Strategies for Traumatically Brain Injured Adults*. Rehabilitation Institute of Chicago, 1983.

Levin, H.S., Benton, A.L. & Crossman, R.G. *Neurobehavioral Consequences of Closed Head Injury*. New York: Oxford University Press, 1982.

Lezak, M. "The Problem of Assessing Executive Functions." *International Journal of Psychology*. 17, 1982, 281-297.

Rimel, R.W., Giordani, B., Barth, J.T., Boll, T.J. & Jane, J.A. "Disability Caused by Minor Head Injury." *Neurosurgery*. 1981, 9, 221-228.

Weddell, R., Oddy, M. & Jenkins, D. "Social Adjustment After Rehabilitation: A Two-Year Follow-up of Patients with Severe Head Injury." *Psychological Medicine*. 10, 1980, 257-263.

Chapter 31

What Private Insurance Coverages Apply to People with Traumatic Brain Injuries?

Brain injuries often result in astronomical medical bills, particularly for individuals with severe injuries who spend a long time in the hospital and in rehabilitation. Hospital care for people with brain injuries is paid for by a wide variety of insurance policies, depending on the origin of the accident. People injured in motor vehicle accidents, the most common cause of brain injuries, may be covered by no-fault or automobile liability insurance. Workers' compensation covers job-related injuries. Health insurance may cover medical care for injuries related to falls, sports accidents, and other causes.

However, significant gaps exist in the insurance safety net. There are a large number of uninsured drivers on the roads, averaging about 10 to 20 percent in most states. (See figure 31. 1 for a state-by-state breakdown.) More than 35 million Americans have no health insurance. That number will continue to increase as premiums skyrocket and put coverage out of reach of many working Americans. The group most at-risk for brain injuries—men between the ages of 15 and 24—is also the group least likely to have insurance (see figure 31.2). A shocking 71.2 percent of all people without health insurance—approximately 25.2 million people—are under the age of 34. The state and federal governments ultimately bear the responsibility for people who have no insurance through Medicaid or uncompensated care.

Even people with adequate private insurance face problems. Third-party insurance coverage often does not apply to long-term

Excerpted from *What Legislators Need to Know about Traumatic Brain Injury*, ©1993 National Council of State Legislatures, reprinted with permission.

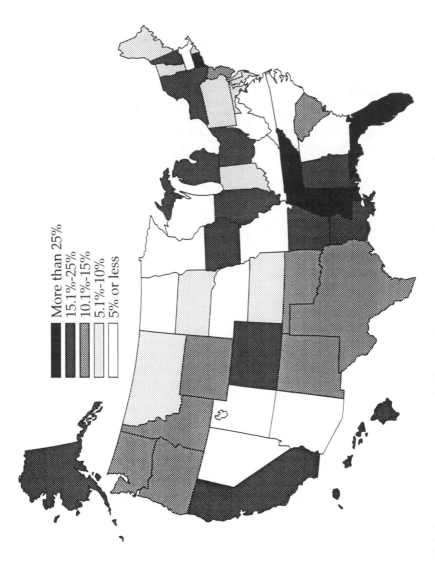

Figure 31.1. *Average percentage of drivers who are uninsured (by state). Source: Best's Insurance Management Reports, Release No. 5, February 26, 1990.*

More than 25%
15.1%–25%
10.1%–15%
5.1%–10%
5% or less

rehabilitation, long-term care or community support services so critical to people recovering from a brain injury.

Following is a list of private insurance policies and gaps that exist for people with brain injuries.

Workers Compensation

Work-related injuries, including vehicle accidents during work hours, are covered by workers' compensation. The full cost of this insurance is covered by the employer. Every state requires workers' compensation, and each state has its own laws. One of the most comprehensive of all insurance coverages, workers' compensation covers medical care, extended rehabilitation, and partial wage replacement, typically two-thirds of the employee's average weekly wage. Some states provide retraining and job placement services when the injured employee is not able to return to work. Workers' compensation offers the greatest opportunity for a person with a brain injury to regain a full and active life. However, statistically, not many brain injuries are caused on the job.

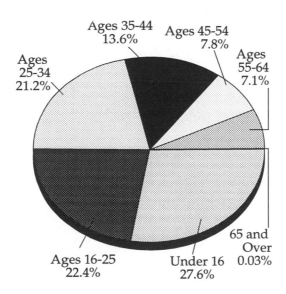

Figure 31.2. Percentage of those not covered by health insurance. Source: U.S. Bureau of Census and "Struggling to Save Our Kids," Fortune, August 10, 1992, p. 37.

Health Insurance

Health insurance policies vary widely in terms of deductibles, co-insurance, life-time maximums, exclusions, and coverage. Often there is no coverage for home health care, outpatient services, and long-term care services. Some hospitals limit the number of hospital days, skilled nursing facility days, or the number of therapy sessions. This can pose a financial problem for people with brain injuries who require extensive services.

Health insurance policies rarely specify benefits for rehabilitation. In catastrophic situations, companies negotiate an "extra contractual agreement." This is an agreement among the payer, the provider of services, and the insured client that the third party payer will reimburse for certain services, such as rehabilitation, even though the services do not qualify for reimbursement under strictly defined contract provisions. There are usually time limitations (at least 90 days), with reporting, extensions, and termination requirements.

Because rehabilitation gains for people with brain injuries often occur slowly, traditional insurance cost containment mechanisms, such as length of stay reviews, may in some cases result in early discharge to less costly environments that may be inappropriate and actually delay the recovery process. Other practices used by health insurers which adversely affect patients with traumatic brain injuries, include: the denial of benefits for cognitive rehabilitation and neuro-behavioral therapies, which are deemed by insurers to be "investigational or experimental" or "not medically necessary"; the classification of treatment therapies as "maintenance services," leading to denial of benefits; the establishment of unrealistic annual limits for specific services, such as mental health and psychiatric services; and the exclusion of coverage for durable medical equipment, other assistive technology devices and services, and prescription drugs.

The Consolidated Omnibus Budget Reconciliation Act (COBRA)

People who suffer severe brain injuries can no longer work and must confront the problem of what to do when the health insurance through their employer expires. COBRA, implemented by Congress in 1986, requires employers with a health benefits program to allow their employees to continue health coverage for 18 months when they terminate employment. The employee must pay the premium. In other circumstances the coverage can be continued for 36 months. An amendment to COBRA in 1989 extends the 18 month term to 29 months for individuals determined disabled by Social Security, at which time the individual would qualify for Medicare. Many Social Security disability determinations take longer than 29 months, thereby severely limiting this approach as a reliable source of health care benefits.

Health Maintenance Organizations and Preferred Provider Organizations

In a health maintenance organization (HMO), a provider group agrees to accept a fixed monthly premium payment for an individual enrolled in the organization in return for providing a predetermined medical care benefit package to the purchaser. A preferred provider organization (PPO) is an arrangement between a medical provider guaranteeing a certain discounted rate for services and an insuring group/company guaranteeing a patient case load in return. In a PPO, the person can see any doctor but is offered a financial incentive to seek care from participating doctors.

HMOs and PPOs are often very limited in their coverage of acute and long term rehabilitation services for the catastrophically injured. Federal law requires only those HMOs that are federally qualified to provide 60 days of rehabilitation care. There is evidence that many of them are not even providing that amount. With the growth of HMOs and PPOs across the country, this poses an increasing problem for people with traumatic brain injuries. Some HMOs and PPOs are looking into re-insurance to provide coverage for people who suffer from catastrophic illnesses.

Re-Insurance

Re-insurance is the insurance company's insurer. A primary insurance company can purchase a contract that requires the re-insurance company to cover health care costs above a predetermined threshold. This allows the original health insurance company to protect itself from the risks of catastrophic injuries. Re-insurance companies have developed expertise in dealing with traumatic brain injury because of its catastrophic nature.

Self-Insurance

Many large corporations choose to self-insure. This means that the organization directly bears the risk and cost of providing health care coverage rather than purchasing coverage from an insurance company. Most of these employers contract with insurance companies to administer claims. Consequently, employees are often unaware that their employer is, in fact, acting as their health care provider. At present, a majority of insured persons under 65 years old have their health insurance through self-insured employers. Many self-insured organizations protect themselves from catastrophic loss by purchasing reinsurance or stop-loss insurance, a type of coverage available from commercial liability carriers that covers losses or claims above a certain stated amount.

The federal Employee Retirement Income and Security Act (ERISA) limits the ability of state government to regulate self-insured organizations. This means that over half of all insured Americans under 65 are not protected by any state regulation, such as minimum benefit laws, unfair trade practices, or a state insurance fund to back up insurance plans that become financially insolvent.

Automobile Liability Insurance

In this traditional type of insurance, car owners buy insurance to protect themselves from lawsuits in case they cause an accident that injures someone else. A major problem with this form of insurance is that the driver or the person found to be at fault is not covered, nor are passengers in the vehicle at fault or injured pedestrians. These people must rely on their private health insurance. Another problem with liability insurance is that, in many cases, the injured parties must wait for several years for the damages to be settled in court. This is especially true of people involved in single motor vehicle accidents. At the end of the wait, the injured party may or may not get a large settlement. If the driver at fault has no assets and little insurance, the injured party might get nothing. People with traumatic brain injury cannot afford to wait for years for a settlement, since rehabilitation therapies are most effective immediately following the onset of injury.

Uninsured Motorist Insurance Coverage

In states that do not offer no-fault insurance, consumers can purchase uninsured motorist insurance coverage. This protects people injured by a driver who is uninsured or flees the scene of the accident. The coverage will also apply if a person is struck by a driver who is not carrying enough insurance to cover the costs of the injuries.

No-Fault Insurance

No-fault benefits are paid through the individual's own insurance company, regardless of who is at fault. The no-fault concept was designed to provide prompt payment for lost wages and medical expenses as they are incurred and to eliminate long delays in recovering economic losses in court.

At present, the District of Columbia and 14 states have no-fault insurance: Colorado, Connecticut, District of Columbia, Florida, Hawaii, Kansas, Kentucky, Massachusetts, Michigan, Minnesota, New Jersey, New York, North Dakota, Pennsylvania, and Utah. An additional 12 states are add-on states, meaning that no-fault coverage is available, but consumers can pursue a third party claim through the tort system. Those states are Arkansas, Delaware, Maryland, Nevada, New Hampshire, Oregon, South Carolina, South Dakota, Texas, Virginia, Washington, and Wisconsin. In the states where parties are able to sue, no-fault has limited effectiveness, and the system exists as a kind of hybrid of liability grafted onto no-fault, with none of the advantages.

For no-fault insurance not to result in higher premiums, the number of lawsuits must be restricted. However, most of the no-fault states have watered-down versions allowing victims to sue after a certain dollar threshold in medical bills is reached, ranging from a low of $400 in Connecticut to a high of $4,000 in Minnesota. Other states have a descriptive threshold, allowing victims to sue if they meet certain criteria, such as a severe, permanent disability. Active lobbying by the trial lawyers associations has contributed to weak no-fault laws.

Most no-fault states place a cap—$50,000, for example—on the amount paid for medical care and rehabilitation. This will not begin to cover the astronomical costs involved in severe brain injuries. Michigan is the only state that offers unlimited medical coverage. Widely acknowledged to have the best no-fault insurance plan in the country, Michigan limits the right to sue. Car owners must buy coverage that reimburses them for their own medical and rehabilitation expenses and for lost wages. It also covers family members hurt in car accidents even if they are in someone else's car or traveling out of state. Michigan's law pays medical and rehabilitation expenses for the life of the victim.

In Michigan, the results of rehabilitation are dramatic. In the mid 1980s, the Automobile Club Insurance Association in Michigan, a major auto insurer in that state, had 623 cases of catastrophically injured victims on its books. Of those, only 15 were in nursing homes.

—by Barbara Wright

Chapter 32

What Federal Assistance Is Available?

Many federal programs exist, but have not been adequately tapped, by persons who are disabled due to a brain injury. With careful planning, states can put together a system to make the most of federal support and stretch state dollars. The federal programs listed here are divided into categories of health care, home- and community-based services, housing, job training and placement, income support, and education.

Health Care

Medicaid

Medicaid is a federally matched, state-run medical assistance program for eligible low-income persons. The program often is referred to as Title XIX because of its authorizing legislation. The federal government establishes guidelines for the program and pays a portion of each state's medical assistance payments, ranging from a low of 50 percent to a high of 80 percent.

States are required to include nine mandated services and have the option of covering an additional 34 services. Optional services that states may use for people with traumatic brain injuries include personal care services, comprehensive day rehabilitation, and targeted

Excerpted from *What Legislators Need to Know about Traumatic Brain Injury*, ©1993 National Council of State Legislatures, reprinted with permission.

case management. Federal Medicaid restrictions require covered services to be available statewide and to be of equal amount, duration, and scope across all groups of Medicaid-eligible persons. Unlike other state plan options, targeted case management can be applied to a specific subpopulation of potentially eligible recipients, such as people with traumatic brain injuries, and does not have to be offered statewide.

Medicare

Medicare is a federal health insurance program covering services to persons aged 65 and older, persons with end stage renal disease (ESRD) of any age, and to adults under 65 and their offspring who have been receiving Social Security Disability benefits for at least 24 months. Medicare has two parts. Part A is hospital insurance and helps pay for inpatient hospital care and related care provided by a certified skilled nursing facility or by home health care and hospice care professionals. Part B is medical insurance and covers physician services, outpatient hospital care, and lab services. There is a monthly premium for Part B coverage, which is either billed quarterly or deducted from the individual's Social Security check. There is also an annual deductible and a 20 percent co-insurance charge. In addition, the individual is responsible for paying the difference between the Medicare-approved amount and the provider's actual bill.

Civilian Health and Medical Program of the Uniformed Services (CHAMPUS)

This health benefit program for the uniformed services has a program that helps pay for attendant care for seriously handicapped persons who are dependents of active duty members. CHAMPUS also helps pay for durable medical equipment, such as wheel chairs. A co-payment is required.

Technology-Related Assistance for Individuals with Disabilities Act of 1988 (P.L. 100-497)

This act is intended to expand the availability of assistive technology services for people with disabilities, enabling them to live more independently. States may apply to the secretary of the Department of Education for three-year grants to provide training and assistance and to establish model consumer-responsive service delivery systems to help individuals with disabilities use technology or devices. Assistive technology and devices that may benefit people with brain injury include wheelchairs, environmental control systems, and computers to serve as memory aids. More information may be obtained from the RESNA Technical Assistance Project (see Chapter 37).

Home- and Community-Based Services

Medicaid Home- and Community-Based Services (HCBS) Waiver

Although originally intended to provide mainly medical services, Medicaid dollars may be used for a variety of nonmedical home- and community-based support services for recipients who otherwise would need more costly institutional care.

Medicaid Model Waiver Option

This waiver allows a state to cover optional services that are not otherwise in its Medicaid state plan for a small targeted group of persons, such as children who are ventilator-dependent. Up to 200 people may be served at one time.

Rehabilitation Act of 1973 (P.L. 93-112)

Known primarily for vocational rehabilitation, this act also contains Title VII, parts A and B, pertaining to independent living. Part A offers case services for severely disabled people who do not have job potential. This includes personal care attendants. Part B sets up independent living centers serving people with all disabilities. More than 400 of these programs exist across the country. The centers do not provide housing but offer a wide range of services that could benefit people with traumatic brain injury. These include housing referral, training of personal assistants, training in independent living skills, assistive technology, and peer counseling. The more people with traumatic brain injury make use of these centers, the more the centers will cater to their specific needs.

Housing

Department of Housing and Urban Development (HUD) Section 8 Rent Subsidies

People who earn up to 80 percent of the median income in their area are eligible for Section 8 rent subsidies. In many supported living programs, rent subsidies have proved to be a vital part of helping people with disabilities find affordable housing.

Section 811 Supportive Housing for People with Disabilities

This HUD program provides 100 percent direct federal loans for constructing, renovating or acquiring housing to serve people who are disabled.

Fair Housing Amendments Act of 1988 (FHAA) (P.L. 100-430)

The FHAA prohibits discrimination in the sale, rental, or financing of housing to persons with disabilities and also sets standards of accessibility for newly constructed multifamily housing.

Job Training and Placement

Americans with Disabilities Act of 1990 (ADA) (P.L. 101-336)

The ADA prohibits employers from discriminating against a qualified individual with a disability because of the disability. Employers who have 25 or more employees must make "reasonable accommodations" for people with disabilities. Starting in July 1994, employers who have between 15 and 25 employees will also be required to comply.

ADA Tax Credit

The Omnibus Budget Reconciliation Act of 1990 provides a small business tax credit for expenses associated with providing "reasonable accommodation" in employment or accessibility under the Americans with Disabilities Act. Businesses with gross receipts under $1 million or with 30 or fewer full-time employees may receive a credit equal to 50 percent of the "eligible access expenditures" between $250 and $10,250 that are incurred for the purpose of complying with ADA.

Targeted Jobs Tax Credit (TJTC)

An important incentive to encourage employers to hire people with disabilities, the TJTC allows employers to claim a tax credit of 40 percent of the first $6,000 of qualified wages per eligible employee, with a maximum credit of $2,400 per employee during the first year of employment.

Rehabilitation Act of 1973 (P.L. 93-112)

This state-federal match program, known in most states as the vocational rehabilitation program, helps people with mental or physical disabilities find jobs. Amendments in 1986 (P.L. 99-506) created Title VI, which recognizes that all people regardless of the nature or extent of their disability, should have the opportunity to work in competitive jobs in the community. Title VI establishes a new funding stream devoted solely to supported employment programs, although these funds represent only a small portion of the dollars states currently are spending on such programs. Title VI provides funds for a limited amount of time. One of the federal requirements for participation in the supported work program is that states provide long-term support to take over after the federal financial participation stops. State participation is particularly important for people with traumatic brain injury, who need vocational support longer than most people with disabilities. The Rehabilitation Act was reauthorized in 1992, with a special emphasis on competitive employment.

Job Training Partnership Act (JTPA) (P.L. 97-300)

The JTPA provides monies for job training for people who are economically disadvantaged. Persons with disabilities are targeted under the JTPA, and funds may be used to educate private employers as well as provide training and support services. In FY 1990, JTPA-sponsored services helped 31,301 adults and 37,073 youth with disabilities.

Income Support

Supplemental Security Income (SSI)

This 100 percent federally funded program provides income assistance to low-income elderly, blind, and disabled individuals. Eligibility is limited to people who are not capable of "substantial gainful employment." No restrictions are placed on how this money may be spent. As of January 1992, the benefit award was $422 for an individual and $633 for a couple living independently, and $281.34 for an individual and $422 for a couple living in a house with others. Upon reaching the age of 18, children become eligible based on their own financial picture, whether they are living at home or on their own. SSI automatically entitles the recipient to Medicaid in most states.

Many people who receive SSI would like to work but are afraid of losing their monthly payments and Medicaid coverage. Today, special Social Security work incentives offer these people ways to continue receiving benefits. Those include:

Section 1619 Work Incentives, Parts A and B. Section 1619 (a) allows beneficiaries to receive SSI cash payments even when earned income exceeds the substantial gainful activity level. Medicaid coverage is continued under Section 1619 (b).

Plan for Achieving Self-Sufficiency (PASS). Individuals receiving SSI are permitted to set aside income and/or resources to obtain occupational training or education, purchase occupational equipment, or establish a business. The income and resources set aside under the plan are excluded from the SSI income and resource test.

Impairment-related work expenses (IRWE). SSI recipients can deduct the costs of certain expenses from income. These expenses include: a personal care attendant in the home to help the disabled person bathe, dress, and prepare for work; the cost of structural modifications to a vehicle needed to get to work; the cost of a driver or taxicabs to get to work; and the cost for computers or other devices necessary to help the person with a brain injury do the job. This work incentive applies to people who receive SSDI as well.

Social Security Disability Income (SSDI)

SSDI provides monthly benefits to workers who have paid into the Social Security system for at least 10 quarters but are unable to continue working because of a physical or mental impairment. The program is funded totally by the federal government from payroll deductions. Recipients are eligible for Medicare benefits after two years. This is a problem for people with brain injuries since the crucial time for rehabilitation is immediately following the injury, and waiting two years could significantly affect a person's chances to lead a productive life.

SSDI is not based on need. Individuals can have assets and unearned income. The amount awarded to the injured party is calculated on the time the person has been employed, age at disability, the amount of money paid into the system, and the period of time the award is to be paid.

Workers in nonprofit organizations are covered under SSDI. Potentially, this means that persons working in sheltered workshops or supported employment and earning as little as $400 per quarter could qualify for disability insurance and be entitled to cash benefits, Medicare coverage, and retirement income.

Medical requirements for SSI and SSDI are strict, and only about one-fourth of the initial claims received each year are allowed. People with brain injuries may have difficulty qualifying for SSI and SSDI because Social Security has no separate code for traumatic brain injury. Cognitive disabilities may not be readily apparent after a brief interview. To counteract this problem, some head injury foundations and federally funded centers are training Social Security eligibility staff to recognize and understand people with traumatic brain injuries.

Food stamps and Aid to Families with Dependent Children (AFDC)

Food stamps and AFDC provide eligible persons who have mental and physical handicaps with resources needed to survive in the community. Food stamps are provided with federal funding to supplement consumer cash income. AFDC authorizes federal matching payments to states for providing aid and services to families with children who meet the state's eligibility criteria.

Education

Individuals with Disabilities Education Act (IDEA) (P.L. 101-476)

In 1990, Congress reauthorized the Education of the Handicapped Act and renamed it the Individuals with Disabilities Education Act. At that time, traumatic brain injury was added as a separate category under the definition of children with disabilities. IDEA guarantees that all children ages five to 21 who have handicapping conditions, including those with brain injury, be offered a free, appropriate education in the least restrictive environment.

Prevention

Centers for Disease Control

The National Center for Injury Prevention and Control in the Centers for Disease Control makes available to state and local health departments cooperative agreements and grants to fund surveillance systems (registries). The national center also funds comprehensive grants that include components of prevention and surveillance, such as registries. Since 1988 the center has funded 33 grants.

The National Center for Environmental Health in the Centers for Disease Control makes available to states disability prevention grants that address surveillance and prevention of traumatic brain injury, developmental disabilities, fetal alcohol syndrome, and other disabilities.

The National Highway Traffic Safety Administration (NHTSA)

NHTSA funds state highway safety offices in each of the 50 states to conduct highway and traffic safety education and enforcement programs.

—by Barbara Wright

Chapter 33

What Are States Doing to Provide Care for People with Traumatic Brain Injuries?

Innovative state and private nonprofit agency efforts demonstrate that quality, consumer-responsive services can help people with traumatic brain injuries live productive lives in the community. The programs discussed in this chapter include comprehensive statewide programs, home- and community-based services, housing, supported employment, education programs, and central registries for people with traumatic brain injury.

Comprehensive Services for People with Traumatic Brain Injury

Although no state has developed a completely comprehensive continuum of care addressing all service needs for people with brain injury, several states, notably Massachusetts and Minnesota, have created statewide systems that provide quality care for people with brain injuries. Other states, such as Missouri and Florida, have made special efforts to meet the needs of people with brain injuries.

Massachusetts

This state has made great strides towards developing comprehensive services for people with brain injuries through its Statewide Head

Excerpted from *What Legislators Need to Know about Traumatic Brain Injury*, ©1993 National Council of State Legislatures, reprinted with permission.

Injury Program (SHIP). The program is administered under the Independent Living Division of the Massachusetts Rehabilitation Commission. It is funded entirely with state funds. The budget for FY 1993 is $6.4 million and include the following services:

Case management. Five case managers, called case coordinators, help coordinate services for clients. Case managers are expected to develop knowledge and expertise in the field of brain injury. Case managers help identify each client's needs in areas such as supervised housing, vocational or pre-vocational services, transportation, specialized therapies, respite care, and recreational/leisure time activities. When clients are placed in a program, the case manager monitors their progress. For clients receiving multiple services, the case manager acts as the coordinator to prevent fragmentation and promote communication and coordination among all parties involved.

Day treatment. Five programs across the state are available to help the individuals with memory, concentration, initiation, independent living skills, work readiness, leisure management, and personal/social development.

Supported employment. Collaborating with the Massachusetts Rehabilitation Commission's Office of Employment Services, SHIP offers supported employment opportunities to people with traumatic brain injury. The programs include job development and intensive job coaching services that help the person with a brain injury get and keep a job in an integrated work setting. Job coaching services are also available on a long-term basis to ensure that the individual is receiving whatever follow-up supports are necessary to maintain his or her employment status. Supported employment staff educate and assist program participants in accessing Social Security work incentives that allow them to sustain their benefits while working.

Substance abuse treatment. SHIP has developed affiliations with three residential substance abuse recovery programs. These programs have been willing to modify their model of treatment to better address the unique needs of people with traumatic brain injury. In exchange, SHIP provides intensive training and consultation to their staff. SHIP also trains staff at other substance abuse programs across the state in an effort to help them better understand the problems associated with brain injury.

Technical assistance and training. SHIP provides training to families, providers and other professionals, and the general public. The goal is to provide these people with the knowledge and skills necessary to serve people with brain injuries more effectively and to expand the programmatic/service options available on a local level to people with traumatic brain injuries.

A neurobehavioral unit. SHIP collaborated with the Greenery Rehabilitation Group and Middlesex County Hospital to develop a secure inpatient treatment program for people with severe behavioral and psychiatric problems. SHIP has access to nine beds that can serve individuals who are a threat to themselves and/or the community.

Ancillary support services. SHIP is actively involved in the identification and development of community-based support services that will allow people with brain injuries to live more independently in their homes and communities, ultimately preventing institutionalization. SHIP purchases services such as short-term case management, respite care, recreation, transportation, home modifications, adaptive devices, homemaker services, one-to-one emergency support, cognitive retraining, individual therapy, and group counseling.

SHIP coordinates with other public and private human services agencies and organizations and has a close, ongoing relationship with the Massachusetts chapter of the National Head Injury Foundation (now known as the Brain Injury Association, Inc.).

The demand for services has been high. Since the program opened its doors in 1985, SHIP has received nearly 2,000 referrals and averages 20 to 25 referrals each month. SHIP served 250 to 300 clients in 1992. Because of budget constraints, services cannot be provided to everyone who needs them. There is a waiting list of about 1,800.

Contact: Debra S. Kamen, Director, Statewide Head Injury Program (SHIP), Massachusetts Rehabilitation Commission, Fort Point Place, 27-43 Wormwood Street, Boston, Massachusetts 02210; (617) 727-8732.

Minnesota

In 1989, the Minnesota Legislature passed the "Services for Persons with Traumatic Brain Injury" legislation which mandated the Department of Human Services to take a lead role in coordinating and supervising health care services for people with traumatic brain injury and to develop an administrative case management system for Medicaid-eligible clients with brain injuries. The program also serves people who have acquired brain injury through near drowning, brain tumors, drug overdose, or infections such as encephalitis.

Minnesota's Traumatic Brain Injury Program supervises and coordinates health care policy and service development in the Department of Human Services. This includes working with other divisions within the department, including chemical dependency, mental health, developmental disabilities, the medical assistance state plan, long-term care management, home care services, and other appropriate divisions. The yearly administrative cost for the program includes $375,000 from the state budget and $100,000 of dedicated funds from the DWI (driving while intoxicated) Driver's License Reinstatement Fund.

Minnesota's administrative case management program has been recognized as exemplary. In addition, Minnesota has made creative use of Medicaid's home- and community-based waivers to serve people with brain injuries.

Contact: Allan Weinand, Supervisor, Traumatic Brain Injury Program, Department of Human Services, 444 Lafayette Road, St. Paul, Minnesota 55155; (612) 297-3711.

Rehabilitation

Approximately 11 states provide post-acute rehabilitation, transitional living, and vocational rehabilitation services at state facilities established specifically for such purposes. Many states have changed the missions of facilities established for tuberculosis or polio to a focus on brain injury, spinal cord injury, and stroke. For example, the Missouri State Chest Hospital was changed by state statute and funding to the Missouri Rehabilitation Center, operated by the Missouri Department of Health. In Virginia, the Woodrow Wilson Rehabilitation Center, owned by the Department of Rehabilitation Services, was converted from a veteran's hospital. Georgia's rehabilitation facility, described in this section, formerly served people with polio.

Georgia

Each year, the Roosevelt Warm Springs Institute for Rehabilitation serves approximately 3,000 individuals with brain injuries, spinal cord injuries and stroke. In FY 1991-92, the patients came from 148 Georgia counties, 24 states, and five foreign countries. In the medical unit, 15 beds are reserved for people with brain injuries. The average length of stay is 31 days. In FY 1991-92, 169 patients with brain injuries were served in the inpatient unit, and 245 in the outpatient unit. The institute also has a vocational and transitional living unit with three levels. Level one offers the highest degree of supervision, and each subsequent level offers less supervision.

Organizationally, the institute falls under Georgia's Department of Human Resources, Division of Rehabilitation Services. The institute receives 25.2 percent of its funding from Medicaid, 13.2 percent from Medicare, 22.3 percent from federal vocational funds, 18.3 percent from state allocations, and 21 percent from private insurance and other funds.

Contact: Sharon W. Short, Program Director, Roosevelt Warm Springs Institute for Rehabilitation, P.O. Box 1000, Warm Springs, Georgia 31830; (706) 655-5361.

Home- and Community-Based Services

The burden of long-term care for people with brain injuries falls mainly on the family. California has developed a statewide program designed to provide support for families who care for a person with a brain injury. Other states or private agencies have developed services to help people with brain injuries remain in the community. These include behavioral management programs, drug and alcohol treatment programs, and consumer training programs.

California

California is the only state that provides services for caregivers of adults with brain impairments. The 1984 Comprehensive Act for Families and Caregivers of Brain-Impaired Adults sets up a statewide system of 11 regional centers, called Caregiver Resource Centers (CRCs), to serve families of individuals whose brain impairments occurred after the age of 18 and were the result of traumatic brain injury, Alzheimer's disease, stroke, Parkinson's disease, AIDS, and dementia. People with brain injuries represent 8 percent of the people served. The centers are administered by the Department of Mental Health, which contracts with nonprofit agencies to deliver services. The program is supported by state general funds.

The legislation grew out of the Family Survival Center demonstration project in San Francisco, which now serves as one of the 11 Caregiver Resource Centers. The CRCs offer specialized information and referral, assessment, family consultation on care planning, legal consultation, in-home and out-of-home respite services, counseling, and support groups to make it possible for families to care for family members with a brain injury at home. The support services families most request are information, emotional support, and respite care.

Families caring at home for a brain-damaged adult can receive in-home support, day care, or transportation for up to 40 hours per month. Each resource center can authorize up to a maximum of $425 per month in respite care for each client. The CRCs make creative use of existing local resources to provide respite care. These include in-home care, adult and social day care, foster and group care, temporary placement in a community health facility, and transportation. During FY 1990-91, 882 families received an average of nine hours of respite care per week. The average monthly cost of respite voucher services per family clients was $267, of which $242 was provided by the state. Family clients contributed, on average, a $25 copayment. At the end of FY 1990-91, 2,251 families were on respite waiting lists at Caregiver Resource Center in California.

Contact: Kathleen Kelly, Executive Director, Family Survival Project, 425 Bush Street, Suite 500, San Francisco, California 94109; (415)-434-3388.

Michigan

Training and Treatment Innovations, Inc., (TTI) in Berkley, Mich., provides in-home training to families who take care of a person with severe behavioral problems. This private nonprofit agency serves families in the southeastern Michigan area who are caring at home for a person with traumatic brain injury, developmental disability, or mental illness. The family unit is the focus of the training. A staff member goes to the home from 10 to 30 hours a week and works with the child or adult who is experiencing behavioral difficulties. The staff member also works with family members to show them how to deal with problems, which may include threatening behaviors, property destruction, violence directed inwardly or toward other family members, or inappropriate, overt sexual behavior. Most interventions are six months in duration. With training in dealing with behavioral problems themselves, families can often avoid having to send a brain-injured relative to an institution.

Contact: Sandra Lindsey, Executive Director, Training and Treatment Innovations, Inc., 2766 W. Eleven Mile Road, Suite W, Berkley, Michigan 48072; (810) 544-9354.

Minnesota

Vinland National Center in Loretto, Minn., offers substance abuse treatment tailored to people with traumatic brain injury. Most people in the program had a pre-existing problem with drugs or alcohol that was related in some way to the injury. Funded by federal and state grants, Vinland mainly serves people who do not have private insurance but are eligible for medical assistance, SSI, and SSDI. Both in- and outpatient treatment are available.

Inpatient. The facility, licensed for 15 beds, is client-centered. Staff members make sure the inpatient facility treats only those individuals who absolutely need to be there. The traditional Alcoholics Anonymous concepts are often too abstract for people with brain injuries. At Vinland, information is repeated in a variety of forms to accommodate the different ways people with brain injury assimilate information. The length of individual sessions is shorter to accommodate the fatigue common among people with brain injuries. Breaks between sessions are longer to allow individuals to assimilate information. Classes are taught using constant repetitions. Recreational therapy is an important part of the program. The average length of stay is 30 to 45 days. The program serves from 70 to 90 clients a year.

Outpatient. Similar teaching techniques are used in the outpatient program. Drug and alcohol treatment is integrated with independent living skills to help the person re-enter the community. After the 13-week program, clients go into a six-month aftercare program and meet one night a week with a social worker who helps them through difficult times and intervenes early if problems arise. The program serves approximately 230 to 250 people.

Contact: Greg Jones, Program Director, Chemical Health Program, Vinland National Center, 3675 Ihduhapi Road, Loretto, Minnesota 55357; (612) 479-4555.

New York

The Partners in Policymaking (PIP) training program, cosponsored by the New York State Developmental Disabilities Planning Council and the Head Injury Services Coordination Council, is designed to train consumers to become more effective advocates for the services and supports they need. The group is composed of 50 individuals from around the state who are either family members of people with traumatic brain injury or individuals who have survived a traumatic brain injury. Sessions focus on the legislative and budget process, education, housing, family and individual supports, and general advocacy skills.

Contact: Barbara Delaney, Coordinator, New York State Head Injury Services Coordinating Council, Bureau of Standards Development, Department of Health, Corning Tower, The Governor Nelson A., Rockefeller Empire State Plaza, Albany, New York 12237; (518) 476-1433.

Housing

Housing is a critical component of community services for individuals who are unable to return to their families to live or prefer to live independently. Housing arrangements range from individuals living in their own apartments with the help of support services, to transitional living, where people with brain injuries live together or in another person's home and receive intensive training in cooking, budgeting, taking transportation, and other skills that will allow them to return to the community to live. Private agencies or corporations in Massachusetts, Minnesota, Oregon, Wisconsin, and Wyoming offer innovative approaches to housing people with brain injuries.

Massachusetts

Looking for a more cost-effective way to purchase postacute rehabilitation services for people with brain injuries, the Medicaid Division of the Massachusetts Department of Public Welfare has contracted with Mentor Clinical Care to provide residential rehabilitation services as an alternative to costly care in rehabilitation hospitals and facilities. The Mentor model involves the placement of a person with a brain injury into the home of a carefully selected rehabilitation technician, known as a mentor, who provides one-on-one training and therapeutic intervention in the natural home environment. Each client and mentor is supported by an interdisciplinary team of rehabilitation professionals who are responsible for client assessment, development of an individualized rehabilitation plan, case coordination, 24-hour backup and support to the mentor homes, and direct service with the client and his or her family. The mentor is responsible for implementing portions of the rehabilitation plan in the home and in the community, thereby allowing the client to relearn the practical skills of daily living, such as caring for oneself, working, socializing, and using community resources. By practicing skills and behaviors in the natural setting of a home and community, and with the assistance of a personal rehabilitation technician, learning is accelerated and generalization to post-discharge settings is facilitated.

Although the Mentor program uses a noninstitutional and individualized model, a full array of services is available to each client, including neuro-psychological services, behavioral management, vocational and educational services, physical, occupational and speech therapies, life skills tutoring, physiological services, respite care services, and clinical case coordination. Because these services are provided in a home and community setting, utilization of existing community resources is maximized, and the high capital and overhead costs related to facility-based models are avoided. As a result, the net cost of a client's rehabilitation program is dramatically reduced.

The Massachusetts Medicaid Division used the Medicaid Personal Care Services Optional Benefit and the Foster Care Option to establish the financing mechanism for this innovative approach to brain injury rehabilitation. No federal waivers were required.

In addition to the individualized residential rehabilitation model described above, Mentor Clinical Care provides a continuum of care for persons who have sustained a brain injury, including day treatment, supported living, and in-home services. Mentor Clinical Care serves a total of 80 persons with brain injuries in its rehabilitation programs. Another 850 clients of all ages are served in specialized programs for persons with emotional and behavioral problems, developmental disabilities, and chronic medical illnesses and disabilities.

Contact: Joyce Lorman, Clinical Liaison, Mentor Clinical Care, 101 Arch Street, Boston, Massachusetts 02110; (800) 947-0071, ext. 46.

Minnesota

Accessible Space, Inc., (ASI) is a nonprofit organization that offers accessible, affordable housing and support services to people with disabilities in 32 sites primarily in Minnesota, with additional sites in Montana, Nevada, and North Dakota. ASI provides cooperative living residences (group homes limited to four to eight people) or individual apartments for 300 people, including 150 with traumatic brain injury. Close to 98 percent of the clients are on some sort of public assistance (SSI, SSDI, medical assistance). New units are developed through cooperative agreements with public housing or through new construction, funded through HUD's Section 811 Supportive Housing for People with Disabilities Program. Over a seven-year period, ASI has developed 200 units through Section 811.

By sharing services, ASI is able to make more cost-effective use of Medicaid personal care dollars. In most states, individuals can get only four to six hours of personal care assistance through Medicaid. This is a problem for people with brain injuries who often need access to 24-hour care. By developing congregate housing, ASI creates the density that allows consumers to share services. Through economies of scale, ASI can deliver homemaker and health aide services 24 hours a day on a shared basis.

ASI has developed a consumer-friendly model that combines housing with a managed care approach to support services. The philosophy is that services should fit the people, rather than making people fit the services. In all programs, the consumer has a choice. Individuals are not required to take part in the services as a condition of their residency.

For individuals with brain injury, ASI has three programs, graduated to meet individual needs. The Shared Living Program serves people with behavioral problems on a residential basis. New Beginnings serves people with brain injuries whose behavior has stabilized but who need 24-hour care. The Independent Living program is for people who don't need 24-hour care, but would benefit from the independent living skills training offered. The program deals with such needs as physical wellness, family adjustment, transportation, financial management, socialization, advocacy, adult sexuality, safety, assistive devices, homemaking, prevocational resources, and communication skills.

Contact: Stephen Vander Schaaf, President, Accessible Space, Inc., 2550 University Avenue West, Suite 301-North, St. Paul, Minnesota 55114; (800) 466-7722 or (612) 645-7271.

Oregon

The Uhilhorn Apartments in Eugene, Ore., offer 20 units exclusively for people with traumatic brain injuries. Residents receive assistance with daily living and can attend classes during the day on memory training, life skills, and vocational training. Recreational activities include a weekly barbecue and trips in the van. Peer support groups and Alcoholics Anonymous are also available. Most behavioral problems are handled in-house. The staff includes four advocate counselors, a program manager, an assistant program manager, and a residential manager. The apartments are subsidized by HUD Section 8 housing subsidies. Each resident pays according to his income, including SSI and SSDI. Approximately 30 percent of participants have a job, usually supported employment. The goal of this transitional housing project is to get people ready for independent living. The apartments are funded by a $917 payment per month per client from Medicaid funds, provided through Senior Disabled Services (Oregon's agency serving people with disabilities). Some funding is also provided by United Way.

Contact: Wally Earl, Program Manager, 689 W. 13th Avenue, Eugene, Oregon 97404; (503) 345-4244.

Wisconsin

Options in Community Living, a private nonprofit agency in Madison, Wisc., supports people with disabilities in their own homes. Out of the 100 people served, six have brain injuries. The philosophy of the agency is to provide whatever it takes to help the person live in the community. Each client is assigned a case manager who sees that client's needs are met and works as an advocate. Supports include help in finding an apartment and a roommate, help managing money, shopping, and cooking. Options will also act as repre-sentative payer and take care of the paperwork for people receiving SSI or SSDI. Mental health services are an important component of support services to people with brain injury, many of whom are still adjusting to the disability and are angry and frustrated. If a personal care assistant is needed, the client helps choose the person. Flexibility and choice are stressed in this innovative model. Options believes that brain-injured people should have a voice in the decisions that affect their lives.

Contact: Gail Jacob, Director, Options in Community Living, 22 N. Second Street, Madison, Wisconsin 53704; (608) 249-1585.

Wyoming

The Double P Ranch in Riverton, Wyo., is an innovative supported living project for people with brain injuries run by the nonprofit Rocky Mountain ReEntry Services. The leased ranch is on the Wind River Indian Reservation. It serves six men with brain injuries. Formerly, two were living in nursing homes, one was in the state mental hospital, another young man was in an institution for behavioral disorders, and two were living at home. The focus on the ranch is on quality of life and independence. Recreational activities, such as backpacking trips to wilderness areas, help build confidence and give the men a chance to focus on the things they can do. Counseling occurs around the campfire. At the ranch and at neighboring ranches, the men feed the horses and work on fences and irrigation. Entrepreneurial projects are encouraged. A man who was injured in a rodeo accident has started his own business refurbishing saddles. Another man has his own sign painting business. Round-the-clock staffing at the ranch includes a life skills specialist, a case manager, and four former football players who help the men dress, cook, feed the horses, and organize their rooms, among other things.

The $30,000 cost per person, while high, is significantly less than maintaining the person in an institution. The costs are covered by workers' compensation, private insurance, self-pay, Wyoming's Division of Vocational Rehabilitation, and a grant from the Rocky Mountain Regional Brain Injury Center.

Contact: Jennifer Johnson, Director, Rocky Mountain ReEntry Services, 2441 Peck Avenue, Riverton, Wyoming 82510; (307) 856-5576.

Supported Employment

Training and employing persons with brain injury serves to both give meaning and structure to their lives and also decrease their reliance on public funds. Large numbers of people with moderate and mild brain injuries can return to work with relatively simple supports. Most brain-injured people have the same intelligence as before, but have certain problems with memory, decision making, and judgment. To compensate, employers can institute some minor, inexpensive supports, such as designating someone to call every morning to see that the person is up because he or she may have forgotten to set the alarm.

Even people with serious disabilities can work successfully. Previously, these individuals were thought to require training at sheltered workshops before entering the work force. However, many professionals question the benefit of pretraining, particularly for people with brain injury who have trouble translating a skill from one environment to another. Increasingly, states and private nonprofit agencies are stressing newer approaches, such as supported employment, where brain-injured people work in jobs side by side with people who do not have disabilities. California, Missouri, North Dakota, and Virginia offer creative approaches to supported employment for people with traumatic brain injury.

California

The private nonprofit Betty Clooney Center in Long Beach approaches job training from a holistic perspective. People with brain injuries become lifetime members of the clubhouse. Members and professional staff work side by side to carry out activities at the center, including daily maintenance and meal preparation. In the mornings, people work in units, including a horticultural unit that raises organically grown herbs and vegetables, a clerical unit that puts out a newsletter, and a creative arts unit. The herbs, vegetables, and crafts are sold to the public at the country store on the campus. Members gain self-esteem through responsibility and, at the same time, gain important life, vocational, and social skills. From 25 to 30 people participate in the day program.

Supported employment is provided outside the center for nine club members. Job developers seek out jobs in the community. Increasingly, the club's job developers are finding that employers are interested in hiring someone with a brain injury, because they get federal tax credits and recognition from the community. In addition, the employer gets a reliable employee. The center's success rate—it has had no job failures for a year—is attributed to the safety net and sense of community provided by the clubhouse model. Not only does the employee have the support of the job coach, he also has the clubhouse, which serves as a central point of reference and a place to return for friendship and peer guidance. The Betty Clooney Center is based on New York's Fountain House prevocational services for people with chronic mental illness. The Betty Clooney Foundation, which operates the center, runs on an annual budget of approximately $750,000. The center also receives funds from California's Traumatic Brain Injury Trust Fund. Additional funding is obtained through public and private grants, benefits, and proceeds from product sales.

Contact: Pat Digre, Director, The Betty Clooney Center, 2951 Long Beach Boulevard, Long Beach, California 90806; (310) 492-6488.

Minnesota

In operation for four years, TBI Metro in Minneapolis placed 180 people with brain injuries in competitive jobs over three and one-half years. Services are strictly individualized. Six employment specialists do whatever it takes to help clients find and keep a job. The specialists do creative footwork to find employers willing to hire someone with a brain injury. A selling point for the service is the fact that TBI Metro offers job coaching for the client, as well as education about brain injury for the employer and, in some cases, other employees. The employer is also informed about the federal Targeted Jobs Tax Credit, which allows employers who hire people with disabilities a tax credit of up to $2,400 per employee during the first year. Any client on the job is expected to arrive on time, follow company policy, and do the work. TBI Metro guarantees that the job will get done, either by the client or by the employment specialists. A private nonprofit agency, TBI Metro receives most of its referrals from the state Division of Rehabilitation Services.

Contact: Cleone Griep, Traumatic Brain Injury Employment Services Coordinator, TBI Metro Services, 123 N. Third Street, Suite 804, Minneapolis, Minnesota 55401; (612) 339-9331.

Missouri

Missouri was the first state in the country to secure long-term funding for brain-injured people in supported employment. Approximately $225,000 from state general revenue is available after the end of time-limited federal financial participation in vocational rehabilitation. This occurs when the client has been in supported employment for nine months, or when the job coach has been phased out to 25 percent of the time, whichever comes first. People in supported employment with a job coach earn an average of $4.51 an hour and work an average of 26 hours a week. The average cost per client is $5,518 for each successfully employed individual. In FY 1991-92, out of 180 people who were "closed" (on the job nine months or using a job coach only 25 percent of the time), 140 were successfully employed. These figures include all disabilities: brain injuries, mental illness, and developmental disabilities. For FY 1991-92, the program served 59 clients with brain injuries.

Contact: Greg Solum, Director of Rehabilitation Facilities, 2401 E. McCarty Street, Jefferson City, Missouri 65101; (314) 751-3251.

North Dakota

Housing, Industry, Training, Inc., (HIT) a private nonprofit agency in Mandan, makes use of natural supports in the work place to help brain-injured people return to the company they worked for before their injury. In this demonstration project, it is essential to reach the people as early as possible after the injury, when they still have family support, an employer familiar with their work, and co-workers who care about them. To accomplish this, HIT staff members have become part of the discharge planning team at general hospitals with rehabilitation units in the Bismarck and Mandan area. HIT staff contact former employers and see if there is some portion of the injured person's job he or she can still do for a limited time each day. Co-workers are taught simple ways to help people with brain injuries when they return to work, such as prompting them about break times and reminding them where to hang their coats. After the person is on the job, HIT staff members check back with employers and co-workers to discuss problems and solutions. If it is not possible for people to return to their previous positions, another job is sought, using the same philosophy of natural supports. At any given time, HIT works with from five to 12 people in jobs. The project is funded by a grant from the Rocky Mountain Regional Brain Injury Center.

Contact: Pat Knudson, Director of Vocational Services, Housing, Industry, Training Inc., 201 Missouri Drive, Mandan, North Dakota 58554; (701) 663-0047.

Virginia

The Rehabilitation, Research and Training Center at Virginia Commonwealth University has placed approximately 90 people with brain injuries in supported employment. At any given time, the caseload is usually 30 to 40 people. Funded by federal grants and the state Department of Rehabilitation Services, the center has job coaches, called staff employment specialists, who do job placement and case management. Clients are placed in a wide range of jobs, including clerical, warehouse, and human services jobs. For people with brain injuries returning to their former place of employment, the specialists act as consultants and help the former employer make adjustments, such as putting cues into the environment to enable the person to operate independently. Researchers at the center have published a number of articles on the cost, outcomes, and critical factors of success in placing people with brain injuries in supported employment.

Contact: Pam Sherron, Program Director, Virginia Commonwealth University Rehabilitation, Research and Training Center, 1314 W. Main Street, Box 2011, Richmond, Virginia 23284; (804) 367-1851.

Education

Children with brain injuries present special challenges for school systems. Common side effects of brain injury are problems with memory, information processing, organization, and visual/perceptual skills; the child may be intelligent but unable to translate codes from the visual mode. Iowa has addressed the unique problems of brain-injured students with special services tailored to their needs.

Education of the brain-injured person does not have to stop at the elementary and secondary level. California has developed an innovative program to use the community college system to offer courses to help individuals with brain injury gain the skills they need to live independently. Many of the students also take regular courses at the community college.

Iowa

This state's Educational Services for Students with Head Injuries grew out of recommendations by a 1988 state task force formed by the Bureau of Special Education. Iowa is divided into 15 area education agencies (AEA) that oversee services for all special education services. Each of these agencies has a team specializing in school-aged children with brain injuries. Rehabilitation hospitals in Iowa have a contact number for each area education agency and inform them of any admitted children. Team members and family members meet with the hospital staff to discuss what the child was like before the injury. Team members are also involved in discharge planning. At school, the team members work with the child's teachers as well as meet with the child's classmates, to let them know what to expect. Hospitals share the child's latest tests with the school so there is no duplication. A case manager is appointed for each child returning to school. The case manager may be a teacher, a guidance counselor, or an administrator. Parents are involved in all decisions made for the child.

Educational Services for Students with Head Injuries is also in the process of setting up support groups for parents and school-aged children with brain injuries. The children meet in one group while the parents meet in another. Educational Services is active in prevention activities, such as encouraging the use of helmets by giving them as prizes in bike races.

Contact: Sue Pearson, State Consultant, Educational Services for Students with Head Injuries, 257 University Hospital School, University of Iowa, Iowa City, Iowa 52242; (319) 356-1172.

California

The San Diego Community College system offers a core curriculum for adults with brain injury. Every semester, approximately 120 students attend the Head Injury Program for four afternoons a week. Students choose from an offering of 25 courses, including memory strategies, communication skills, social and interpersonal skills, vocational readiness, career development, and study skills and notetaking. Most students take two years to get through the program. At the end of that time, students are usually placed in a job or mainstreamed into the regular community college. All courses are offered to students at no cost.

Learning in Natural Community Settings (LINCS) is an important part of the Head Injury Program. LINCS is funded through a three-year grant from the U.S. Office of Education-Rehabilitation Services Administration. This program offers independent living skills training in natural settings. Students learn to use public transportation by getting a bus schedule, boarding the bus, and using the system until they become self-sufficient. Students shop at grocery stores and go to the bank to open a checking account and learn how to use the automatic teller machines. Training is personalized and designed to meet the student's needs at home and at work. At the end of the program, people are set up in apartments or helped to move from a group home to the community. Students are able to participate in LINCS in the morning and attend the regular classes in the afternoon.

The Head Injury Program's vocational training is offered in conjunction with California's Department of Rehabilitation. Program personnel help people with brain injuries to find jobs. A job coach offers support services until the individuals can do the job independently, and employers are educated about the Americans with Disabilities Act.

The San Diego Community College program offers students with brain injuries an upbeat mainstream environment in which to learn to live independently. Problems of loneliness and isolation are alleviated by the presence of a large peer support group. The record is impressive. Approximately 80 percent of people placed on a job are still working at the same job a year later. Most people who move into their own apartments are still living in the same place a year later.

Contact: Wanda Windsor, Project Director, Learning in Natural Community Settings (LINCS), San Diego Community College Head Injury Program, 3375 Camino del Rio South, Suite 275, San Diego, California 92108; (619) 584-6983.

Central Registry System

A registry is a reporting system that collects information about people with brain injuries and the care they receive. Reports to the registry are made by hospitals and, in some states, public/private health and social agencies, physicians, clinics, public health nurses, and emergency medical services staff.

Lawmakers use the information in registries to guide their decision making. For example, knowing how many people are injured each year in auto accidents could influence voting on seat belt and helmet laws. Information from the registries also provides valuable data to guide prevention efforts, planning for health care, and other services.

At present, 12 states have statewide registries for traumatic brain injury: Arkansas, Florida, Georgia, Iowa, Maine, Maryland, Missouri, North Dakota, Rhode Island, Utah, Virginia, and West Virginia.

Illinois, Kentucky, Louisiana, Michigan, and Texas have passed legislation to create a central registry but have not yet started collecting data.

States that have registries all use different criteria for collecting information, making it impossible to compare information among states. The National Center for Injury Prevention and Control in the Centers for Disease Control is working toward standardizing the registries in order to collect national statistics. States considering registry legislation should contact the Centers for Disease Control. Missouri is widely regarded as having one of the best trauma registry systems in the country.

Missouri

In 1986, the Missouri legislature passed a law requiring hospitals to report all head and spinal cord injuries to the Department of Health. Missouri's head and spinal cord injury registry was instituted in July 1987. Missouri is unique in that the state has five data systems that other states do not have: Missouri Head and Spinal Cord Injury Registry, Statewide Trafficway Accident Reporting System, Missouri Ambulance Reporting System, Hospital Admissions System and the Death Certificates System. The accident reporting system is administered by the State Highway Patrol; the other systems are administered by the Department of Health. The trauma registry allows Missouri to have at its fingertips the following information about people with brain injuries: age, race, source of insurance, cause of injury, severity, discharge summary, problems resulting from the brain injury, services required. The information allows the state to address the extent of injury in Missouri and the effectiveness of laws and educational programs directed toward the prevention of injuries.

Contact: Garland Land, Director, Division of Health Resources, Department of Health, 1738 E. Elm Street, P.O. Box 570, Jefferson City, Missouri 65102; (314) 751-6272.

Veterans Services

The Defense Veterans' Head Injury Project

A research study is being conducted jointly by the Department of Defense and the Department of Veterans' Affairs, in conjunction with the Brain Injury Association, Inc., to provide information and services to people sustaining traumatic brain injuries in the military and the veterans' affairs system. Three military hospitals and four veterans' hospitals will be designated as model treatment centers offering rehabilitation programs. The centers are scheduled to begin operation in 1993. Each center will have a registry to collect data. People with brain injuries using the facilities will be tracked for several years. The Brain Injury Association, Inc.'s role is to provide assistance and educational materials, through a toll-free number, and to provide technical assistance in training case managers and setting up the rehabilitation programs and support groups.

Contact: Brain Injury Association, Inc., Information and Resource Service, 1776 Massachusetts Avenue, NW, Suite 100, Washington, D.C. 20036: (202) 296-6443 or (800) 444-6443.

—by Barbara Wright

Part Five

Further Help and Information

Chapter 34

Basic Questions about Head Injury and Disability

What is Traumatic Brain Injury (TBI) or a Head Injury?

There are two basic types of head injury: "closed head injury" (CHI) and "open head injury" (OHI). CHI is usually caused by a rapid acceleration and deceleration of the head during which the brain is whipped back and forth, thus bouncing off the inside of the skull. The stress of this rapid movement pulls apart nerve fibers and causes damage to the activated system of neuro-fibers which send out messages to all parts of the body.

This type of injury often occurs as a result of motor vehicle crashes, and places extreme stress on the brain stem—the part which connects the large areas of the brain to the spinal cord. A large number of functions are packed tightly in the brain stem, e.g. controls of consciousness, breathing, heart beat, eye movements, pupil reactions, swallowing and facial movements. All sensations going to the brain, as well as signals from the brain to the rest of the body, must pass through the brain stem.

CHI may individually or collectively cause physical, intellectual, emotional, social, and vocational difficulties for the injured person. These problems may affect both the present and future life and personality of the head injury survivor. Indeed, it frequently means that the person, as you know him/her, may never again be quite the same.

The second category of TBI is usually referred to as "open head injury." This is a visible injury and may be the result of an accident, gun-shot wound or a variety of other outside factors. OHI differs from CHI in that the injury is usually located at a focal point in the brain. Thus, very specific problems will result. For example, the individual may experience difficulties with forming speech, but show no problem with writing those words on paper.

Finally, cardiac arrest, stroke, accidents such as drowning, etc. all can cause anoxia (loss of oxygen to the brain), and thus may result in TBI. In these cases all of the brain cells may be affected, thus there may be an overall change in the behavior and personality of the individual.

What are the Symptoms of Traumatic Brain Injury?

"The Silent Epidemic" is a phrase frequently used to describe TBI as this injury often is not physically visible. Symptoms can vary greatly depending upon the extent and location of the brain injury. Physical disabilities, impaired learning ability, and personality changes are common.

Physical Impairments—speech, vision, hearing and other sensory impairments; headaches; lack of coordination; spasticity of muscles; paralysis of one or both sides and seizure disorders.

Cognitive Impairments—memory deficits: short and long term, concentration, slowness of thinking, attention, perception, communication, reading and writing skills, planning, sequencing and judgment.

Psycho-Social-Behavioral-Emotional Impairments—fatigue, mood swings, denial, self-centeredness, anxiety, depression, lowered self-esteem, sexual dysfunction, restlessness, lack of motivation, inability to self-monitor, difficulty with emotional control, inability to cope, agitation, excessive laughing or crying and difficulty in relating to others.

When Do We Know How Serious the Traumatic Brain Injury Is?

Usually it is difficult to predict the outcome of TBI during the first hours, days or weeks. In fact, the outcome may remain unknown for many months or years. For loved ones, a physician's comment that "we'll just have to wait and see" can be very frustrating. Nonetheless, it is often the most accurate answer. During this time, the patient's loved ones should become advocates for him/her in order to ensure that he/she is receiving the best possible care (including the current advances in treatment and rehabilitation for traumatic brain injury) so that the patient can reach his/her maximum potential. But what does it mean to be an advocate? It means asking questions of doctors, nurses, and other health professionals, and learning as much as possible about the issues which surround head injury.

A severe brain injury is typified by a period of time in coma and a myriad of remaining disabilities. Some statistical information has shown that the longer coma lasts, the greater the disability is likely to be. However, recent studies have reduced the degree to which these facts are directly correlated. For patients with moderate brain injury (surviving six hours or less of coma) over half will be able to return to school, jobs, and independent living within a year after injury. Many of these individuals will have some residual cognitive (thinking and reasoning) problems. The process of recovery often takes much longer than family and friends expect. Furthermore, it is a source of great frustration to all involved when professionals do not have enough information to give a definite prognosis.

What Is Coma?

Coma can be thought of simply as a prolonged state of unconsciousness. Although individuals in coma may have sleep and wake cycles, there is no speech, the eyes usually are closed (but may be open and not focused) and there is no meaningful response to external stimuli. When this sleep-like state lengthens to an hour or more, the term "coma" is used. There are several levels of coma defined by the person's increasing awareness in response to his/her surroundings. Professionals measure levels of coma by the *Glasgow Coma Scale* or the *Rancho Los Amigos* levels of cognitive functioning.

What about Minor Traumatic Brain Injury?

Minor head trauma is the temporary disruption of brain functioning due to an insult to the head. Usually, head trauma is called "minor" if the injury is not judged serious enough to require formal rehabilitation, and the patient is sent directly home from the hospital.

Most people who suffer mild bumps to the head will not experience permanent problems. Only when enough brain cells have been damaged—or if there are repeated minor injuries—will persons experience permanent changes in the way they think, feel, and act. Minor head trauma should not be dismissed lightly. The BIA can provide information and resources to people with head injuries, their families and professionals.

What about Rehabilitation?

Rehabilitation should begin as soon as possible following a head injury, even while the person is in coma. Early intervention by a rehabilitation facility that has expertise with TBI increases the possibility of maximum recovery—medically, physically, cognitively and psychologically.

As families plan for the future, they should retain and organize information in a detailed manner. A loose-leaf notebook including different categories of information needed on the multiple aspects of TBI, rehabilitation centers, resources, and services available will ease the difficulty of coping with the flow of information. In addition, families can prepare for the difficult decisions they will face as a person requires different treatment options. The BIA has a written guide which lists questions to ask when visiting potential programs for their loved one. This, and other resources available from the BIA can help the family plan for the best possible care and treatment over the lifetime of their family member.

The catastrophic effect of TBI is very stressful for all those involved. It is important for each person to maintain his own well-being and to reach out and ask for help or support when needed—from family, friends, medical staff or clergy. A critical resource is your BIA State Association and local support group of the Brain Injury Association, Inc. which can provide information on appropriate rehabilitation settings as well as emotional support for persons who have survived TBI and for their families.

What Are the Different Types of Programs for Survivors of Head Injury?

The following categories are used to describe the various types of facilities involved in the rehabilitation of persons who have experienced TBI. These categories are not mutually exclusive and programs may overlap. The descriptions are intended to serve only as a guide and it is up to each individual (or family) to determine what program is suitable to his/her needs.

The following definitions have been designated by BIA to classify the continuum of head injury rehabilitation programs available in the 1989 edition of the *National Directory of Head Injury Rehabilitation Services*. Call the BIA today for details on ordering a directory.

Coma Treatment. Primary emphasis is on active intervention with a person described as being in Ranchos Los Amigos scale levels I-IV. A coma treatment program will accept a person for active intervention even though the person is unable to actively participate in therapy.

Acute Rehabilitation. Primary emphasis is on the early rehabilitation phase which usually begins as soon as a person is medically stable. The program is individually designed and based in a medical facility with a typical length of stay lasting 3-4 months. Treatment is provided by an identifiable team in a designated unit.

Subacute Rehabilitation. Primary emphasis is on the post acute phase of rehabilitation. This type of program has the capacity to keep an individual from 6-24 months if necessary and does not have to be hospital based. Treatment is provided by an identifiable team in a designated unit.

Behavior Disorders. Primary emphasis is on intervention with the person who exhibits destructive behavior to self and others. These patterns of behavior prevent active participation in rehabilitation and are treated through a continuum of controlled settings.

Transitional Living. Primary emphasis is to provide training for an environment of greater independence. There is a greater focus on compensating for skills that cannot be restored and an emphasis on the functional skills needed to live in the community. The typical length of stay is usually from 4 to 18 months.

Day Treatment. Primary emphasis is on a program based in an outpatient setting with intervention across all disciplines.

Lifelong Living. Primary emphasis is for persons discharged from rehabilitation who need ongoing lifetime support. Structured activities are provided on both an individual and group basis usually in a residential skilled nursing environment.

Independent Living. Primary emphasis is on community based services to maximize a person's ability to be empowered and self-directed. An independent living program allows an individual to live in his or her own home with maximum personal control over how services are delivered, combined with the opportunity to work as much as possible.

Homecare. Primary emphasis is on a team integrated home program. A comprehensive program is designed with training and case management services in place before an individual returns home.

Educational. Primary emphasis is on primary, secondary, and higher education programs. Realistic academic goals are set based upon professional knowledge of deficits resulting from head injury.

Employment. Primary emphasis is on vocational rehabilitation services that are designed to lead to an employment goal. Services can range from assessment to basic on-the-job supports.

Respite/Recreation. Primary emphasis is on a program which allows the person and family to adapt psychologically and environmentally to the residual deficits of head injury. This non-interventional model addresses socialization, recreation and respite needs.

What are the Different Specialty Services for Survivors of Head Injury?

Categories identified by the BIA to classify frequently requested services. These services include respirator dependent, substance abuse, driver education, evaluation, visually impaired and Spanish translation.

Evaluation. A service offered by a program to assess and make recommendations about an individual's course of treatment and program design.

Substance Abuse. A service offered by a program to deal with chemical dependency of an individual. The dependency may have occurred prior to the head injury or as a result of the head injury.

Visually Impaired. A service offered by a program to deal with an individual who is blind, either prior to a head injury or as a result of a head injury.

Respirator Dependent. A service offered by a program to care for people who are dependent on a ventilator for breathing.

Driver Evaluation. A service offered by a program to assess an individual's functional ability to drive after a head injury.

Spanish Translation. A service offered by a program to assure that both the Spanish speaking person and his/her family have access to someone who can translate all program information into Spanish.

Where Can I Find Help?

There is an increasing amount of information available on all facets of head injury. If you have specific questions about head injury, information is available from the Brain Injury Association, Inc., State Associations. Additionally, you can have direct family-to-family contact with others who may have experienced similar situations through one of the BIA support groups or local chapters.

For more information on all aspects of life after head injury, [consult the list of resources in the next chapter or] write to: The Brain Injury Association, Inc., 1776 Massachusetts Ave, NW, Suite 100, Washington, DC 20036, or call (202) 296-6433.

Chapter 35

Help from the National Rehabilitation Information Center

Introduction

This guide contains information that persons with head injury, their families, and friends can use to adjust to life after head injury. It includes resources to enhance one's knowledge of head injury, coping and caregiving skills, and the general quality of life for the person with a head injury.

The resources listed are in a variety of forms, including telephone hotlines, magazines, newsletters, pamphlets, booklets, and books. Resources were selected based on their usefulness to people without medical backgrounds and availability through clearinghouses, libraries, or publishers.

For user convenience, most of the listings include a phone number. In some cases the caller will be routed through a system, which may put the caller on hold, or request the caller to explain the need or question more than once. Patience and persistence will pay off. Some of the organizations have answering machines that will record messages when staff members are not available.

This guide was produced by the National Rehabilitation Information Center (NARIC), a project funded by NIDRR under contract #HN93029001. For additional copies or for more information, contact

NARIC, 8455 Colesville Road, Suite 935, Silver Spring, MD 20910-3319. (800) 346-2742; (301) 588-9284. (Both lines are Voice/Text Telephone). Hours: 8 A.M. to 6 P.M. Eastern Time.

National Resources

The organizations listed below provide resources in one or more of the following ways: they answer requests for information over the phone; they direct persons with head injury and their families to services and support groups; or they distribute printed publications such as brochures, booklets or books. Some are membership organizations, some are not. All hours listed are for Monday to Friday.

A Chance to Grow. 3820 Emerson Avenue North, Minneapolis, MN 55412. (612) 521-2266. Legal information hotline: (612) 339-1290. Hours: 8 a.m. to 5:30 p.m. Central time.

A self-help group for parents of people with brain injury. Maintains a library on head injury, which includes legal information. Operates the Sandler rehabilitation program, which uses physical movement, an exercise regimen, spinal fluid regulation, and proper nutrition to improve the physical and cognitive skills of head injury survivors. Publishes a newsletter called *Growing Times* (quarterly).

Coma Recovery Association. 377 Jerusalem Avenue, Hempstead, NY 11550. (516) 486-2847. Hours: 10 a.m. to 3 p.m. Eastern time.

Provides information relating to coma, including information on treatment techniques. Offers legal consulting services.

The Family Caregiver Alliance (FCA). 425 Bush Street, Suite 500, San Francisco, CA 94108. (415) 434-3388; (800) 445-8106 (California only). Hours: 9 a.m. to 5 p.m. Pacific time.

The Family Caregiver Alliance (FCA) is a nonprofit organization founded to assist families of adults with chronic or progressive brain disorders (stroke, head injury, Alzheimer's disease, etc.). Its goals include public advocacy for those with financial and emotional distress and the national distribution of information on the care of people with brain injuries. Information for families is available on adult brain disorders. Available publications include 23 fact sheets on brain disorders and caregiving issues. A publications list is available upon request.

National Head Injury Foundation, Inc. (NHIF), now known as **Brain Injury Association, Inc.** 1776 Massachusetts Avenue NW, Suite 100, Washington, DC 20036. (800) 444-6443; (202) 296-6443; (202) 296-8850 (fax). Hours: 9 a.m. to 5 p.m. Eastern time.

BIA is the leading, national, advocacy and support organization for persons with head injuries and their families. BIA is actively involved in legislation at the federal and state level. BIA offers a toll-free "Family Helpline," as well as brochures describing head injury; prevention programs; a national directory of resources for persons with head injury and their families; national conferences for rehabilitation professionals, trial lawyers, and people with head injuries and their families; and a catalog of educational materials. BIA publishes a national newsletter as well as films and videos. These products are available through Information and Resources at BIA.

The National Institute of Neurological Disorders and Stroke (NINDS). Office of Information and Scientific Health Reports, 9000 Rockville Pike, Building 31, Room 8A-16, Bethesda, MD 20892. (800) 352-9424; (301) 496-5751. Contact: Information Specialist. Hours: 9 a.m. to 4:30 p.m. Eastern time.

This office, part of the National Institutes of Health, provides pamphlets written for nonprofessionals about various neurological disorders, including brain injury. One such publication is *Head Injury: Hope Through Research* (37 pages, free). They also publish fact sheets, special reports, and other documents. A list of free publications is available.

The Perspectives Network (TPN). 7205 Pullman Place, Mobile, AL 36695-4321. (800) 685-6302; (205) 639-5037; (205) 639-5037 (fax). Hours: 10 a.m. to 6 p.m. Eastern time.

The Perspectives Network is a nonprofit, service organization which provides various forums and opportunities wherein persons with brain injury, family members and friends, professionals, and community members are encouraged to discuss the issues relating to treatment, recovery, and reentry. TPN also provides peer communication networks for adults, teenagers, youth, and parents with brain injury, as well as spouses, children, parents, and siblings. These networks may be joined by writing to TPN, Attention: Networks (specifying the appropriate network).

TPN publishes a quarterly magazine with an international circulation. TPN also produces the following brochures: *Brain Injury: Prevention IS Worth a Pound of Cure but Sometimes It Happens Anyway!* and

From Bump on the Head to Coma: We Are All Interlinked (available by sending a stamped, self-addressed envelope to TPN, Attention: Fact Brochures).

Research and Training Center on Rehabilitation and Childhood Trauma. Tufts University, New England Medical Center, Department of Rehabilitation Medicine, 750 Washington Street, 75K-R, Boston, MA 02111. (617) 956-5036; (617) 956-5513 (fax). Hours: 9 a.m. to 5 p.m. Eastern time.

The Research and Training Center on Rehabilitation and Childhood Trauma, which is funded by the National Institute on Disabilities and Rehabilitation Research (NIDRR), conducts research to increase knowledge about the causes, treatment, and outcomes of injuries among children. The project also includes a training and dissemination program to make its information available to those most directly affected by childhood trauma—children, their families or guardians, and the providers of services. A special program is dedicated to addressing the unique needs of minority populations. Emphasis will be given to developing informational packages, training programs, and effective interventions that can be replicated nationally. Journal articles, a directory, a newsletter, conference proceedings, books, monographs, curricula, and audiovisuals are produced by the center. The RTC also provides information and referral services, develops curricula/training materials, conducts conferences and surveys, and provides technical assistance.

Well Spouse Foundation (WSF). P.O. Box 801, New York, NY 10023. (212) 724-7209; (212) 724-5209 (fax). Hours: 10 a.m. to 5 p.m. Eastern time.

The Well Spouse Foundation is a nationwide organization that provides support for the husbands, wives, and partners of people who are chronically ill or have disabilities. Regional support groups, a newsletter, and round robin letters help members cope with the difficulties they face as spousal caregivers.

Independent Living Centers

Independent living centers are local organizations administered and staffed by people with disabilities. They provide peer counseling, advocacy, and information about local services. The name, address, and phone number of the closest independent living center is available through a NARIC Information Specialist at (800) 346-2742 (V/TT) or (301) 588-9284 (V/TT). (301) 587-1967 (fax).

NIDRR-Funded Projects

The National Institute on Disability and Rehabilitation Research (NIDRR) contributes to the independence of persons of all ages who have disabilities by seeking improved systems, products, and practices in the rehabilitation process. NIDRR funds research and training centers (RTCs), rehabilitation engineering research centers (RERCs), field-initiated research, research and demonstration projects, research fellowships, and dissemination and utilization grants. Many of the projects are of interest to persons with head injury and their families.

As a repository for their projects' newsletters, research results, and final reports, NARIC can provide more information about the projects currently funded by NIDRR.

Other Government-Funded Head Injury Projects

The Rehabilitation Services Administration (RSA) funds other projects that may be of interest to persons with head injury and their families. More information about the services of these projects can be obtained from NARIC.

Periodicals

The following publications may be of interest to persons with head injury and their families. All prices listed are for individuals living in the United States.

Cognitive Rehabilitation. NeuroScience Publishers, 6555 Carrollton Avenue, Indianapolis, IN 46220. (317) 257-9672.

A publication for therapists, families, and patients, designed to provide information relevant to the rehabilitation of impairment resulting from brain injury; includes techniques, programs, and new methods. Published six times per year. Cost: $35 per year.

Exceptional Parent. Psych-Ed Corporation, 1170 Commonwealth Avenue, Boston, MA 02134-4646. (617) 730-5800. New subscriptions: (800) 247-8080. Customer service: (800) 562-1973.

Publication for parents of children with disabilities. Articles provide ideas, guidance, personal experiences, and practical information. Published eight times a year. Cost: $18 per year (individuals); $24 per year (parents); $70 per year (institution).

NHIF Newsletter. National Head Injury Foundation, (now known as Brain Injury Association, Inc.) 1776 Massachusetts Avenue NW, Suite 1100, Washington, DC 20036. (202) 296-6443.

Contains news and articles for families and professionals concerned with head injury. Information on BIA activities are also included. Quarterly. Cost: $35 per year (individual membership); $200 (corporate membership).

Documents

The NARIC library currently contains more than 1,400 documents pertaining to head injuries. The following books and journal articles have been singled out as being useful for people with head injury and their families.

Copyright law prevents NARIC from photocopying some documents; some are found in a local library, or the local library may be able to get them through the interlibrary loan program. Purchasing information has been provided as well; many of the books are available by special order from book stores—others are available only from the publisher.

Lash, M. (1990). ***When Your Child is Seriously Injured in an Accident.*** Boston: Tufts University/New England Medical School, RTC in Rehabilitation and Childhood Trauma, in collaboration with the Kiwanis Pediatric Trauma Institute. Available from the RTC in Rehabilitation and Childhood Trauma, Department of Rehabilitation Medicine, Tufts-New England Medical Center, 750 Washington Street, #75K-R, Boston, MA 02111. (800) 535-1910; (617) 956-5036. Contact: B. Saunders in the publications department. Cost: $4.50.

This booklet offers support and assistance for families of injured children, including information about the hospital stay, loss and what it means for the parent and child, helping brothers and sisters, getting help and coping, and planning for discharge from the hospital. Also included is a Parents' Bill of Rights, samples of a family log or notebook, resources, and suggested reading.

Anderson, J., & Parente, F. (1985). **Training Family Members to Work with the Head Injured Patient.** *Cognitive Rehabilitation.* (*3*)4, 12-15. NARIC Accession Number: XJ4632.

Describes exercises that families of people with head injuries can use to assist in a person's cognitive rehabilitation. The exercises included are designed to increase the person's attention span and to help the person remember information by organizing it for better retention. Topics discussed include verbal mediation, mnemonics, and imagery. Discusses the relationship between memory and attention, types of organizational strategies, methods to remember disassociated information using mnemonics, and teaching the concept of mental imagery as a precursor to memory training. Includes references.

Angle, Deborah K., & Buxton, Julie M. (1991). *Community Living Skills Workbook for the Head Injured Adult.* Gaithersburg, MD: Aspen Publishers, Inc. Available from: Aspen Publishers, Inc. 200 Orchard Ridge Drive, Gaithersburg, MD 20878. (800) 638-8437 (orders only); (301) 417-7500. Cost: $83.

Presents a manual of treatment activities for persons with head injury. Eight modules are presented with the first module describing the role occupational therapy takes and the remaining modules outlining specific treatment activities that address functional skill areas. Areas covered by the modules include the role of the occupational therapist, family education, home management, money management, interpersonal skills, leisure, transportation, and prevocational and vocational skills.

Aronow, H. U., Desimone, B. S., & Wood, R. L. (1987). **Traumatic Brain Injury: Discharge and Beyond: The Discharge and Recovery Process.** *Continuing Care.* (*6*)3, 26-29. NARIC Accession Number: XJ7526.

Discusses factors involved in rehabilitation of persons with head injury, focusing on the person's reactions following discharge, early emotional and behavioral obstacles, issues surrounding early discharge to the community versus transitional programs, factors that influence the speed of recovery, and effects of rehabilitation. Describes the benefits of early rehabilitation.

DeBoskey, D. S. Hecht, J. S., & Calub, C. J. (1991). *Educating Families of the Head Injured: A Guide to Medical, Cognitive, and Social Issues.* Gaithersburg, MD: Aspen Publishers, Inc. Available from: Aspen Publishers, Inc., 200 Orchard Ridge Drive, Gaithersburg, MD 20878. (800) 638-8437 (orders only); (301) 417-7500. Cost: $70 (plus postage).

While the cost of this document may be prohibitive for individuals, its comprehensive scope may make it a useful reference tool for support groups and patient libraries. The topics covered include the medical issues in head injury, inpatient rehabilitation, preparing for home, outpatient options, mild-to-moderate head trauma, funding sources, how to choose an appropriate treatment facility, long-term placement considerations, cognitive and behavioral problems and how to manage them, emotional problems experienced by families, long-term medical and psychological problems, substance use/abuse and the person with TBI, medications and side-effects, the family as educator, special considerations for children and the elderly, and community reintegration. Includes glossary, bibliography, and index.

HEATH Resource Center. (1988). *The Head Injury Survivor on Campus: Issues and Resources.* Washington, DC: Author. Available from: Heath Resource Center, One Dupont Circle NW, Suite 800, Washington, DC 20036-1193. (800) 544-3284; (202) 939-9320. Free.

This publication offers encouragement and information resources to college students with head injuries, their families, school administrators, and faculty members. Included is information about the types of programs that are available, tips for setting up a program, and questions that should guide program planning (for students, family members, and professionals). Includes descriptions of successful programs, including addresses and phone numbers of people to contact for more information.

Hoffman, M., Lehmkuhl, D., Probst, D., & Sawicki, R., (Eds.). (1989). *Brain Injury Rehabilitation: a Manual for Families.* Houston, TX: The Institute for Rehabilitation and Research, Texas Medical Center. Available from the Brain Injury Program, The Institute for Rehabilitation and Research, 1333 Moursund, Houston, TX 77030-3405. (713) 797-5945. Cost: $60 (plus $3 shipping).

Manual developed to help families of persons with traumatic brain injury understand the effects of the injury, participate in the rehabilitation process, adjust to changes in roles and relationships, and become aware of the resources that are available for assistance.

Lehmkuhl, L. D. (Ed.). (1991). ***Brain Injury Glossary.*** Houston, TX: The Institute for Rehabilitation and Research (TIRR). Available from HDI Publishers. (713) 682-8700. Cost: $7.50.

Subtitled "A Glossary of Terms and Definitions of Interest to Family Members and Survivors of Head Injury, Case Managers, Insurance Representatives, Staffs of Health Care Facilities, Staffs of Governmental Agencies, Local, State, Regional, and National Head Injury Associations." Compiled by the manager of the Head Injury Rehabilitation Research Project at TIRR, this glossary briefly defines approximately 400 terms. It was originally compiled to improve communication between researchers, but is understandable to readers without medical backgrounds.

Miller, C., & Campbell, K. (1987). ***From the Ashes: A Head Injury Self-Advocacy Guide.*** Seattle, WA: Phoenix Project. Available from the Phoenix Foundation, P.O. Box 84151, Seattle, WA 98124. (206) 329-1371; (206) 621-8558. Cost: $20 (plus $5 shipping).

A handbook written by two women with brain injuries for fellow persons with brain injuries. It addresses what happens functionally and psychologically when the brain is injured, recognizing the changes in behavior caused by head injury, ways to recognize what triggers reactions like a sense of separateness, irritability, headache, disorientation, and disinhibition, and self-management principles to help detect, analyze, correct, and adjust responses to the on-going problems people with head injury experience. Also discussed is finding the right doctor, medical tests, psychic losses, psychic pain, and life changes. Includes a glossary and bibliography.

Miller, L. (1993). **When the Best Help is Self-Help, or, Everything You Always Wanted to Know about Brain Injury Support Groups.** *The Journal of Cognitive Rehabilitation*, (*10*)6, 14-17. NARIC Accession number: XJ24596.

This article discusses the benefits of brain injury support groups to persons with brain injury and their families, and outlines steps towards forming a support group.

National Head Injury Foundation. (1994). (Now known as Brain Injury Association, Inc.) ***National Directory of Head Injury Rehabilitation Services.*** Washington, DC: Author. Available from the Brain Injury Association, Inc. (BIA), 1776 Massachusetts Avenue NW,

Suite 100, Washington, DC 20036. (800) 444-6443; (202) 296-6443; (202) 296-8850 (fax). Cost: $40.

The 1994 directory lists thousands of detailed descriptions and services, and includes a comprehensive indexing system that lists rehabilitation programs, as well as individual service providers.

Pi Lambda Theta National Honor and Professional Association in Education, San Jose Area Chapter. (1983). *Helping Head Injury and Stroke Patients at Home: A Handbook for Families.* San Jose, CA: Author. Available from: Mary Ellen Dierks, 5266 Cribari Heights, San Jose, CA 95135. Cost: $20 (CA residents need to add $1.65 sales tax).

This self-help handbook gives specific examples of cognitive skills which injury may have impaired, and describes retraining techniques for cognitive skill improvement. Topics discussed include: memory, visual-spatial relationships, language-communication, slow responses, judgment-reasoning, planning-follow-through, rights, and do's and don'ts. Includes bibliography, glossary, suggested progress chart, and two resource sections.

Pieper, B. (1991). *For Families from Families: What They Told Us About Having a Child with a Traumatic Brain Injury.* Albany, NY: New York State Head Injury Association. Available from: New York State Head Injury Association, 855 Central Avenue, Albany, NY 12206. (518) 459-7911. Cost: $3.

Report from a survey of families in which a child under the age of 16 had experienced a traumatic brain injury. The survey was designed to elicit information about the impact of head injury in the families' lives, the families' service needs, and availability of services. Families were asked about their most important needs: responses centered on the need for complete, honest, accurate, and understandable information about their child's condition, changes in his condition, and the care provided.

Pieper, B. (1991). *Sisters and Brothers, Brothers and Sisters in the Family Affected by Traumatic Brain Injury.* Albany, NY: New York State Head Injury Association, under a grant from NIDRR. Available from: New York State Head Injury Association, 855 Central Avenue, Albany, NY 12206. (518) 459-7911. Cost: $3.

This paper discusses the family stress that often accompanies TBI, how parents can identify the unspoken concerns of uninjured brothers and sisters, and methods parents have used to reduce the concerns.

The methods included are strengthening communications, finding people who can provide emotional support, and arranging sibling support group meetings guided by a professional. Includes resource listing.

PSI International. (1986). **The Silent Epidemic: Rehabilitation of People with Traumatic Brain Injury.** *Rehab BRIEF.* (*9*)4. Washington, DC: National Institute on Disability and Rehabilitation Research. Available from NARIC at (800) 346-2742. Single copies are free.

Defines traumatic brain injury and describes the patterns of damage caused by closed head injury, specific brain functions that can be affected, residual deficits, myths of recovery versus factors in improvement, vocational rehabilitation intervention, and the role of head injury rehabilitation professionals. While this document provides good introductory information about head injury, a few of the listings in the resource section are no longer current.

PSI International. (1991). **Aphasia.** *Rehab BRIEF.* (*13*)5. Washington, DC: National Institute on Disability and Rehabilitation Research. Available from NARIC at (800) 346-2742. Single copies are free.

Contains a review of the clinical perspectives on aphasia and areas of concern in the delivery of services to people with aphasia. The first section examines changing views of the nature of aphasia and the implications for clinical practice. The second section explores issues of concern in service delivery, including support for aphasic people and their families, specialized personnel trained to meet the needs of aphasic people, service delivery in rural areas, cultural and linguistic diversity, and responses to needs in service delivery.

Sachs, P. R. (1986). **Family Guide to Evaluating Transitional Living Programs For Head-Injured Adults.** *Cognitive Rehabilitation.* (*4*)6, 6-9. NARIC Accession Number: XJ7246.

This guide tells how family members can evaluate transitional living programs. These programs generally include speech, cognitive memory, and behavioral therapies for people with a head injury and are often an essential step between inpatient treatment for the injury and living independently after the medical problems have diminished. Differentiates transitional living from other types of head injury treatment.

Spanbock, P. (1992). **Children and Siblings of Head Injury Survivors: A Need to Be Understood.** *Journal of Cognitive Rehabilitation.* (*10*)4, 8-9. NARIC Accession Number: XJ22967.

This article discusses issues to consider when dealing with children and siblings of individuals who have sustained head injuries.

Willer, B. S., Allen, K. M., Liss, M., & Zicht, M. S. (1991). **Problems and Coping Strategies of Individuals with Traumatic Brain Injury and Their Spouses.** *Archives of Physical Medicine and Rehabilitation.* (*72*)7, 460-464. NARIC Accession Number: XJ20398.

This document examines the problems and coping strategies of people with head injury and their uninjured spouses. Researchers gathered information from 20 men and 11 women, at least one and a half years after the injury. The report discusses the resulting list of the top five or six problems and coping strategies of wives with head injury, wives whose husbands have head injury, husbands with head injury, and husbands whose wives have head injury.

Ylvisaker, M., Hartwick, P., & Stevens, M. (1991). **School Reentry Following Head Injury: Managing the Transition from Hospital to School.** *Journal of Head Trauma Rehabilitation.* (*6*)1, 1-22. NARIC Accession Number: XJ19408.

This journal article examines elements involved in the successful return to school for children and youth following a head injury. Topics discussed include goals of school reentry programming, the initial steps in reentry planning, activities during rehabilitation admission that are directed toward reentry into the school system, reentry activities undertaken shortly before discharge from rehabilitation, transitional classrooms, head injury consultants, and special school reentry problems such as summer discharge, children unable to attend school, mild injuries with good recovery, preschoolers, transportation, and funding.

The National Rehabilitation Information Center Home Page

Information for Independence

The National Rehabilitation Information Center (NARIC) is a library and information center on disability and rehabilitation. Funded by the National Institute on Disability and Rehabilitation Research

(NIDRR), NARIC collects and disseminates the results of federally-funded research projects. The collection, which also includes commercially published books, journal articles, and audiovisuals, grows at a rate of 300 documents a month.

NARIC currently has more than 46,000 documents on all aspects of disability and rehabilitation, including:

- Physical disabilities
- Mental retardation
- Psychiatric disabilities
- Independent living
- Medical rehabilitation
- Special education
- Employment
- Assistive technology (including information from the ABLEDATA project)
- Law and public policy

These materials are indexed in NARIC's bibliographic literature database, REHABDATA. NARIC's information specialists and users search REHABDATA to obtain citations for materials that suit the user's needs and interests. A nominal fee is required for some searches; unless otherwise protected by copyright law, photocopies of documents that are difficult to obtain elsewhere are also available for a nominal charge.

NARIC is committed to serving anyone, professional or lay person, who is interested in disability and rehabilitation, including consumers, family members, health professionals, educators, rehabilitation counselors, students, librarians, administrators, and researchers. We offer a variety of services, and there are several ways to use NARIC services.

Publications Available from NARIC

- NARIC resource guides introduce the reader to organizations, resources, and documents pertaining to a specific disability or condition.
  - *Spinal Cord Injury: A NARIC Resource Guide for People with SCI and Their Families*
  - *Head Injury: A NARIC Resource Guide for People with Head Injuries and Their Families*

- *Home Modification: A NARIC Resource Guide*
- *Stroke: A NARIC Resource Guide for Stroke Survivors and Their Families*
- *The NARIC Guide to Resources for the Americans with Disabilities Act (ADA)*
- *"Coverage of the Internet in the Disabilities Press."*

- *NIDRR Program Directory for 1995.* This directory is available in hard copy and online. It is divided into 16 chapters and indexed by subject, state, grantee, principal investigator, and NIDRR officer. Contact NARIC for information on how to get your own hard copy for just $5!

- *The 1994-95 Directory of National Information Sources on Disabilities.* This user-friendly, keyword-searchable version of the sixth edition of the NIS was compiled by NARIC for NIDRR, and is posted on the CODI (Cornucopia Of Disability Information) gopher. Contact NARIC [(800) 346-2742, or see bottom of this page] for information on how to get your own hard copy/ alternative format version. This consumer's guide, professional's handbook, and marketing tool includes more than 700 organizations, more than 100 other resource directories, and 42 databases. And the U.S. price for the hard copy is only $15—try before you buy!

- *The 1994 Compendium of Products by NIDRR Grantees and Contractors.* This Compendium provides researchers, rehabilitation professionals, and others in the field of disability with practical information on the spectrum of research, demonstration, training, engineering, and technical assistance materials produced with NIDRR support. NARIC encourages use of these products to improve policies, programs, and services for people with disabilities.

- *NARIC Calendar of Events* in Disability, Rehabilitation, and Assistive Technology. The calendar is updated the first week of every month to provide information on conferences, training, and symposia in the disability field.

- *The Fiscal Year 1994 NIDRR Program Directory.* The full text of one of the most utilized and important publications produced by

NARIC—a listing of all projects funded by NIDRR during the NIDRR fiscal year. This directory assists the rehabilitation community in locating pertinent research related to particular areas of expertise.

- *REHAB BRIEF: Bringing Research Into Effective Focus*

- *REHABDATA Thesaurus* ($25), a listing of descriptors used to search REHABDATA

NARIC is operated by KRA Corporation and is funded by the National Institute on Disability and Rehabilitation Research (NIDRR) under contract number HN93029001.

NARIC
8455 Colesville Road, Suite 935
Silver Spring, MD 20910-3319
(800) 346-2742 (V)
(301) 588-9284 (V)
(301) 495-5626 (TT)
(301) 587-1967 (fax)
(301) 589-3563 (BBS)
Home Page: http://www.naric.com/naric

Chapter 36

Head Injury Clinical Research Centers

The NINDS head injury research program supports a broad spectrum of studies by investigators at leading biomedical research institutions across the country. Key components of the program are regional head injury clinical research centers. Information on research activities at these centers, possible clinical trials, and patient eligibility may be obtained from the principal investigators listed below:

Donald P. Becker, M.D.
Department of Surgery (Neurosurgery)
UCLA Medical Center
Room 74-140 CHS
10833 LeConte Avenue
Los Angeles, California 90024-6901
(213) 825-5111

Eugene Flamm, M.D.
Tracy K. McIntosh, Ph.D.
Department of Surgery (Neurosurgery)
Hospital of the University of Pennsylvania
3400 Spruce Street
Philadelphia, Pennsylvania 19104
(215) 662-3487

National Institute of Neurological Disorders and Stroke (NINDS), January 24, 1996.

Robert G. Grossman, M.D.
Department of Neurosurgery
Baylor College of Medicine
One Baylor Plaza
Houston, Texas 77030
(713) 798-4696

Myron D. Ginsberg, M.D.
Department of Neurology
University of Miami School of Medicine
Miami, Florida 33101
(305) 547-6449

H. Richard Winn, M.D.
Department of Neurological Surgery
Harborview Medical Center ZA-86
325 Ninth Avenue
Seattle, Washington 98104
(206) 223-3497

Harold F. Young, M.D.
Division of Neurological Surgery
Medical College of Virginia
Virginia Commonwealth University
Richmond, Virginia 23298
(804) 786-9165

A. Byron Young, M.D.
Department of Surgery
University of Kentucky Medical Center
800 Rose Street, MN 268
Lexington, Kentucky 40536-0084
(606) 323-6013

Donald W. Marion, M.D.
Department of Neurological Surgery
9402 Presbyterian-University Hospital
230 Lothrop Street
Pittsburgh, Pennsylvania 15213
(412) 647-0956

Chapter 37

Resource List of Organizations

Accreditation

Commission on Accreditation of Rehabilitation Facilities (CARF)
2500 North Pantano Road
Tucson, AZ 85715
(602) 748-1212

Advocacy

National Organization on Disability (NOD)
910 16th Street NW, Suite 600
Washington, DC 20006
(202) 293-5960
(800) 248-2253

Alcoholism and Substance Abuse

National Clearinghouse for Alcohol and Drug Information
P.O. Box 2345
Rockville, MD 20852
(301) 468-2600

Excerpted from *Resource List of Organizations* prepared by the Brain Injury Association, Inc. 1776 Massachusetts Ave. N.W., Suite 100, Washington, DC 20036-1904, reprinted with permission; with additions from NIH Pub. No. 94-3825.

349

Assistive Devices

ABLEDATA
Newington Children's Hospital
Adaptive Equipment Center
181 East Cedar Street
Newington, CT 06111
(800) 344-5405
(203) 667-5405

Request Rehabilitation Engineering Center
National Rehabilitation Hospital
102 Irving Street NW
Washington, DC 20010
(202) 877-1932

RESNA: Association for the Advancement of Rehabilitation
Technology
1101 Connecticut Ave., NW, Suite 700
Washington, DC 20036
(202) 857-1199

Ataxia

Friedreich's Ataxia Group in America
P.O. Box 11116
Oakland, CA 94611
(415) 655-0833

National Ataxia Foundation
600 Twelve Oaks Center
Wayzata, MN 55391
(612) 473-7666

Brain Injuries and Brain Tumors

Family Survival Project
425 Bush Street, Suite 500
San Francisco, CA 94108
(415) 434-3388
(800) 445-8106 (CA only)

Cerebral Palsy

American Academy for Cerebral Palsy and Developmental Medicine
2315 Westwood Ave.
P.O. Box 11083
Richmond, VA 23230
(804) 282-0036

United Cerebral Palsy Association
7 Penn Plaza, Suite 804
New York, NY 10001
(212) 268-6655
(800) 872-1827 (Out of state only)

Child Advocacy

American Bar Association Child Advocacy Center
1800 M St. NW, Suite 200
Washington, DC 20036
Phone: 202-331-2250

Association for the Care of Children's Health
7910 Woodmont Ave., Suite 300
Bethesda, MD 20814
(301) 654-6549

Children's Defense Fund
122 C Street, NW, Suite 400
Washington, DC 20001
(800) 424-9602

Coordinating Council for Handicapped Children (CCHC)
20 East Jackson Blvd., Room 900
Chicago, IL 60604
(312) 939-3513
(312) 939-3519 (TDD)

Council for Exceptional Children
1920 Association Drive
Reston, VA 22091
(703) 620-3660

Federation for Children with Special Needs
95 Berekley, Suite 104
Boston, MA 02116
(617) 482-2915
(800) 331-0688 (MA only)

National Association of Private Schools for Exceptional Children
7926 Jongu Branch Drive, Suite 1100
McClean, VA 22102
(800) 999-5599

National Easter Seal Society
2023 West Ogden Avenue
Chicago, IL 60612
(312) 243-8400
(312) 243-8000 (for deaf)

National Information Center for Handicapped Children and Youth (NICHCY)
P.O. Box 1492
Washington, DC 20013
(703) 893-6061
(800) 999-5599

National Institute of Child Health and Human Development
National Institute of Health
900 Rockville Pike
Building 31, Room 2A03
Bethesda, MD 20892
(301) 496-3454

Consumer Safety

Consumer Product Safety Commission
(800) 638-2772

Education

Disability Rights Education and Defence Fund
2212 6th Street
Berkeley, CA 94710
(415) 644-2555

HEATH Resource Center
Higher Education and Adult Training for People with Handicaps
One Dupont Circle, Suite 800
Washington, DC 20036-1193
(202) 939-9320 (Voice and TDD)
(800) 544-3284 (Voice and TDD)

Employment

President's Committee on Employment of the Handicapped
1111 20 Street NW, Suite 636
Washington, DC 20036-3470
(202) 653-5044
(202) 653-5050 (TDD)

Epilepsy

Epilepsy Foundation of America
4351 Garden City Drive
Landover, MD 20785
(301) 459-3700
(800) 332-1000

Epilepsy Information Line
University of Washington
Seattle, WA
(800) 426-0660 (WA only)

Epilepsy Information Service & Comprehensive Epilepsy Program
Bowman Gray School of Medicine
300 South Hawthorne
Winston Salem, NC 27013
(919) 748-2319
(800) 642-0500 (NC only)

Grant Information

The Foundation Center
79 Fifth Avenue
New York, NY 10003
(800) 424-9836
(212) 620-4230

Handicapped Access

Architectural and Transportation Barriers Compliance Board
1111 18th Street, NW, Suite 501
Washington, DC 20036-3894
(202) 653-7834

Head Injury and Brain Trauma

Brain Trauma Foundation
555 Madison Avenue, Suite 2001
New York, New York 10022-3303
(212) 753-5003
(212) 753-0149 Fax

Coma Recovery Association
377 Jerusalem Avenue
Hempstead, New York 11550
(516) 486-2847

National Brain Injury Research Group, Inc. (JMA Foundation, Inc.)
5667 Stone Road
Department 555
Centreville, Virginia 22020
(703) 818-0078
(800) 447-8445

Phoenix Project
Box 84151
Seattle, Washington 98124
(206) 621-8558 (Head Injury Hotline)

Vital Active Life After Trauma (VALT)
53 Linden Street
Brookline, Massachusetts 02146
(617) 277-6327

Headache

National Headache Foundation
5252 North Western Ave.
Chicago, IL 60625
(312) 878-5558
(800) 843-2256

Health Information

National Center for Health Statistics
3700 East-West Highway
Hyattsville, MD 20782
(301) 436-8500

National Health Information Center
P.O. Box 1133
Washington, DC 20013
(301) 565-4167
(800) 336-4797

Hearing Impaired

Alexander Graham Bell Association for the Deaf
3417 Volta Place, NW
Washington, DC 20007
(202) 337-5220

National Association of the Deaf
814 Thayer Avenue
Silver Spring, MD 20910
(301) 587-1788

National Center for Law and the Deaf
800 Florida Ave., NE
Washington, DC 20002
(202) 651-5373

National Information Center on Deafness
Gallaudet College
800 Florida Avenue, NE
Washington, DC 20002
(202) 651-5109
(202) 651-5976 (TDD)
(800) 672-6720 (Voice or TDD)

Hospital Associations

American Hospital Association
840 North Lake Shore Drive
Chicago, IL 60611
(312) 280-6459

Independent Living

Independent Living Research Utilization Project (ILRU)
Institute for Rehabilitation and Research
P.O. Box 20095
Houston, TX 77225
(713) 797-0200

Mental Illness

National Institute of Mental Health
5600 Fisher's Lane, Room 15C-05
Rockville, MD 20857
(301) 443-4513

National Mental Health Association
1021 Prince Street
Alexandria, VA 22314-2971
(703) 684-7722
(800) 969-NMHA
(800) 684-6642

Neurological Disorders

National Institute of Neurological Disorders and Stroke (NINDS)
Office of Scientific and Health Reports
National Institutes of Health
Building 31, Room 8A-06
Bethesda, MD 20892
(301) 496-5924
(301) 496-4000 (general info.)

Occupational Therapy

American Occupational Therapy Association
1383 Piccard Dr., Suite 301
Rockville, MD 20850
(301) 948-9626
(800) 843-2682

Physical Therapy

American Physical Therapy Association
1111 North Fairfax Street
Alexandria, VA 22314
(703) 684-2782

Product Safety

National Injury Information Clearinghouse
Westwood Towers
5401 Westbard Ave. Room 625
Washington, DC 20207
(301) 492-6424
(800) 638-2772

Registry

National Athletic Head and Neck Injury Registry
University of Pennsylvania Sports Medicine Center
235 South 33rd Street
Philadelphia, PA 19104

Rehabilitation

National Association of Rehabilitation Facilities (NARF)
P.O. Box 17675
Washington, DC 20041
(703) 648-9300

National Association of Rehabilitation Professionals in Private
Sector (NARPPS)
P.O. Box 870
Twin Peaks, CA 92391
(714) 336-1531

National Institute on Disability and Rehabilitation Research (NIDRR)
400 Maryland Ave., SW
Washington, DC 20202-2572
(202) 732-1186

National Rehabilitation Information Center (NARIC)
8455 Colesville Road, Suite 935
Silver Spring, MD 20910
(301) 588-9284
(800) 346-2742

Office of Special Education and Rehabilitation Services (OSERS)
Clearinghouse on Disability Information
U.S. Dept. of Education
Switzer Bldg., 330 C Street SW
Washington, DC 20202-2524
(202) 732-1723
(202) 732-1245

Rehabilitation and Education

National Clearinghouse of Rehabilitation Training Materials
Oklahoma State University
115 Old USDA Building
Stillwater, OK 74078
(405) 624-7650

Research

Sunny Von Bulow Coma and Head Trauma Research Foundation
11 Park Place, Suite 1601
New York, NY 10007
(212) 732-8767

Sibling Support

Sibling Information Network
991 Main Street, Suite 3A
East Hartford, CT 06108
(203) 282-7050

Speech and Hearing

American Speech-Language-Hearing Association
10801 Rockville Pike
Rockville, MD 20852
(301) 897-5700
(800) 638-8255

National Association for Hearing and Speech Action
10801 Rockville Pike
Rockville, MD 20852
(301) 897-8682
(800) 638-8255

Stroke

National Stroke Association
300 East Hampden Street, Suite 240
Englewood, CO 80110
(303) 762-9922

Traffic Safety

National Highway Traffic Safety Administration (NHTSA)
(202) 366-9550 (Public Info.)
(202) 366-2588 (Publications Info.)

Trauma

American Trauma Society
P.O. Box 13526
Baltimore, MD 21203
(301) 328-6304

Victim Assistance

National Organization for Victims Assistance
1757 Park Road, NW
Washington, DC 20010
(202) 232-6682

Sunny Von Bulow National Victim Advocacy Center
307 West 7th Street, Suite 1001
Fort Worth, TX 76102
(817) 877-3355

Vocational Rehabilitation

Materials Development Center
Stout Vocational Rehabilitation Institute
University of Wisconsin-Stout
Menomonie, WI 54751
(715) 232-1342

—Prepared by Claudia Jensen, RPT, MS

Chapter 38

Glossary of Medical Terms Related to Head Injury

A

Abstract Concept. A concept or idea not related to any specific instance or object and which potentially can be applied to many different situations or objects. Persons with cognitive deficits often have difficulty understanding abstract concepts.

Acute Rehabilitation Program. Primary emphasis is on the early phase of rehabilitation which usually begins as soon as the patient is medically stable. The program is designed to be comprehensive and based in a medical facility with a typical length of stay of 1-3 months. Treatment is provided by an identifiable team in a designated unit.

Adiadochokinesia. Inability to stop one movement and follow it immediately with movement in the opposite direction.

Agnosia. Failure to recognize familiar objects although the sensory mechanism is intact. May occur for any sensory modality.

Akinetic Mutism. A condition of silent, alert-appearing, immobility that characterizes certain subacute or chronic states of altered

Definitions in this chapter were excerpted and compiled from *Brain Injury Glossary*, ©1996 HDI Publishers and *Mild Head Injury: Care of the Child at Home*, © 1990 by Children's National Medical Center; both reprinted with permission.

consciousness. Sleep-wake cycles have been retained, but no observable evidence for mental activity is evident; spontaneous motor activity is lacking; person appears to be aware but inactive. Exhibited by persons with high brain stem lesions.

Alexia. Inability to read.

Amnesia. Difficulty remembering new information after the injury (antegrade), or loss of memory for events immediately before the injury (retrograde).

Anomia. Loss of ability to recall the specific names or words for objects, people, or actions.

Anoxia. A lack of oxygen. Cells of the brain need oxygen to stay alive. When blood flow to the brain is reduced or when oxygen in the blood is too low, brain cells are damaged.

Anterograde Amnesia. Inability to consolidate information about ongoing events. Difficulty with new learning.

Aphasia. Inability to understand what is said (receptive), or inability to express thoughts into words (expressive).

Aphemia. The isolated loss of the ability to articulate words without loss of the ability to write or comprehend spoken language.

Apraxia. Inability to carry out a complex or skilled movement; not due to paralysis, sensory changes, or deficiencies in understanding.

Arousal. Being awake. Primitive state of alertness managed by the reticular activating system (extending from medulla to the thalamus in the core of the brain stem) activating the cortex. Cognition is not possible without some degree of arousal.

Ataxia. Inability to coordinate muscle movements, or irregular muscle movements, especially with walking.

Automatic Speech. Words said without much thinking on the part of the speaker. These may include songs, numbers, and social communication; or, can be items previously learned through memorization.

Spontaneous swearing by individuals who did not do so before their injury is another example.

Awareness, Deficit. The patient's inability to recognize the problems caused by impaired brain function.

B

Brain Death. A state in which all functions of the brain (cortical, subcortical, and brain stem) are permanently lost.

Brain Injury, Closed. Occurs when the head accelerates and then rapidly decelerates or collides with another object (for example the windshield of a car) and brain tissue is damaged, not by the presence of a foreign object within the brain, but by violent smashing, stretching, and twisting, of brain tissue. Closed brain injuries typically cause diffuse tissue damage that results in disabilities which are generalized and highly variable.

Brain Injury, Mild. A patient with a mild traumatic brain injury is a person who has had a traumatically-induced physiological disruption of brain function, as manifested by at least one of the following: 1) any period of loss of consciousness, 2) any loss of memory for events immediately before or after the accident, 3) any alteration in mental state at the time of the accident (e.g., feeling dazed, disoriented, or confused), 4) focal neurological deficit(s) which may or may not be transient; but where the severity of the injury does not exceed the following: a) loss of consciousness of approximately 30 minutes or less; b) after 30 minutes, an initial Glasgow Coma Scale score of 13-15; c) Post Traumatic Amnesia not greater than 24 hours.

Brain Injury, Moderate. A Glasgow Coma Scale score of 9 to 12 during the first 24 hours post injury.

Brain Injury, Penetrating. Occurs when an object (for example a bullet or an ice pick) fractures the skull, enters the brain and rips the soft brain tissue in its path. Penetrating injuries tend to damage relatively localized areas of the brain which result in fairly discrete and predictable disabilities.

Brain Injury, Severe. Severe injury is one that produces at least 6 hours of coma; Glasgow Coma Scale score of 8 or less within the first 24 hours.

Brain Plasticity. The ability of intact brain cells to take over functions of damaged cells; plasticity diminishes with maturation.

Brain Scan. An imaging technique in which a radioactive dye (radionucleide) is injected into the blood stream and then pictures of the brain are taken to detect tumors, hemorrhages, blood clots, abscesses or abnormal anatomy.

Brain Stem. The lower extension of the brain where it connects to the spinal cord. Neurological functions located in the brain stem include those necessary for survival (breathing, heart rate) and for arousal (being awake and alert).

C

Cerebellum. The portion of the brain (located at the back) which helps coordinate movement. Damage may result in ataxia.

Cerebral Angiography. A medical test involving injection of dye into an artery so that the vascular system of the brain can be studied through an x-ray; can detect aneurysms, tumors, or circulation problems.

Cerebral Compression. The brain substance is pushed aside and compressed by the presence of a brain tumor, aneurysm, swelling or hematoma.

Cerebral Infarct. When the blood supply is reduced below a critical level to a specific region of the brain and the brain tissue in that region dies.

Cerebral-spinal Fluid (CSF). Liquid which fills the ventricles of the brain and surrounds the brain and spinal cord.

Circumlocution. Use of other words to describe a specific word or idea which cannot be remembered.

Cognition. The conscious process of knowing or being aware of thoughts or perceptions, including understanding and reasoning.

Cognitive Impairment. Difficulty with one or more of the basic functions of the brain: perception, memory, attentional abilities, and reasoning skills.

Cognitive Rehabilitation. Therapy programs which aid persons in the management of specific problems in perception, memory, thinking and problem solving. Skills are practiced and strategies are taught to help improve function and/or compensate for remaining deficits. The interventions are based on an assessment and understanding of the person's brain-behavior deficits and services are provided by qualified practitioners.

Coma. A state of unconsciousness from which the patient cannot be awakened or aroused, even by powerful stimulation; lack of any response to one's environment. Defined clinically as an inability to follow a one-step command consistently; Glasgow Coma Scale score of 8 or less.

Coma Vigil. A patient who has no meaningful interaction with his or her environment but exhibits sleep and wake cycles, spontaneous respiration and heart beat. See Persistent Vegetative State.

Community Skills. Those abilities needed to function independently in the community. They may include: telephone skills, money management, pedestrian skills, use of public transportation, meal planning and cooking.

Concrete Thinking. A style of thinking in which the individual sees each situation as unique and is unable to generalize from the similarities between situations. Language and perceptions are interpreted literally so that a proverb such as "a stitch in time saves nine" cannot be readily grasped.

Concussion. Blow to the head in which the brain in "shaken" inside the skull, but there is no obvious bruise or bleeding noticed on x-ray.

Confabulation. Verbalizations about people, places, and events with no basis in reality. May be a detailed account delivered.

Consciousness. The state of awareness of the self and the environment.

Contusion. A blow to the head which bruises the brain.

Core Therapies, Brain Injury. Basic therapy services provided by professionals on a brain injury rehabilitation unit. Usually refers to nursing, physical therapy, occupational therapy, speech-language pathology, neuropsychology, social work and therapeutic recreation.

Cortical Blindness. Loss of vision resulting from a lesion of the primary visual areas of the occipital lobe. Light reflex is preserved.

Coup-Contracoup. A blow to the head with enough energy to bounce the brain on both sides of the skull, causing injury to two areas of the brain. The degree of injury to both areas depends on the force of the blow.

CT Scan. A series of x-rays taken through different levels of the brain to detect injury.

D

Diaschisis. A theoretical state following brain injury in which healthy areas connected to the damaged area show a temporary loss of function.

Diffuse Axonal Injury (DAI). A shearing injury of large nerve fibers (axons covered with myelin) in many areas of the brain. It appears to be one of the two primary lesions of brain injury, the other being stretching or shearing of blood vessels from the same forces, producing hemorrhage.

Diffuse Brain Injury. Injury to cells in many areas of the brain rather than in one specific location.

Diplegia. Paralysis of corresponding parts on both sides of the body, such as both arms.

Diplopia. Seeing two images of a single object; double vision.

Discrimination, Auditory. The ability to differentiate and recognize sounds. This involves distinguishing between words, noises, and sounds that might be similar. A person with poor auditory discrimination might answer the phone in his room although the actual ringing came from an alarm clock.

Discrimination, Visual. Involves the differentiation of items using sight. An individual with impaired visual discrimination may not be able to distinguish between a red and green light while driving or may have difficulty distinguishing between the letter "E" and the letter "F".

Doll's Eye Maneuver. The eyes appear to move in the direction opposite to the motion of the head, when the head is gently rotated.

Dysarthria. Difficulty in forming words or speaking them because of weakness of muscles used in speaking or because of disruption in the neuromotor stimulus patterns required for accuracy and velocity of speech.

Dysmetria. Inability to stop a movement at the desired point; also known as past-pointing.

E

Echolalia. Imitation of sounds or words without comprehension. This is a normal stage of language development in infants, but is abnormal in adults.

Edema. Swelling in the brain (or other body part) caused by a collection of fluid.

Electrocardiogram(ECG/EKG). The recording made by electrode pads located on the patient's chest to monitor heart rate and rhythm. These are connected to a monitor and used routinely in the intensive care unit.

Electroencephalogram (EEG). A procedure that uses electrodes on the scalp to record electrical activity of the brain. Used for detection of epilepsy, coma, and brain death.

Electromyography (EMG). An insertion of needle electrodes into muscles to study the electrical activity of muscle and nerve fibers. It may be somewhat painful to the patient. Helps diagnose damage to nerves or muscles.

Embolism. The sudden blocking of an artery or a vein by a blood clot, bubble of air, deposit of oil or fat, or small mass of cells deposited by the blood flow.

Emotional Lability. Exhibiting rapid and drastic changes in emotional state (laughing, crying, anger) inappropriately without apparent reason.

Encephalography. Non-invasive use of ultrasound waves to record echoes from brain tissue. Used to detect hematoma, tumor, or ventricle problems.

Error Recognition. Refers to a person's awareness that a response is inappropriate for a task. Return of this ability may be reflected by a patient stating, for example, "I know this is wrong," or show a confused, quizzical look after making an inappropriate response.

Evoked Potential. Registration of the electrical responses of active brain cells as detected by electrodes placed on the surface of the head at various places. The evoked potential, unlike the waves on an EEG, is elicited by a specific stimulus applied to the visual, auditory or other sensory receptors of the body. Evoked potentials are used to diagnose a wide variety of central nervous system disorders.

Evoked Responses, Brain Stem. Auditory brain stem responses provoked by discreet sounds delivered to the ears through headphones. These sound waves are convened to nerve impulses by receptors in the ear. A machine is used to test whether the brain stem has received the signals. The quality of the brain stem's response in a comatose patient is thought to be an important indicator of the degree and site of brain injury. Because this test requires very specialized and expensive equipment, it is not available in all hospitals. A more common test is the EEG.

Executive Functions. Planning, prioritizing, sequencing, self-monitoring, self-correcting, inhibiting, initiating, controlling or altering behavior.

F

Frontal Lobe. Front part of the brain; involved in planning, organizing, problem solving, selective attention, personality and a variety of "higher cognitive functions."

Frustration Tolerance. The ability to persist in completing a task despite apparent difficulty. Individuals with a poor frustration tolerance will often refuse to complete tasks which are the least bit difficult. Angry behavior, such as yelling or throwing things while attempting a task is also indicative of poor frustration tolerance.

G

Gait Training. Instruction in walking, with or without equipment; also called "ambulation training."

Glasgow Coma Scale. A standardized system used to assess the degree of brain impairment and to identify the seriousness of injury in relation to outcome. The system involves three determinants: eye opening, verbal responses and motor response all of which are evaluated independently according to a numerical value that indicates the level of consciousness and degree of dysfunction. Scores run from a high of 15 to a low of 3. Persons are considered to have experienced a 'mild' brain injury when their score is 13 to 15. A score of 9 to 12 is considered to reflect a 'moderate' brain injury and a score of 8 or less reflects a 'severe' brain injury.

Glasgow Outcome Scale. A system for classifying the outcome of persons who survive. The categories range from 'Good Recovery' in which the patient appears to regain the pre-injury level of social and career activity (even if there are some minor residual abnormal neurological signs); 'Moderate Disability' in which the patient does not regain the former level of activity but is completely independent with respect to the activities of daily life; 'Severe Disability' is defined as a state wherein the conscious, communicating patient is still dependent on the help of others. The original scale had five outcome categories, the newest scale has eight outcome categories. This scale relates to functional independence and not residual deficits.

H

Hematoma. The collection of blood in tissues or a space following rupture of a blood vessel. Regarding Brain:

- Epidural: Outside the brain and its fibrous covering, the dura, but under the skull.
- Subdural: Between the brain and its fibrous covering (dura).
- Intracerebral: In the brain tissue.
- Subarachnoid: Around the surfaces of the brain, between the dura and arachnoid membranes.

Hemiplegia. Paralysis of one side of the body as a result of injury to neurons carrying signals to muscles from the motor areas of the brain.

Hemiparesis. Weakness of one side of the body.

I

Impulse Control. Refers to the individual's ability to withhold inappropriate verbal or motor responses while completing a task. Persons who act or speak without first considering the consequences are viewed as having poor impulse control.

Incontinent. Inability to control bowel and bladder functions. Many people who are incontinent can become continent with training.

Intermittent Catheterization Program (ICP). Bladder training program where a catheter is inserted to empty the bladder at regular time intervals.

International Classification of Disease (ICD-9). A three digit "N" code used to indicate the pathological nature of an injury. The ninth revision of this classification (ICD-9) has been in use for several years. Unfortunately, the term "brain injury" does not appear as a category. There are ten rubrics which cover most brain/head injuries. The ICD is less useful than desired because rubrics are not mutually-exclusive. Differences occur in coding from one institution to another. A new version, ICD-10, is under preparation.

Intracranial Pressure (ICP). Cerebrospinal fluid (CSF) pressure measured from a needle or bolt introduced into the CSF space surrounding the brain. It reflects the pressure inside of the skull.

Intracranial Pressure Monitor. An ICP monitor. A monitoring device to determine the pressure within the brain. It consists of a small tube (catheter) attached to the patient at the skull by either a ventriculostomy, subarachnoid bolt, or screw and is then connected to a transducer, which registers the pressure.

Intracranial Insult. Something that causes injury to the brain. Includes hematomas (intraparenchymal and extraparenchymal; immediate or delayed) elevations of intracranial pressure (ICP), brain swelling, edema, and vasospasm.

K

Kinesthesia. The sensory awareness of body parts as they move (see Position Sense and Proprioception).

L

Lability. State of having notable shifts in emotional state (e.g., uncontrolled laughing or crying).

Locked-in Syndrome. A condition resulting from interruption of motor pathways in the ventral pons, usually by infarction. This disconnection of the motor cells in the lower brain stem and spinal cord from controlling signals issued by the brain leaves the patient completely paralyzed and mute, but able to receive and understand sensory stimuli; communication may be possible by code using blinking, or movements of the jaw or eyes, which can be spared.

Lucid Interval. A period shortly after injury when the patient was reported to have talked.

M

Magnetic Resonance Imaging (MRI). An x-ray procedure which uses magnetic fields to create a picture of the brain's soft tissue and identify specific injuries.

371

Medically Stable. Reaching a point in medical treatment where life-threatening injuries and disease have been brought under control.

Memory, Audio-Visual. Auditory memory is the ability to recall a series of numbers, lists of words, sentences, or paragraphs presented orally. Visual memory requires input of information through visuo-perceptual channels. It refers to the ability to recall text, geometric figures, maps, and photographs. A brain-injured survivor with impaired visual memory may have to refer to a road map numerous times to reach a nearby destination. A brain-injured inpatient may need frequent assistance from staff to locate his room. A patient with impaired auditory memory will likely require frequent reminders of orally presented task instructions from staff. Notably, information may be encoded in memory using words or visual images independent of the mode of presentation.

Memory, Delayed. Recall of information after a delay, often with other information presented to prevent active rehearsal. There is no particular specification of the required time interval; typically it is ten minutes or more.

Memory, Episodic. Memory for ongoing events in a person's life. More easily impaired than semantic memory, perhaps because rehearsal or repetition tends to be minimal.

Memory, Immediate. The ability to recall numbers, pictures, or words immediately following presentation. Patients with immediate memory problems have difficulty learning new tasks because they cannot remember instructions. Relies upon concentration and attention.

Memory/Learning. Change in a person's understanding or behavior due to experience or practice. Often thought of as acquisition of new information. For example, a person who learns quickly will likely remember an entire set of instructions after hearing them a single time. A patient with severely impaired learning ability will show little gain in recall after numerous repetitions. Learning and memory are interdependent. If immediate memory is poor, learning will be poor because only a portion of the information will be available for rehearsal/repetition. It is important to note that patients may have intact learning ability, but poor delayed memory. For example, a brain-injured patient may learn a set of instructions after several repetitions, but forget them the next day.

Memory, Long Term. In neuropsychological testing, this refers to recall thirty minutes or longer after presentation. Requires storage and retrieval of information which exceeds the limit of short term memory.

Memory, Recall. Ability to retrieve information without renewed exposure to the stimulus.

Memory, Recognition. Ability to retrieve information when a stimulus cue is presented. Free recall of the information is often deficient if cues must be provided.

Memory, Remote. Information an individual correctly recalls from the past, stored before the onset of brain injury. There is no specific requirement for the amount of elapsed time, but it is typically more than six months to a year. Preserved information from delayed memory becomes part of remote memory.

Memory, Semantic. Memory for facts, usually learned through repetition.

Memory, Short Term. Primary or 'working' memory; its contents are in conscious awareness. A limited capacity system that holds up to seven chunks of information over periods of 30 seconds to several minutes, depending upon the person's attention to the task.

Mental Competence. The quality or state of being competent; having adequate mental abilities; legally qualified or adequate to manage one's personal affairs. An individual found by a court to be mentally incompetent has a guardian appointed to make personal and/or economic decisions on their behalf.

Metacognition. Insight into accurately judging one's own strengths and limitations, particularly with regard to cognitive skills.

Monoplegia. Paralysis of one arm or one leg.

Motivation. Requires initiative and refers to the extent to which an individual desires to reach a goal and demonstrates actual follow-through. A greater level of motivation is required for completion of difficult tasks. A brain-injured person with reduced motivation may need frequent cueing to finish dressing even though being able to verbalize the complete procedure.

Motor Control. Regulation of the timing and amount of contraction of muscles of the body to produce smooth and coordinated movement. The regulation is carried out by operation of the nervous system.

Motor Control, Fine. Delicate, intricate movements as in writing or playing a piano.

MRI *see* **Magnetic Resonance Imaging (MRI)**

Muscle Tone. Used in clinical practice to describe the resistance of a muscle to being stretched. When the peripheral nerve to a muscle is severed, the muscle becomes flaccid (limp). When nerve fibers in the brain or spinal cord are damaged, the balance between facilitation and inhibition of muscle tone is disturbed. The tone of some muscles may become increased and they resist being stretched—a condition called hypertonicity or spasticity.

N

Neologism. Nonsense or made-up word used when speaking. The person often does not realize that the word makes no sense.

Neuro Developmental Treatment (NDT). A therapeutic approach based on the development of movement and emphasizing the restoration of normal movement in performing functional activities.

Neurologist. A physician who specializes in the nervous system and its disorders.

Neuropsychologist. A psychologist who specializes in evaluating (by tests) brain/behavior relationships, planning training programs to help the survivor of brain injury return to normal functioning and recommending alternative cognitive and behavioral strategies to minimize the effects of brain injury. Often works closely with schools and employers as well as with family members of the injured person.

O

Obtunded. Mental blunting; mild to moderate reduction in alertness.

Occipital Lobe. Region in the back of the brain which processes visual information. Damage to this lobe can cause visual deficits.

Occupational Therapy. Occupational Therapy is the therapeutic use of self-care, work and play activities to increase independent function, enhance development and prevent disability; may include the adaptation of a task or the environment to achieve maximum independence and to enhance the quality of life The term occupation, as used in occupational therapy, refers to any activity engaged in for evaluating, specifying and treating problems interfering with functional performance.

Organization, Cognitive. Using selective attention skills, the individual correctly perceives stimulus attributes or task elements, selects a strategy, monitors use of the strategy and reaches a correct solution.

- Low Level: Those individuals who can sustain attention and appropriately switch sets. Persons with low level organization ability usually "fall apart" in high stress situations.

- High Level: Those individuals who can deal with multiple pieces of information and integrate them for accomplishing relatively complex tasks. Some persons demonstrating high level cognitive organization may still "fall apart" in high stress situations.

Orientation, Situational. The ability to accurately describe present circumstances. For example, in the acute stages of injury, brain-injured patients may be unable to respond accurately to questions such as, "Why are you in the hospital?" Situational disorientation is commonly observed during the period of post-traumatic amnesia (PTA).

P

Palliative Care. A program designed to reduce the severity of symptoms and/or decrease their impact on the individual, and to improve the quality of life.

Paraparesis. Weakness of the lower limbs.

Paraphasic Error. Substitution of an incorrect sound (e.g., tree for free) or related word (e.g., chair for bed).

Paraplegia. Paralysis of the legs (from the waist down).

Parapnasias. Use of incorrect words or word combinations.

Parietal Lobe. One of the two parietal lobes of the brain located behind the frontal lobe at the top of the brain.

Parietal Lobe, Right. Damage to this area can cause visuo-spatial deficits (e.g., the patient may have difficulty finding their way around new, or even familiar, places).

Parietal Lobe, Left. Damage to this area may disrupt a patient's ability to understand spoken and/or written language.

Persistent Vegetative State (PVS). A long-standing condition in which the patient utters no words and does not follow commands or make any response that is meaningful. See Persistent Unawareness.

Persistent Unawareness. The transition of a person who remains unconscious from a state of 'coma' to one of 'vegetative behaviors' reflects subtle changes over a period of several weeks from a condition of no response to the internal or external environment (except reflexively) to a state of wakefulness but with no indication of awareness (cortical function). A patient in this state may have a range of biological responses at the sub-cortical level such as eye opening (with sleep and wake rhythms) and sometimes the ability to follow with their eyes. Normal levels of blood pressure and respiration (vegetative functions) are maintained automatically. The label 'persistent' is not applicable until the person has been unconscious for a year or more. Also called Coma Vigil.

Physiatrist. Pronounced Fizz ee at' rist. A physician who specializes in physical medicine and rehabilitation. Some physiatrists are experts in neurologic rehabilitation, trained to diagnose and treat disabling conditions. The physiatrist examines the patient to assure that medical issues are addressed; provides appropriate medical information to the patient, family members and members of the treatment team. The physiatrist follows the patient closely throughout treatment and oversees the patient's rehabilitation program.

Physical Therapist. The physical therapist evaluates components of movement, including: muscle strength, muscle tone, posture, coordination, endurance, and general mobility. The physical therapist also evaluates the potential for functional movement, such as ability to move in the bed, transfers and walking and then proceeds to establish an individualized treatment program to help the patient achieve functional independence.

Posey Vest/Houdini Jacket. A vest worn to keep the person in bed or in the wheelchair. This is for the person's safely.

Position Sense. The sensory awareness of the location and orientation of body parts without moving them. See Kinesthesia and Proprioception.

Post-concussive Syndrome. A combination of symptoms which lasts four to six weeks following a concussion or mild head injury.

Post Traumatic Amnesia (PTA). A period of hours, weeks, days or months after the injury when the patient exhibits a loss of day-to-day memory. The patient is unable to store new information and therefore has a decreased ability to learn. Memory of the PTA period is never stored, therefore things that happened during tha period cannot be recalled. May also be called Anterograde Amnesia.

Proprioception. The sensory awareness of the position of body parts with or without movement. Combination of kinesthesia and position sense.

Prosody. The inflections or intonations of speech.

Proximal Instability. Weakness of muscles of the trunk, shoulder girdle or hip girdle which causes poor posture, abnormal movement of the arms or legs and the inability to hold one's head up. Strength of muscles of the hands or legs may be normal.

Psychologist. A professional specializing in counselling, including adjustment to disability. Psychologists use tests to identify personality and cognitive functioning. This information is shared with team members to assure consistency in approaches. The psychologist may provide individual or group psychotherapy for the purpose of cognitive retraining, management of behavior and the development of coping skills by the patient/client and members of the family.

Psychometric Instruments. Standardized tests (utilizing paper and pencil) which measure mental functioning.

Psychomotor Skills. Skills that involve both mental and muscular ability such as playing sports or other activities where practice or concentration is involved.

Psychosocial Skills. Refers to the individual's adjustment to the injury (and resulting disability) and one's ability to relate to others. Includes feelings about self, sexuality and the resulting behaviors.

Q

Quadriparesis. Weakness of all four limbs.

Quadriplegia. Paralysis of all four limbs (from the neck down). British authors often use the prefix "tetra" to mean four, so they may describe a patient as having tetraplegia.

R

Random Movement. An action or process of moving without obvious aim, purpose, or reason.

Reasoning, Abstract. Mode of thinking in which the individual recognizes a phrase that has multiple meanings and selects the meaning most appropriate to a given situation. The term "abstract" typically refers to concepts not readily apparent from the physical attributes of an object or situation.

Reasoning, Association. A skill dependent on a person's ability to determine the relationship between objects and concepts. A patient with impairment may touch a hot stove, failing to realize that pain is associated with touching a heated burner. Similarly, a patient given a knife, spoon, fork, and baseball may not be able to discriminate which of the objects "does not belong."

Reasoning, Cause and Effect. The ability to perceive and anticipate the consequences of a given action or statement. For example, a patient may sit for a long period in a darkened room without realizing that flipping a light switch will cause the light to turn on. A patient may turn the oven up to make a cake cook faster, not realizing that the increased heat will simply cause the food to burn.

Reasoning, Concrete. The ability to understand the literal meaning of a phrase.

Reasoning, Deductive. Drawing conclusions based upon premises or general principles in a step-by-step manner.

Reasoning, Generalization. The ability to take information, rules and strategies learned about one situation and apply them appropriately to other, similar situations. For example, a patient who learns to lock his wheelchair brakes in physical therapy may not lock the brakes while sitting in his room.

Reasoning, Inductive. Awareness of one's behavior and the accuracy or appropriateness of one's performance. Usually automatic and on-going.

Reasoning, Problem-Solving. The ability to analyze information related to a given situation and generate appropriate response options. Problem-solving is a sequential process that typically proceeds as follows: identification of problem; generation of response options; evaluation of response option appropriateness; selection and testing of first option; analysis as to whether solution has been reached. A patient/client may discontinue making a cup of coffee because the sugar bowl is empty, even though sugar is readily available in a nearby cabinet. A patient/client may easily navigate his way into a room crowded with furniture, but request staff assistance to navigate his way out.

Recreation Therapist. Individual within the facility responsible for developing a program to assist persons with disabilities plan and manage their leisure activities; may also schedule specific activities and coordinate the program with existing community resources.

Rehabilitation. Comprehensive program to reduce/overcome deficits following injury or illness, and to assist the individual to attain the optimal level of mental and physical ability.

Remediation. The process of decreasing a disability by challenging the individual to improve deficient skills.

Respirator/Ventilator. A machine that does the breathing work for the unresponsive patient. It serves to deliver air in the appropriate percentage of oxygen and at the appropriate rate. The air is also humidified by the respirator.

Respite Care. A means for taking over the care of a patient temporarily (a few hours up to a few days) to provide a period of relief for the primary caregiver.

Retrograde Amnesia. Inability to recall events that occurred prior to the accident: may be a specific span of time or type of information.

S

Secondary Condition. People with disabling conditions are often at risk of developing secondary conditions that can result in further deterioration in health status, functional capacity, and quality of life. Secondary conditions are causally related to a primary disabling condition and include, among others, contractures, physical deconditioning, mental depression, cardiopulmonary conditions and decubitus ulcers.

Secondary Insult. Secondary or delayed brain injury; for traumatic brain injury, includes all events other than the mechanical injury sustained at the time of impact. Secondary phenomena may be divided into systemic and intracranial insults. Systemic insults include hypoxemia, anemia, hypotension, hypercarbia, hyperthermia, and electrolyte imbalance.

Seizure. An uncontrolled discharge of nerve cells which may spread to other cells nearby or throughout the entire brain. It usually lasts only a few minutes. It may be associated with loss of consciousness, loss of bowel and bladder control and tremors. May also cause aggression or other behavioral change.

Selective Attention. Ability to focus on the most important aspect of a situation without becoming distracted.

Sequencing. Reading, listening, expressing thoughts, describing events or contracting muscles in an orderly and meaningful manner.

Shock, Circulatory. A clinical condition characterized by signs and symptoms which arise when the cardiac output is insufficient to fill the arterial tree with blood under sufficient pressure to provide organs and tissues with adequate blood flow.

Shunt. A procedure to draw off excessive fluid in the brain. A surgically-placed tube running from the ventricles which deposits fluid into either the abdominal cavity, heart or large veins of the neck.

Skull Fracture. The breaking of the bones surrounding the brain. A depressed skull fracture is one in which the broken bone exerts pressure on the brain.

Social Adjustment Training. Structured program designed to assist the disabled individual to interact with individuals and groups within the community in an acceptable manner.

Somatic. Relating to, or affecting the body.

Somatosensory. Sensory activity having its origin elsewhere than in the special sense organs (such as eyes and ears) and conveying information to the brain about the state of the body proper and its immediate environment.

"Space Boots" (Spenco Boots). Padded support devices made of lamb's wool used to position the feet and ankles of the patient. Without this support and alignment, patients who are unconscious for long periods may develop deformities limiting future movement.

Spasm. An involuntary and abnormal muscular contraction; also, a sudden violent and temporary effort or emotion.

Spasticity. An involuntary increase in muscle tone (tension) that occurs following injury to the brain or spinal cord, causing the muscles to resist being moved. Characteristics may include increase in deep tendon reflexes, resistance to passive stretch, clasp knife phenomenon, and clonus.

Spatial Ability. Ability to perceive the construction of an object in both two and three dimensions. Spatial ability has four components: the ability to perceive a static figure in different positions, the ability to interpret and duplicate the movements between various parts of a figure, the ability to perceive the relationship between an object and a person's own body sphere, and the ability to interpret the person's body as an object in space.

Spontaneous Recovery. The recovery which occurs as damage to body tissues heals. This type of recovery occurs with or without rehabilitation and it is very difficult to know how much improvement is spontaneous and how much is due to rehabilitative interventions. However, when the recovery is guided by an experienced rehabilitation team, complications can be anticipated and minimized; the return of function can be channeled in useful directions and in progressive steps so that the eventual outcome is the best that is possible.

Status Epilepticus. Continuous seizures: may produce permanent brain damage.

Stimulus. That which causes sensation (i.e., light for vision, salt for taste, sound for hearing, etc.). When a patient begins to emerge from coma, an organized program of controlled stimulation is sometimes used to begin "exercising" the brain. However, when a patient becomes agitated, the amount and intensity of stimulation should be limited (e.g., only one task for one sense at a time).

Stupor. Deep sleep; unresponsive but can be awakened with repeated, noxious stimulation. Awareness is depressed but present.

Subarachnoid Screw. Also Subarachnoid Bolt. A device for measuring intracranial pressure which is screwed through a hole in the skull and rests on the surface of the brain.

Subdural. Beneath the dura (tough membrane) covering the brain and spinal cord.

T

Tactile Defensiveness. Being overly sensitive to touch; withdrawing, crying, yelling or striking when one is touched.

Tactile Discrimination. The ability to differentiate information received through the sense of touch.

- Sharp/dull discrimination: ability to distinguish between sharp and dull stimuli;

- Two-point discrimination: the ability to recognize two points applied to the skin simultaneously as distinct from one single point.

Telegraphic Speech. Speech which sounds like a telegram. Only the main words of a sentence (nouns, verbs) are present; the small words (ifs, ands, buts,) are missing. This type of speech often gets the message across.

Temporal Lobes. There are two temporal lobes, one on each side of the brain located at about the level of the ears. These lobes allow a person to tell one smell from another and one sound from another. They also help in sorting new information and are believed to be responsible for short-term memory.

- Right Lobe: Mainly involved in visual memory (i.e., memory for pictures and faces).

- Left Lobe: Mainly involved in verbal memory (i.e., memory for words and names).

Tracheostomy. A temporary surgical opening at the front of the throat providing access to the trachea or windpipe to assist in breathing.

Tremor, Intention. Course, rhythmical movements of a body part that become intensified the harder one tries to control them.

Tremor, Resting. Rhythmical movements present at rest and may be diminished during voluntary movement.

U

Unilateral Neglect. Paying little or no attention to things on one side of the body. This usually occurs on the side opposite from the location of the injury to the brain because nerve fibers from the brain typically cross before innervating body structures. In extreme cases, the patient may not bathe, dress or acknowledge one side of the body.

V

Vegetative State. Return of wakefulness but not accompanied by cognitive function; eyes open to verbal stimuli; does not localize motor responses; autonomic functions preserved. Sleep-wake cycles exist. See Persistent Vegetative State.

Ventricles, Brain. Four natural cavities in the brain which are filled with cerebrospinal fluid. The outline of one or more of these cavities may change when a space-occupying lesion (hemorrhage, tumor) has developed in a lobe of the brain.

Ventriculostomy. A procedure for measuring intracranial pressure by placing a measuring device within one of the fluid-filled, hollow chambers of the brain.

Verbal Apraxia. Impaired control of proper sequencing of muscles used in speech (tongue, lips, jaw muscles, vocal cords). These muscles are not weak but their control is defective. Speech is labored and characterized by sound reversals, additions and word approximations.

Vestibular. Pertaining to the vestibular system in the middle ear and the brain which senses movements of the head. Disorders of the vestibular system can lead to dizziness, poor regulation of postural muscle tone and inability to detect quick movements of the head.

Visual Field Defect. Inability to see objects located in a specific region of the field of view ordinarily received by each eye. Often the blind region includes everything in the right half or left half of the visual field.

Visual Perception. The ability to recognize and discriminate between visual stimuli and to interpret these stimuli through association with earlier experiences. For example, to separate a figure from a background, to synthesize the contents of a picture and to interpret the invariability of an object which is seen from different directions.

Vocational Counseling. Process of assisting a person to understand vocational liabilities and assets, provide occupational information to assist one in choosing an occupation suitable to one's interests and liabilities.

W

Wagner O'Day. Common name for Public Law 92-28 which directs the purchase by the Federal Government of selected commodities and services from qualified workshops serving blind and other severely disabled individuals, with the objective of increasing the employment opportunities for these individuals.

Work Tolerance. Ability to sustain a work effort for a prolonged period of time; ability to maintain a steady flow of production at an acceptable pace and acceptable level of quality; ability to handle a certain amount of pressure.

Index

Index

Page numbers shown in *italic* type refer to references in graphics and/or tables; page numbers followed by the letter n refer to references found in notes.

A

AAN *see* American Academy of Neurology (AAN)
Abbreviated Injury Scale (AIS) 131, 132-34
ABLEDATA 350
abstract reasoning 378
abstract thinking, head injuries 76-77, 219, 361
Accessible Space, Inc. 310
acoustic reflex tests 108, 109
acute rehabilitation 327, 361
ADA *see* Americans with Disabilities Act
adiadochokinesia 361
adolescents, memory problems 76
adrenaline and fainting 80
advocacy groups, traumatic brain injury 21-22
AFDC *see* Aid to Families with Dependent Children (AFDC)

age factor
  brain 9
  head injuries 59-60
  inner ear operations 98-99
  traumatic brain injury 12
agitated states 206
agnosia 361
Aid to Families with Dependent Children (AFDC) 299
airbags 231
AIS *see* Abbreviated Injury Scale
akinesia 206
akinetic mutism 147, 149, 361-62
Alabama, helmet laws 38, 45
Alaska, helmet laws 45, 46
alcohol abuse 349
  traumatic brain injury 213-24
  see also drug abuse
Alcohol World: Health & Research 213n
Alexander Graham Bell Association for the Deaf 355
alexia 362
Allen, K. M. 342
all terrain vehicles (ATV)
  head injuries 48
  pediatric trauma related deaths 25, 27, 28, 29-30
alprazolam 200

389

household accidents, traumatic brain
injury 13-14
Housing, Industry, Training, Inc. 315
housing assistance 296
states 308-12
Howard, M. 284
HUD *see* Department of Housing and
Urban Development (HUD)
hypersexuality 205
hypothalamus 6
hypothermia therapy 241
hypoxia 98, 211, 273
hypoxic-ischemic brain injury 153-54

I

ICD *see* International Classification
of Disease (ICD)
Idaho, helmet laws 45
IDEA *see* Individuals with Disabilities Education Act (IDEA)
Illinois, helmet laws 45
imagery 193-94
imaging techniques 10, 55, 242
see also computerized axial
tomography scan; magnetic
resonance imaging; X-rays
impaired mental functions, head injuries 76-77, 215, 324
impairment-related work expense
(IRWE) 298
impatience 164, 254
impotence 205
see also sexual difficulties
impulse control 370
impulsive control disorders 205
impulsivity 166
inappropriate behavior, head injuries
76-77
inappropriate care, traumatic brain
injury 20-21
inappropriate social behavior 167-68,
216
self-stimulation 227-28
incidence rates, traumatic brain injury 11-13
income support assistance 298-99

incontinence 370
independent living 265-66, 328, 343
independent living centers 334-35
Independent Living Research Utilization Project (ILRU) 356
Indiana, helmet laws 45, 46
Individualized Quantitative Assessment 152
Individualized Written Rehabilitation
Plan (IWRP) 174
Individuals with Disabilities Education Act (IDEA) 300
inductive reasoning 379
infant head injuries 89
infant restraint seats 61
information organization, frontal lobe
92
information transfer, between two
hemispheres of brain 3-4
injury prevention assistance 300
in-line roller skating, helmets 49-50
inner ear injury 98
Institute on Rehabilitation Issues
(IRI) 171-72, 173
insurance, traumatic brain injury 21,
285-92
Insurance Institute for Highway
Safety
"Helmet Laws" 33n, 39n
"Motorcycles" 39n
intellectual handicaps, head injury
69, 73
intelligence 9
intermittent catheterization Program
(ICP) 370
Intermodal Surface Transportation
Efficiency Act (1991) 41
International Classification of Disease (ICD) 11, 370
Internet addresses
Consumer Product Safety Commis-
sion 52
Cornucopia Of Disability Informa-
tion (CODI) gopher 344
National Rehabilitation Information Center 342-43, 345
intracerebral hematoma 70
intracranial hematoma 116

O